HEALTH, ECONOMICS,
AND HEALTH ECONOMICS

CONTRIBUTIONS
TO
ECONOMIC ANALYSIS

137

Honorary Editor
J. TINBERGEN

Editors
D.W. JORGENSON
J. WAELBROECK

NORTH-HOLLAND PUBLISHING COMPANY
AMSTERDAM · NEW YORK · OXFORD

HEALTH, ECONOMICS, AND HEALTH ECONOMICS

*Proceedings of the World Congress on Health Economics,
Leiden, The Netherlands, September 1980*

Edited by

JACQUES VAN DER GAAG
*Institute for Research on Poverty
Madison, Wisconsin*

and

MARK PERLMAN
*Department of Economics
University of Pittsburgh
Pittsburgh, Pennsylvania*

NORTH-HOLLAND PUBLISHING COMPANY
AMSTERDAM · NEW YORK · OXFORD

ISBN: 0 444 86210 2

Publishers:
NORTH-HOLLAND PUBLISHING COMPANY
AMSTERDAM · NEW YORK · OXFORD

Sole distributors for the U.S.A. and Canada:
ELSEVIER NORTH-HOLLAND INC.
52 VANDERBILT-AVENUE
NEW YORK, N.Y. 10017

Library of Congress Cataloging in Publication Data

World Congress on Health Economics (1980 : Leiden,
    Netherlands)
    Health, economics, and health economics.

    (Contributions to economic analysis ; 137)
    Bibliography: p.
    Includes index.
    1. Medical economics--Congresses. I. Gaag, J. van
der. II. Perlman, Mark. III. Title. IV. Series.
[DNLM: 1. Delivery of health care--Congresses.
2. Economics, Medical--Congresses. 3. Insurance, Health
--Congresses. W 74 W926h 1980]
RA410.A2W68 1980   338.4'73621   81-38385
ISBN 0-444-86210-2   AACR2

Printed in the Netherlands

Introduction to the series

This series consists of a number of hitherto unpublished studies, which are introduced by the editors in the belief that they represent fresh contributions to economic science.

The term 'economic analysis' as used in the title of the series has been adopted because it covers both the activities of the theoretical economist and the research worker.

Although the analytical methods used by the various contributors are not the same, they are nevertheless conditioned by the common origin of their studies, namely theoretical problems encountered in practical research. Since for this reason, business cycle research and national accounting, research work on behalf of economic policy, and problems of planning are the main sources of the subjects dealt with, they necessarily determine the manner of approach adopted by the authors. Their methods tend to be 'practical' in the sense of not being too far remote from application to actual economic conditions. In addition they are quantitative rather than qualitative.

It is the hope of the editors that the publication of these studies will help to stimulate the exchange of scientific information and to reinforce international cooperation in the field of economics.

The Editors

CONTENTS

INTRODUCTION

1. HEALTH, ECONOMICS, AND HEALTH ECONOMICS

THE ROLE OF GOVERNMENT

2. ECONOMIC ASPECTS OF THE ROLE OF GOVERNMENT IN HEALTH CARE

3. AN INTERPRETATION OF GOVERNMENT INTERVENTION IN HEALTH:
    THE ITALIAN CASE

4. THIRTY YEARS OF FRUITLESS ENDEAVOR? AN ANALYSIS OF
    GOVERNMENT INTERVENTION IN THE HEALTH CARE MARKET

5. THE COST OF NURSING HOME CARE IN THE UNITED STATES:
    GOVERNMENT FINANCING, OWNERSHIP, AND EFFICIENCY

DEMAND ANALYSES

6. THE DEMAND FOR MEDICAL CARE SERVICES: A RETROSPECT
    AND PROSPECT

LIST OF TABLES

LIST OF FIGURES

Acknowledgments

This volume contains a selection of the more than forty papers presented at the World Congress on Health Economics, a meeting held at the historic University of Leiden, The Netherlands, 8-11 September 1980.

The Congress received generous financial support from the Dutch Health Fund, Ziekenzorg, Amsterdam, as part of the Fund's 85th anniversary celebration. It was both gratifying and encouraging to find such general interest in health economics research within a policy-making agency whose main interest is in the day-to-day management of part of the Dutch health-care system. Ziekenzorg's support, and especially the stimulating interest of its chairman, Dr. Theo de Vries, are gratefully acknowledged.

Yet, if financing is essential, it is not sufficient. Obviously many others were critical to the planning and organization of the Congress.

Chief among these was Professor Bernard M. S. van Praag, Director of the Center for Research in Public Economics at Leiden University. He served as host of the Congress and was a member of the Advisory Board, together with Martin S. Feldstein (President of the National Bureau of Economic Research and Professor of Economics at Harvard University) and Professor Victor R. Fuchs (Stanford University).

Six participants were invited to submit papers, but most of the space on the program was reserved for selection by competition. The program committee consisted of the two editors of this volume, Jacques van der Gaag and Mark Perlman. Well over 100 individuals offered to prepare papers for the Congress. Confronted with such a rich choice, we have made as wise a selection as we could, focusing on four broad topics: the role of government, measurement of health status, the demand for medical services, and physician behavior. Inevitably there was an effort to include among the papers breadth, as illustrated by reports from a variety of countries, and analytical rigor. Naturally, there were trade-offs involved and the results were, no doubt, just as naturally subject to some criticisms.

On the basis of this selection process, about three dozen people from 15 countries were asked to submit papers, which were then presented to the approximately 350 individuals who attended the Congress. The format was generally to allow the author(s) to describe the paper briefly and then have the paper formally discussed by a critic. Generally there was time for questions and comments from the floor.

At the end of the Congress, the two editors selected for publication the papers that appear in this volume. What resulted represents a general, though not complete, consensus. Some papers which were otherwise excellent had to be rejected because they were too long. Others, also quite excellent, ran into stiff competition because they dealt with topics which were the same as those handled by still more excellent papers. Inevitably, the selection presented has been influenced by our own taste, though we have made every effort to be objective. In any event, we think that what follows in this volume is a representative, if not balanced, selection of the best work presented at the Congress.

Professor van Praag and the program committee are thoroughly indebted to Miss Manon G. F. van Voorst tot Voorst, Secretary to the Congress. Her capacity to match van der Gaag's attention to detail (a point made by Perlman, not van der Gaag) cannot be too highly praised. Her invariable good humor and reassuring sense of responsibility is something which everyone connected with the Congress quickly perceived. The enthusiastic cooperation of the affiliates of the Center for Research in Public Economics is also gratefully acknowledged. Their involvement and hard work made it possible to finish many last minute chores in time.

We are also indebted to the Board of the University of Leiden, to Dr. P. Siderius (Secretary-General of the Ministry of Health and Environmental Protection), and to the Burgomasters of both Leiden and Amsterdam for their cooperation, generosity, and sympathetic interest.

We have made every effort to prepare the Conference papers for publication within three months of the date of the Conference, without sacrificing the quality of the papers or of their preparation. To the extent that we have succeeded, we owe much to the highly skilled editorial and technical typing staff of the Institute for Research on Poverty at the University of Wisconsin-Madison, in particular to Jan Blakeslee, Alice Clark, Joyce Collins, Elizabeth Evanson, Marie Goodman, Ginger Ohrmundt, Nancy Weber, and Joann Zick. Their ability to maintain a good-humored approach under great pressure of time is exemplary.

In our opinion, this collection of papers is not only informative today, but it also reflects major areas of health economics research, and research progress, prevalent in the period 1970-1980. By their very nature, the papers will become dated. This will reflect not only changes in the substance of the findings, but, more importantly, in the refocusing of objectives and concerns. Perhaps it is this awareness of the dynamic nature of what health economics is all about (or, better yet, what it is about to become) which has been the most rewarding and exciting part of our function as members of the program committee.

Having thanked so many individuals specifically, we must also thank the many people who attended the Congress and whose contributions to the discussion we and everyone else there found so stimulating.

J.v.d.G.
M.P.

INTRODUCTION

HEALTH, ECONOMICS, AND HEALTH ECONOMICS
J. van der Gaag and M. Perlman (editors)
© *North-Holland Publishing Company, 1981*

HEALTH, ECONOMICS, AND HEALTH ECONOMICS

A. J. Culyer

Viewed from my side of the Atlantic, health economics is 21 years old in 1981 (dating its inception from Lees, 1960) and it is therefore particularly apt to review the state of our art at this time. Viewed from the Americas it is older: a special session of the American Economic Association meetings in 1951 was devoted to the economics of medical care (Ginzberg, 1951). Perhaps we should claim that it all began with William Petty and is 290 years old (dating from the publication of <u>Verbum Sapienti</u> in London). This not only has the advantage of bringing the first application of the notion of human investment to prevention of disease back to my side of the Atlantic, but also reminds us that Petty is held as intellectual father not only by economists but also by epidemiologists and medical statisticians, whose subsequent separate paths of development are long overdue for closer integration. Petty was a classic child of his intellectual times: a professor of anatomy, professor of music, Latin scholar, poet, judge, and occupier of major public positions, as well as economist and statistician. Although that kind of polymathy is beyond even the most able minds of today, few economists today feel constrained to restrict the application of their discipline to its traditional field, "the economy," and economists are increasingly viewed with suspicion by those whose disciplinary territory--like health--they increasingly seem to be invading. Are the suspicions warranted? Do our accomplishments justify our claims? Do the contents of a volume such as this convey adequately both to us and to those from neighboring disciplines what we are about? These are the main questions I propose to discuss in this introductory essay.

Alan Williams (1979) has made a distinction that some of you may think self-evident, but which helps us to tackle the question of "economic imperialism." This distinction is between an "area of study" and a "mode of thinking." The idea of an "area of study" connotes a set of phenomena to be studied, problems "out there" to be tackled, policies to be investigated, issues to be explored. The idea of a "mode of thinking" connotes the conceptual apparatus that is to be brought to bear upon the phenomena, problems, policies, issues, etc. As a shorthand, I shall follow Williams in using the terms "topic" and "discipline" to refer to these two.

"Health" denotes, of course a topic--a set of phenomena amounting to a broad but quite well-defined area of study. It includes conceptual issues (for example, the meaning of "health" itself). It includes behavioral, environmental, and medical causes of health and ill health (compare Selma Mushkin's rather narrow 1958 definition of the task of health economics: "to appraise the efficiency of the organisation of health services, and to suggest ways of improving this organisation"). It includes the study of health services: administration, finance, and the behavior of decision-makers acting under different administrative, financial, and other social constraints. The scope of a topic is, however, conventional. The topic "health" has not always included all the features I have mentioned. The scope is, of course, affected by social institutions, current policy questions, and the prevailing values in society. "Economics" too is a topic, broadly construed as "the economy." The definition of the topic of economics is also conventional. What seems to characterize economics as a topic is a cash nexus: the things that are included in "wealth" are the central things in the topic of economics. Here I want, however, to focus on economics as a discipline. This is not at all characterized by what economists study, but by the way they study it. The hallmark of a discipline is its theory or theories. In the case of economics we are concerned with normative and positive theories of the allocation of scarce resources--whether or not they are associated with any cash nexus and whether or not they are transacted in markets.

You will immediately see that the topic of health and the topic of economics are not the only topics to which the discipline of economics may be applied, nor is the discipline of economics the sole discipline capable of being applied to the topic of health or the topic of economics. This is, I think, an important message for economists to teach noneconomists who may fear "economic imperialism." It is also important for those economists who work, like many Germans, in an academic community of economics that has become excessively compartmentalized according to topic.

Health economics can likewise in principle be viewed as a discipline, a topic (that is, the things that health economists as "disciplinarians" study), or as the discipline economics applied to the topic health. I believe that only the last view makes any sense at all. Health economics as a discipline does not exist independently of economics as a discipline: there are few techniques of economic analysis that are not applicable in the topic of health; moreover, there are few theoretical ideas in health economics that are truly sui generis. Health economics as a topic does not strike a chord either: it has at present no settled bounds of convention, other than those bounding the topic health itself, though there is a striking asymmetry in the distribution of research effort to the topic of health--an asymmetry that varies from place to place. Accordingly, we are left with the discipline of economics applied to the topic of health. We should note, as I have just mentioned, that economics is not the only discipline applicable to this topic, nor is it the only discipline applicable even to the more "economic" topics within the general topic of health: very frequently, therefore, health economists will have to work with students of other disciplines working in this common topic.

The distinction between topic and discipline is useful not only in reminding us that the satisfactory resolution of many health research problems requires more than just economics. It also serves to remind noneconomists that we are neither glorified cost accountants nor students only of the marketplace and market phenomena. It

is also useful in reminding us that the topics of our research are
largely conventional, being determined by contingent elements such
as local circumstances and institutions, personal talents, and personal values, rather than by our discipline itself. It is for this
reason that I set little store by attempts to draw up a research
agenda in the hope that all may subscribe to it: we are all too
diverse and our circumstances too heterogeneous for that to be a
valuable exercise.

I suspect that two major elements underly the suspicions that others
entertain about economists: one relates to a widespread belief that
economists have a naive and rather hard-baked system of underlying
political values; the other relates to the belief that too much of
the activity of economists is erected upon excessively simple concepts both of the determinants of human action regarding health matters and as regards health itself. A careful reading of the
contents of this book should go some way toward dispelling these
beliefs (or at least in suggesting that we are at least as critical
of one another as others may be of us), but since we are often poor
advocates in our own cause, let us pause to explore in greater
detail how an "insider" like myself views these misgivings.

I detect that most economists working in health have their initial
interest aroused through the policy issues of the time or, perhaps,
for more profound political reasons. It is not accidental that the
earliest contributions to health economics were all very directly
concerned with the appropriate roles of markets and the state in
health care provision (recall Mushkin's definition). If one takes
1963 as the year of the real economic watershed in health (it was,
of course, the year of Arrow's classic article in the American
Economic Review) it is striking that nearly all the published work
on health by economists up to and including that year was concerned
with questions of welfare economics. The rest was largely descriptive material: mostly social survey work and international and/or
regional comparisons of this or that.

It was already clear in the late 1950s and early 1960s, and so it
has remained and is evidenced by the papers in this volume, that
there was not within health economics (as there is not within
neoclassical economics in general) any single notion of what welfare
economics applied to the topic health really is. On the one hand
there is the familiar Paretian notion concerned with the evaluation
of alternative states of society (in principle being complete
descriptions of society) by reference to the preferences of individual members of society. The objective of the game played according
to this value judgment is to identify Pareto improvements, actual or
potential; and the practical yardstick of measurement of both cost
and benefit is "willingness to pay" as measured in principle by com-
pensating variations in income.

This framework provides economists with their concept of efficiency
(i.e., a Pareto optimum). Its very limitation as a description of
what the objectives of society are, however, means that few (if any)
of us regard it as either an adequate guide alone for public policy
or as the limit to which economists may go in contributions to
public debate and policy making. Consequently, one is driven to go
further, for example into questions of distributive justice.

Here the broad stream of welfare economics as applied to health
divides into several tributaries, each of which is worthy of
exploration. Explorers along one tributary seek to evolve a system
of weights, derived from a supplementary principle (like desert or
equality) or from a set of supplementary principles (e.g., based on
a Rawlsian conceptual experiment) that can be applied to the benefits and costs of the efficiency analysis. Others, on the grounds,
say, that the principle of distributive justice in health (or
elsewhere) cannot be adequately summarized in terms of the weights
to be applied to costs or benefits or utilities, would follow
another tributary that requires separate treatment of efficiency
questions and questions of justice as distinct and separate
languages of evaluation that it lies not in our competence to combine into some kind of super-ethical Esperanto (Culyer, 1977).

Yet another tributary is followed by those who take the view that
distributional questions need not--at least in part--necessarily be
treated sui generis--that is, having a special value-judgmental
source distinct from the individual preferences that form the basis
of efficiency analysis. These analysts posit that individuals also
have preferences about distributional outcomes and that these distributional externalities (following Hochman and Rodgers, 1969) are conceptually on all fours with the other kinds of externality that
everyone recognizes as a proper consideration to account for in efficiency analysis (provided, of course, one believes they exist).

There is yet another major tributary of the mainstream of welfare
economics which takes on most of the analytical superstructure of
efficiency analysis as described above but replaces individuals'
valuations of costs and benefits (that is, the individuals whose
welfare is affected in any way by a change) with other people's
valuations, in particular, with so-called "expert" decision-makers'
values. Such values, along this tributary, are not only those concerning distributional weights, but may even be valuations of goods
and services, which are considered, in the jargon, as "merit goods."
Alan Williams, in his paper in this volume, is frank about the
potential conflict between the merit-good approach and the traditional Paretian approach when, for example, the source of value for
reckoning benefit is different from that for reckoning cost. Once
again there is ample scope for up-stream exploration and, one may
argue, health economics is a particularly apposite territory in
which these various explorations in welfare economics may be conducted, for it is in this terrain of economics more perhaps than any
other that questions of distributive justice vie for at least equal
status with questions of efficiency (see the papers by Aaron, and
Maynard and Ludbrook in this volume) and here more than in most
other problems of resource allocation that one may plausibly
question the competence and hence relevance of consumer values in
assessing efficiency.

But it seems to me that there are some profound ambiguities of
interpretation here, about which we all need to think further. For
example, it is clear that while I detect a broad consensus that the
organization of and terms of access to health services cannot be adequately either explained or justified by reference to the customary
economic assumption of rational self-interest, there is no consensus
concerning the two principal contenders for both an explanatory and a

normative basis for analysis. These are, on the one hand, the proposition that individuals care about one another--interpersonal utility interdependence--and that this both helps account for, as a
positive exercise, and also helps justify, as a normative exercise,
collectivism in health; and on the other hand that individuals feel
a moral duty to guarantee all citizens certain levels of consumption
of a primary good such as health. Insofar as moral notions may
actually affect behavior, they too have a positive role to play as
well as their more obvious normative one. (Distinctions of this
sort are made in Harsanyi, 1955, and Sen, 1977.) The distinction is
important for several reasons, but chiefly in a welfare economics
context because we tend to take preferences--the basis of the externality view--as data in the system, whereas morals, or concepts of
social justice, are arguable. Thus if caring preferences are
widespread, and are taken into account in the specification of an
efficient allocation of resources to and within the health services,
this cuts out a whole set of debates that those taking the view that
they are not widespread but that moral concerns are important would
want to engage in. Unfortunately, however, what is essentially an
empirical issue concerning why people may act in unselfish ways is
not easily resolvable by empirical observations, for behavior determined by preferences and behavior determined by ethical views
(especially if utilitarian and as subject to trade-off as are
preferences) are not easy--possibly impossible--to differentiate.

Another ambiguity running through the literature relates to the
apparently wide gulf between the Paretians and the advocates of the
merit-good approach. In terms of behavioral implications and the
formulation of a program of empirical research, that distinction
rapidly becomes fuzzy as soon as it becomes plausible to argue that
individuals consider it in their own interest to delegate decisions
to others such as health professionals and politicians as agents who
are to interpret both individual and collective needs.

Thus it seems to me that what at first sight seem to be profound
methodological, even ideological, differences between us have an
exasperating habit of becoming practically hard to maintain and seem
to bring us all to a similar set of concerns as regards access to
services; price and income elasticities of demand; health status
measurement; estimation of health production functions; behavior of
physicians, bureaucrats, and others with decision-making authority;
costs; and so on--albeit by rather different routes. Let me
illustrate by reference to health status.

The view one takes of the competence of consumers to value the services they receive, whether preventive, curative, or caring, and
whether in the sector of the economy designated as the health care
sector or other health-affecting sectors, is one of the central
issues in debates about the finance and organization of health services and must be one of the principal contingent factors determining the kind of research one does. The need for health status
measurement is related to how one interprets the implications of
these debates: for example, not everyone will be equally concerned
about the geographical distribution of health services and hence
with measures designed to inform policy-makers about the consequences of alternative distributional policies.

However, although the range of problems in which health status
measurement may provide helpful monitoring and resource allocation
guidelines is wider or smaller depending on the view one takes, even
the most convinced libertarian must recognize a potentially useful
role for health status measures in clinical management of patients
and in clinical and epidemiological research, while even the most
convinced collectivist recognizes the legitimacy of some sources of
satisfaction that can never (at least I suspect they can never) be
included in any health index (comfort and reassurance are a couple
of obvious ones).

Measurement of health illustrates well the complementary nature of
the various disciplines operating in the topic of health. While
economists have had a useful role to play in identifying the kinds
of value judgment inescapably embodied in a health index and in providing conceptual and experimental methods for eliciting such values
(time trade-offs, standard gambles, and the like), it is remarkable
that much of the genuine innovation seen here in the last decade has
come from outside the ranks of the economics profession, from operations researchers, systems analysts, psychologists, epidemiologists,
and clinical researchers (e.g., Katz et al., 1963; Fanshel and Bush,
1970; Torrance, 1970; Patrick et al., 1973; Rosser, 1979).

Health status measurement has its fans among explorers along each of
the methodological tributaries I have identified; and alongside the
technical contributions economists can make there are no less important contributions at the level of political economy. Good
Paretians see the desirability of such measurement as a direct consequence of the postulate (itself an empirical matter) that the
health status of others enters an individual's utility function--
though there remain questions as to whether it enters as a cardinal
entity in its own right or as a statistic describing a community
distribution of health (again empirical questions). Others argue
that the evidence is thin that health status is a matter of
altruistic preference and is, instead, best seen as an object of
moral concern derived from, say, a Rawlsian or utilitarian system of
ethical imperatives. Yet others see it as a direct outcome of the
merit-good approach, of social importance because it figures in
decision-makers' utility functions or in their ethics.

While there has been progress, it is amply clear that the full implications of alternative postulates about externality relationships
have yet to be worked out, especially when one casts the externality
net wider--as I think one must--than Aaron does in his paper in this
volume (Culyer, 1980, Ch. 7). If one assumes, for example with
Pauly (1971), that the externality takes the form of A's health care
consumption entering B's utility function, and that the demand for
health care is income elastic, it seems to follow that optimal price
subsidies vary inversely with the consumer's income. If one assumes
with Lindsay (1969) that it is differences in consumption of services that matter, we get in addition the implication that access
will be rationed by nonprice factors to the relatively rich. If, on
the other hand, one assumes that A's health status itself enters B's
utility function, then any positive price may be just a nuisance,
for the policy problem is mainly the engineering one of ensuring
that effective services go where they may do most good. That doesn't
mean the engineering problem is value free. It evidently is not

(Culyer, 1978b). But it may well mean that the relevant source of value in any individual case need not be the values of that individual. Depending on which view one takes, the political economy consequences for the design of the system are manifestly very different.

Work on the demand side of the economics of health has gotten a good deal further than that on the supply side. The agency role of physicians, for example, has mostly focused on the ability of the medical profession to shift consumers' demand curves, with obvious implications for the stability of medical markets, control of health care cost inflation, and so on. The ability--and/or willingness--of physicians to act thus is clearly an empirical matter about which there are currently no settled conclusions (e.g., the papers by Newhouse, Richardson, Stoddart and Barer, Wilensky and Rossiter, and Zweifel in this volume). Quite independently of physicians' power to shift demand curves in response to the changing parameters of medical practice (changes in fee schedules and so on) there remains a problem for welfare economics from the agency relationship if we are to interpret this as consisting in at least the partial replacement of consumers' values with the agents' values. This interpretational problem exists even if no demand shifting takes place, for the usual procedures of applied welfare economics (integrating marginal values and so on) will be evaluating at best a set of filtered consumer values. Here we find ourselves on the first tilt of a slippery slope: if values filtered by medical agents are accepted as normatively "legitimate" (as consumer values customarily are), then what of values filtered by hospital administrators, regional planning boards, state and federal politicians, etc. Each may claim to act for his clients. Each may claim his role has been ascribed to him by a legitimate process. Each may claim to be accountable to his clients. Yet clearly many economists feel a profound disquiet as the "distance" between the patient and the agent expressing values on the patient's behalf becomes remoter: the individualistic base of welfare economics shades by gradual degrees into the collectivism of merit wants. This aspect of the agency role of physicians seems to me to warrant more attention than it has received.

There is, it would therefore seem, an active debate in process within the health economics literature that is directly confronting some central issues of value. The fact that there is no consensus as to either the appropriateness of using consumer values or the ability of the medical marketplace to reveal them accurately should be heartening news not only to those of us who value the continued questioning of familiar presumptions but also to those outsiders who fear we are all naive philistines.

Similar heart should be taken from the ways economists have tackled the question of health (for example, its definition), its relationship with human behavior, and its production by health services. A good deal of the contribution here has arisen in the context of specific cost-benefit and cost-effectiveness studies, where the twin problems of outcome measurement and its relationship with inputs via a health service production function cannot be avoided. Although such work is not represented in this volume (but for an excellent review see Drummond, 1980 and 1981), it is probably in work of this sort that multidisciplinary collaboration has gone furthest, which accounts for my belief that the sharing of honors in the development

of measures of health requires more plaudits to collaborating noneconomists than to economists. But at least this demonstrates that
economists <u>can</u> work well with other disciplinary experts (especially
epidemiologists).

More specifically economic is the research program initiated by
Grossman (1972b), which seems to be producing a new economic
etiology of illness (see his paper with Shakotko and Edwards in this
volume, and the paper by Wolfe and van der Gaag also in this
volume). This relatively new tradition of analysis draws on what
seems to be a clear example (possibly the only one to date) of a
genuinely new theoretical idea (viz., the demand for health)
emerging from health economics. It should be of particular interest
to epidemiologists, especially since the level of both theoretical
and statistical sophistication is a good deal higher than that commonly found in "mainstream" epidemiology.

The treatment by economists, then, of values and of models of health
behavior has increased enormously in subtlety, sophistication, and
ingenuity of empirical estimation in the past decade or so. It is
not merely that economists have--as they seem to have--a comparative
advantage in distinguishing value judgments from other kinds of
judgment, nor that their conceptual apparatus for sorting out costs
and benefits, supply and demand, and so on, and for handling
problems associated with the dating of flows of costs and benefits,
and for handling uncertainty, is better developed than others'.
Nor is it only the tremendous strides that have been made in quantifying key parameters constraining public choices (demand elasticities and the like). While all these things must be counted as
substantial achievements, the main contribution made by economists
to the way we now think about health in the community, and the
health services in particular, lies in the kind of perception
characteristically brought to bear by economists: the desire to
specify an unambiguous objective or set of objectives against which
to judge and monitor policy; the desire to identify the production
function; the recognition of the importance of human behavior, as
well as technology and the natural environment, in the causes, prevention, cure, and care of disease.

I should therefore say that the achievement has been substantial and
that it is not to be measured solely in terms of the quantification
of interesting features of the system that previously lacked it.
Although such work is arguably the most conspicuous achievement
(Newhouse's review of the empirical demand literature in this volume
admirably lists the accomplishments), I would reckon of no less
importance the increasing permeation of economic modes of thinking in
neighboring disciplines and in the thinking of private and public
decision-makers in the health and related services. While much of
this is attributable to the published track record of health economists reviewed in various ways in this volume, much is also attributable to the less obvious work of proselytizers, economic advisers,
and those who, at a fairly humdrum level, are able to give practical
help to those facing practical problems, but whose work rarely graces
the pages of even the less prestigious journals. Therefore, while
volumes such as this tend naturally (and not inappropriately) to
focus our gaze upon the work of the high priests of our arcane art,
they by no means tell the whole story either of our achievements or

of the kind of work that mostly occupies those who describe themselves as health economists. (In the United Kingdom, for example--
and I dare say it may be true elsewhere--about one-third of all
research projects currently underway are cost-benefit or cost-
effectiveness studies, but not a single such study is reported in
this volume.)

Twenty-first birthday greetings then seem in order. I detect clear
evidence that we have come of age. Not only has the discipline of
economics proved its fruitfulness in application to the topic health;
it has also shown itself a complement to rather than a substitute for
neighboring disciplines--notably epidemiology and clinical medicine,
but, who knows, possibly even medical sociology. If we are really
mature enough to collaborate, where the topic suggests it would be
fruitful, with those colleagues whom economists used at one time to
label perfunctorily (scathingly?) as "noneconomists," then we have
truly come of age.

THE ROLE OF GOVERNMENT

HEALTH, ECONOMICS, AND HEALTH ECONOMICS
J. van der Gaag and M. Perlman (editors)
© *North-Holland Publishing Company, 1981*

ECONOMIC ASPECTS OF THE ROLE OF GOVERNMENT IN HEALTH CARE

Henry Aaron

Government-promoted health care is one of the growth industries of developing and mature economies.* From modest beginnings in the provision of such traditional public goods as drainage of swamps, clean water, and public sanitation, the scope of government intervention in public health and medical care has continued to expand. Public health activities now include efforts to reduce pollution of air, water, and land. Along with improved nutrition and inoculation against major infectious diseases, these collective activities account for most of the decline in mortality and morbidity rates that have occurred over the past century within today's developed countries, and they explain most of the difference in mortality and morbidity rates between contemporary poor and rich countries. While externalities are sometimes in the eye of the beholder, and judgments differ about whether transactions costs produce market failure or merely create the opportunity for another market to operate efficiently, at least since the time of Adam Smith the collective provision of such goods has been an activity of government approved by economists with even the most single-minded allegiance to free markets.

The role of government extends far beyond the provision of traditional public goods. In his classic article, Kenneth Arrow (1963) explored a variety of reasons why private arrangements for and government participation in the production and allocation of health care services are so different from those attending the production and allocation of most other commodities. He concluded by placing great emphasis on the importance of uncertainty. In the first part of this paper, I shall review the role of uncertainty, and I shall suggest some further differences between health care and other commodities that have led the populations of all developed countries to involve their governments extensively in the provision of health care.

While the special characteristics of health care as an economic good help explain the role and function of government in its provision, I believe it apparent that health care has been treated in considerable degree, like justice and the suffrage, as a right in the regulation and management of which the role of government is treated as natural and primary and the market is regarded as secondary and even illegitimate (Okun, 1975). From this standpoint, an analysis

---

*I want to thank Victor Fuchs, Joseph Newhouse, Uwe Reinhardt, Louise Russell, and William Schwartz for helpful comments and constructive criticism.

of the role of government in the provision of health care demands
the attention of political scientists, social psychologists, and
experts in public management more than that of economists.

In another sense, however, the puzzle simply moves to another part
of the economist's domain: how has a commodity that represents such
a large and growing drain on economic resources come to be treated
as a right, without regard for the resources it uses? In the second
part of this paper, I shall outline the approach to the role of
government that flows from seeing health care as a right. I shall
argue that this approach dominated policy in developed countries
during the first two-thirds of the twentieth century, and that it
continues to explain many elements of the ideology of health care in
all developed countries; that it rests on technological characteristics of health care services destroyed by recent scientific
advances; and that these scientific advances require the reconsideration of the role of government in the production and allocation of health care services.

THE GOVERNMENT AS A CORRECTIVE TO MARKET FAILURE

Economists conventionally approach the role of government in the
provision of any commodity by asking if an unregulated market can
provide the commodity in a manner that is both productively efficient and distributionally just. The burden of proof lies on the
person who would establish a role for government to show that one or
both of the following pairs of conditions is satisfied. On efficiency grounds, the proponent of government intervention must show
(a) that the market in which the commodity is produced or traded
does not satisfy the conditions under which competition can be shown
to produce outcomes such that no one's lot can be improved without
harming someone else's and (b) that the costs of collective intervention to improve the market outcome are smaller than the costs of
market failure. On distributional grounds, the proponent of government intervention must establish that redistribution is desirable
and also that manipulation of the price of a particular commodity is
a more efficient or politically more feasible way of accomplishing
redistributional objectives than direct income supplements or taxes
would be. The absence of purely competitive conditions in large
parts of modern economies is easy to document, but the costs of
collective intervention are not so easy to measure. More basically,
the existence of nonlump-sum taxes and attendant distortions make it
hard to establish whether the efficiency of any particular market
outcome can be improved.

Efficiency

If governments were as uninvolved in the production and distribution
of health care services and research as they are in the production
and distribution of, say, shirts, the markets for health care services and research would tend to suffer from a number of inefficiencies that would make collective intervention seem attractive. Other

justifications for a government role in health care and research flow from imperfections resulting from actions by government themselves. For example, the role of government in ameliorating shortages of health care providers is justified in part by the shortages that government in some degree causes by licensing, a separate action that is justified in principle, if not in specific applications, by a desire to assure the competency of providers whom patients are incompetent to evaluate.

Externalities. In a free market setting there would be too little health care research. Clinical research leading to improved empirical methods, but not keyed to patentable devices or chemical compounds, would yield the investigator only a fraction of the total social benefits generated by any discovery and hence would attract too few resources. Laboratory research into basic science likewise yields results that may be far removed from application and, for reasons too familiar to merit repetition, too little of it would be undertaken in the absence of collective subsidy. Between these two limiting cases would fall research yielding appliances or chemical compounds that are patentable and that in principle could elicit sufficient research.

Even for such research two dilemmas would arise. The first would occur between, on the one hand, preserving incentives for research by protecting secrecy of scientific methods and results, and, on the other hand, sufficiently disseminating knowledge to forestall repetitious research by successive investigators. The second dilemma would occur between the imperative of economic efficiency to price the products of research at marginal cost, and the fact that incentives for future research arise from the promise of being able to produce and sell at a price in excess of marginal cost.

These dilemmas are well known and explain the difficulty in fashioning patent laws and in defining the role of government in support of basic research. The precise institutional arrangements and the amount spent vary widely from one country to another. Even with collective support of research, one could argue that if governments acted like well-informed maximizers of the welfare of their own citizens, too little would be invested in medical research world-wide, because the results of research supported by one country are available to others, even when full compensation is not paid. The incentive of each nation to appropriate the research findings of others is reinforced for small countries to the extent that research is characterized by economies of scale.

Uncertainty, Ignorance, and "Irrationality". The pervasive influence of risk and uncertainty on the market for health care services, long recognized in an informal way, received formal recognition in Arrow's article. Patients do not know when they will demand health care or how much they will demand. Taken alone, such risk does no more than establish the possibility of welfare gains from risk pooling and insurance. In addition, however, patients lack information about the services available under many contingencies, about the probabilities of various outcomes should they obtain particular kinds of care under specified contingencies, and about the relative efficiencies of various health care providers. Most of the services are consumed infrequently,

often at times when the consumer's judgment or ability to gather
information is impaired. Moreover, the consequences of ill-informed
purchase of care include irreversible injury and premature death.
The decision not to collect adequate information sometimes is the
rational response of people to a situation in which information is
both valuable and costly. But much ignorance is unavoidable at
reasonable cost, and even providers can forecast outcomes only
probabilistically.

The results of this combination of risk, uncertainty, and irrationality are respectively insurance, a major problem of moral hazard,
and a desire for what Victor Fuchs (1979) has called "precommitment."
The governments of all developed countries either directly protect,
or encourage the private sector to protect, people from all or most
of the financial risk of hospital care; most also pay for outpatient
services, drugs, and some ancillary social services, and many make
cash payments to protect against earnings loss. The list of services covered is finite (although often broad), but, within an
approved list, provision of services to any single person depends
only on the joint decision of provider and patient, subject to occasional and lenient review by other providers.

Many of the actions governments take to regulate the provision of
health care flow directly from the problem of moral hazard inherent
when consumers of a commodity are insured against the cost of consuming it, so that the "correct" timing, quantity, and quality of
their consumption cannot be specified precisely. These actions now
include controls on the number of health professionals who are
trained, what they study, and how they are licensed, and on what
capital goods are purchased, including buildings and equipment.
Until recently, policy in the United States and in some other
countries promoted the supply of both labor and capital to health
care.

Moral hazard probably explains many aspects of professional ethics
as well. For example, the ethics of noncompetition among providers
of health care, such as the ban on advertising and price competition, may be regarded as evidence of the judgment that any
short-run gain in information would lead to declines over time in
the quality of care that would be hard to monitor, expose, and prevent (Noll, 1975).

Capital Market Imperfections and Moral Hazard. In principle, capital markets could be used to finance a large part of medical care.
If capital markets were not imperfect, young people could borrow to
pay all but the largest medical expenses and amortize their costs
over the remainder of their lives. Catastrophic medical outlays
would require insurance protection even for the young. As people
aged, the size and number of medical outlays for which borrowing
and capital markets would suffice would shrink, and the necessary
scope of insurance would increase. Capital market imperfections
alone would suffice to prevent widespread use of this method of
financing health care, but other factors discussed below would be
even more important.

The fact that medical care services are costly, and are consumed
mostly in large lumps at infrequent intervals that are hard to fore-

cast for individuals but relatively easy to forecast for large groups, would appear to make them ideal candidates for insurance. The object of insurance, of course, is to lift the risk of financial loss from the consumer at the time the service is required.

In principle, such loss can be placed either on providers or on some third party, insurance companies or society as a whole, i.e., the government. If the full cost of any service provided is placed on a third party, then neither the producer nor the consumer of health care services has any incentive to economize on the amounts of the service provided or the methods by which they are provided. The consumer has the incentive to seek all services that produce marginal benefits greater than costs (including, of course, not only out-of-pocket costs and foregone earnings, but also the value of time and inconvenience). Producers of medical care face different incentives depending on the control they exercise over the kinds of care provided and the methods of provision. If the physician is regarded as the decision-maker who sets quantity, quality, and method of production, if he seeks to maximize income, and faces no restriction from government or his profession, he would seek to maximize net revenue subject to any constraint on his working time. The result would be the provision of all services that cost less to produce (including the shadow price of his time) than permitted charges, so that patients have incentives to seek all services, however costly, promising outcomes that improve expected utility, however little. So long as physicians are deterred by professional ethics or some other consideration from producing any services that harm patients, the issue of how many services should be produced must remain a subtle one. Physicians, however, would not face incentives to see that those services are efficiently produced.

If medical services were well defined and produced well-defined benefits with market values, then the incentives to provide excessive amounts of health care and to produce them inefficiently could be curbed.[1] By analogy, fire insurance may cause builders and owners to skimp on safety measures, but the effects of these incentives are reduced, if not suppressed, by building codes, inspections, and requirements written into insurance policies. But many of the physical benefits of medical care are not precisely measurable and the valuation placed upon them is subjective. Many tests, for example, are prescribed in order to rule out remote possibilities considered unlikely at the outset. Under open-ended third-party reimbursement, therefore, medical judgment and professional ethics must bear the burden of limiting care, if any limits are to be imposed.

In fact, medical ethics and patients' desires both call for the provision of all care that is technically beneficial. (See, for example, Schwartz and Joskow, 1978.) In the presence of third-party reimbursement, providers and patients have the incentive to provide all health care that promises any benefits.[2] Unless the benefits of health care fall off abruptly beyond a certain level of service, the decision to ask third parties (insurance companies or governments, the choice is immaterial) to bear the financial risk of medical care will create incentives for health care expenditures to rise to the point where marginal expected benefits approach zero, and will result in pressures for collective intervention to terminate medical care

that yields benefits worth less (by some calculus) than their cost.
These incentives create the need for imposing budget limits or
otherwise regulating the provision of care in ways reviewed below.

If the financial risk of medical care is not borne by patients or by
third parties, then it must be borne by providers. This result
occurs under prepaid group health plans, where a group of health care
providers is responsible for all of the health care provided to a
group. It does not occur under arrangements such as those in the
United Kingdom where only primary care is provided on a closed-panel
basis. Because professional ethics and the natural instinct of
craftsmen to excel technically are placed in opposition to the
financial interests of providers to minimize expenditures, it is
clear that the tendencies of third-party reimbursement to produce
too much care will be muted; but it is possible that the result will
be too little care or care of the wrong kinds. The incentive structure within prepaid plans has received inadequate analysis from
economists. In many respects, a closed-panel system resembles
worker-owned and managed factories. But the impact of different
forms of reimbursement on the quantity of health care and on the
methods chosen for its production (assuming maximizing behavior) has
not been extensively explored. What is clear is that the role of
government in regulating prepaid plans is very different from the
problems of regulating the provision of care under third-party
reimbursement.

Income Distribution

On economic grounds, it is hard, but not impossible, to justify the
use of subsidies tied to the consumption of medical care to
redistribute income (Atkinson and Stiglitz, 1976). If one is prepared to relax the rationality assumptions that underly standard
analysis, it is not hard at all. The standard argument against the
use of commodity subsidies to redistribute income rests on the elementary proof that in a first-best world, commodity subsidies result
in lower welfare than do lump-sum subsidies. In a second-best
world, commodity subsidies may, but need not, be inefficient instruments for altering income distribution. This approach implicitly
treats medical expenditures as "utility-generating, voluntary
consumption."

It might seem reasonable to regard medical expenditures as analogous
to factory maintenance expenditures--in other words, as expenses
incurred to produce net income--or, in Fuchs's analogy, as randomly
distributed, unjust reparations paid to a foreign power. From this
standpoint, medical expenditures by individuals should be deducted
from income to yield an appropriate net income measure on which to
base distributional policy. Although such an approach would affect
the income measure used in determining taxes and transfers, it would
not, if instruments for achieving an optimal income distribution
were at hand and usable, call for a subsidy of medical care.
However, the intense subjectivity of response by different patients
to similar symptoms suggests that any mechanical analogy is
strained.

Subsidies tied to the consumption of medical care would be efficient
devices for redistributing real income if collective concern about
inequality were differentiated and placed greater weight on inadequate consumption of some commodities than on inadequate consumption
of others. Efficient pursuit of such "commodity egalitarianism"
would require the use of full or partial subsidies tied to favored
commodities. But commodity egalitarianism cannot explain why the
same subsidy, full or partial, would be provided to all persons
regardless of their income. Uniform, rather than income-related,
subsidies are frequently supported because the reduction in the
number of income tests is alleged to reduce social and political
fragmentation. Uniform subsidies could be shown to be superior to
income-tested ones as well, if the efficiency losses from
mistargeted subsidies under uniform subsidies were shown to be
smaller than the resource costs of administering income tests.
Because the cost of administering income-tested programs in the
United States is demonstrable--roughly 8 to 10 percent more than the
cost of administering entitlement programs--such a demonstration may
be feasible. But it requires analysts explicitly to balance and
weigh losses from the misallocation of transfers against the
resource costs of allocating them more accurately. I know of no
such effort. Subsidies to the purchase of medical care can also be
justified if one rejects the notion that all or nearly all people
make rational decisions about their demand for medical care,
including insurance. If myopia or the free rider problem causes a
perceptible fraction of the population not to protect itself against
financially major health costs, the remainder of the population has
an interest in compelling the uncovered to pay for their own protection.

THE EMERGENCE OF HEALTH CARE AS AN ECONOMIC COMMODITY

In this section I shall suggest, first, that the medical technology
that existed until recently made relatively cheap the collective
decision to treat health care as a right (like criminal justice,
military service during wartime, and voting privileges) to which the
usual canons of market allocation and distribution were not allowed
to apply and, second, that recent changes in medical technology make
the continuation of that traditional approach very costly. These
changes in technology have led to world-wide interest in medical
cost containment; but they have forced (or soon will force) a popular reexamination of attitudes toward health care delivery in most
developed countries and will probably lead to important changes in
the role of government in financing and regulating the delivery of
health care. In presenting my reasons for these statements, I shall
resort to some oversimplification.

The Traditional View of Medical Care

Until well after the start of the twentieth century, medical care
providers could contribute very little to the cure of chronic and
most acute illnesses, or to otherwise improving the health of

patients, beyond encouraging them to rest in relatively sanitary
surroundings and to eat well. For a limited number of acute
problems, such as broken bones or severe lacerations, physicians
could provide services with clear and obvious benefits. Midwives
and physicians aided in childbirth. Vaccinations reduced the incidence of a number of infectious diseases. Before antibiotics,
however, the methods of treating bacterial infections were
primitive. The causes and cures of chronic diseases were understood
poorly or not at all. Most of the medical benefits of hospital
medical care were related to the "hotel" services provided in hospitals and to the psychological succor provided by physicians.

A number of writers has commented on the quasi-religious role of
medical care, and the priestlike role played by physicians. The
fears and mysteries of birth, illness, and death, processes imperfectly understood or not understood at all that gave rise to shamans
and rituals in much of the world, gave rise to hospitals and physicians in western societies and much of Asia. Also, many authors
have pointed out that the importance of physicians and of hospitals
has increased as the historical processes of industrialization and
attendant urbanization have broken down the familial networks
through which personal care services are provided in agricultural
societies, and as the decline of religion has diminished the capacity of clerics to provide the psychological aid and comfort now
dispensed by psychiatrists, other physicians, or psychologists.

If one concluded on distributional grounds that no sick person,
however poor, should be allowed to languish unattended, unfed, and
unsheltered, the cost of providing all medical services considered
to produce any medical benefits, until recently, was limited and
modest. To put matters slightly differently, once the distributional commitment was made, the waste entailed by an open-ended promise to provide all medically beneficial care was small. The
economic loss in providing services worth less (in some sense) than
their cost certainly was small compared to the political gains of
broad coverage, and in any event, formal attempts to distinguish
between justified and unjustified services would have been
treacherous to administer.

Against this background, the decision taken in most developed
western states during the twentieth century to place health care
outside the market, to treat it as a commodity that should be
available, like the right to vote and the obligation to serve in the
military during wartime, as a concomitant of citizenship irrespective of income or wealth, imposed little inefficiency.

Even so, the movement to comprehensive and universal coverage pro-
ceeded slowly and at different speeds in various countries. Not all
members of society were covered at an early stage. The first health
plans tended to develop along occupational lines, and this legacy is
visible, for example, in the plans of France, Germany, Italy, and
other countries, where coverage still is provided through numerous
employment-based sickness funds. Free or subsidized medical care
first was offered to industrial workers or government employees,
groups concentrated in urban areas. Medical care for these groups
served to mute political unrest among workers whose loyalty incum-
bent governments regarded as vital. Coverage at first was narrowly

limited to hospitalization, but grew broader as more services were
added, until sometime after World War II when most developed western
nations provided comprehensive coverage of inpatient and outpatient
medical services including mental health care and dentistry, and
most also provided income protection against the risk of earnings
loss during periods of illness. Some routinely provided social services such as household help for pregnant mothers.

Provision of health care has never been completely free or equal.
All nations have permitted people to supplement collectively provided health care in order to have such "extras" as private or
semiprivate hospital rooms, the privilege of avoiding waiting lists,
or attendance by physicians reputed to be more capable than the
average.

The point of the foregoing discussion is to assert that the technology of health care until recently contributed a favorable
environment for the development of the ideology that health care
should be available freely to all on an essentially egalitarian
basis. The cost of providing medical care on such terms was perceived to be modest. The availability of such care assuaged
profound human fears in the cold environment of industrializing
or industrialized societies. From an economic standpoint, the cost
of this ideology was modest, and it entailed little waste. As long
as one placed a value that exceeded the cost on the benefits of
minimal medical care for the least favored member of society, there
was little question about the extent of medical need or of how much
it would cost to meet that need, and, by definition, few expenditures yielded benefits worth less than their cost.[3]

Beneath this broad pattern of similar evolution evolved health care
systems and government involvement that differed greatly from one
nation to another. In some nations the government directly employs
most physicians on salary and owns and operates most hospitals. In
others physicians are independent and are paid fees for services
rendered. Some sickness funds are nominally independent of government and enjoy political standing of their own, while the payments
for health care in other countries flow directly from the national
treasury to providers. The source of revenues for health care
includes varying mixes of premiums, payroll taxes, and other revenues. The proportion of medical costs paid directly by patients
varies from nothing for most services to significant fractions for
others. Debates on these aspects of collectively organized care
have been intense, and their resolution has both shaped the effect
of health programs on the distribution of income, and determined or
expressed the locus of political power. But this diversity should
not obscure the startling similarity in the ideology of health care
that has dominated thinking in most developed nations, or the fact
that this similarity flowed from the technical character of health
care.

Changes in Health Care Technology

That a scientific revolution has transformed medical care during the
last generation is well known. Its impact on the role of government

has been multi-faceted, but two effects deserve special notice. The
first is the dramatic increase in total expenditure attributable to
scientific advances. The second and more important for present purposes is the change in the nature of decisions that must be made at
the margin in determining how much more or less to spend on health
care and in deciding what services to provide.

Total Cost. In principle, improvements in health technology can
raise or lower expenditures. A few advances clearly lower
expenditures. Antibiotics, for example, have made possible the
prompt and complete cure of certain infectious diseases that previously had resisted treatment or responded only to costly and
protracted therapies. Most technical advances have boosted expenditures by enabling improvements in expected health outcomes to be
achieved at greater total expenditure. Still others permit replacement of costly therapies with less expensive procedures but so
expand the number of patients who can benefit from treatment that
aggregate expenditures increase. Some improvements represent marginal advances in the effectiveness of previously available forms of
care--intensive care units, for example. Some improvements, such as
renal dialysis, permit treatment where no effective alternative previously existed. The true medical value of some procedures--such as
coronary artery surgery--remains in dispute. (For further examples,
see Russell, 1979.)

Whether future improvements in medical technology in combination
will raise or lower expenditures is unclear. The creation of arti-
ficial organs or developments that permit the proliferation of
transplants would raise expenditures. Other advances, such as a
breakthrough in our understanding of cancer, might lead to less
costly methods of treating it and might tend to reduce medical
expenditures. Even advances that reduce costs of treating one
disease may raise expenditures after all; to cheat death for a
moment on the cheap leaves open the risk of more costly debility.
To put matters conservatively, one should not ignore the possibility
that technical advances will lead to further increases in medical
expenditures.

Marginal Decisions. The preceding paragraphs are based on the tacit
assumption that the traditional ideology of medical care described
above prevails, with its attendant policy of meeting medical need.
From a technical standpoint, all health care that yields any medical
benefits is "needed". From a behavioral standpoint, needed care
will be demanded only if the patient and/or his physician perceives
benefits that exceed the costs the patient must bear. Whether the
service will be provided and whether the technical means of providing it will be efficient depend on the incentives and limits providers face.

The key point is that the technical revolution in medicine not only
has contributed to the growth of medical expenditures but also has
created many actual or potential medical services that produce some,
but often small, benefits. Physicians, for example, have available
an armory of diagnostic weapons many of which are noninvasive and
hence entail negligible risks or none at all to the patient. They
are medically "needed", in the sense defined above, as long as

resulting additions to information have any value at all. Where
once the list of medical needs at zero cost to patient and full
reimbursement to the provider was fairly well defined and limited,
the list is now long and growing, and it is populated at the margin
by many costly procedures of limited medical value. Some of these
procedures are scientifically dramatic and widely discussed: CT
scanners, dialysis, radiotherapy. Less dramatic, individually less
costly but collectively more expensive procedures, such as routine
lab tests, are at least as important (Moloney and Rogers, 1979).

The result is that the policy of meeting medical need, which once
entailed little social waste, now threatens to cause considerable
waste, largely through the provision of services that are medically
needed (the benefit to the patient is positive), demanded (because
marginal cost to the patient is zero or very low), and supplied
(because providers are fully reimbursed or are indifferent between
low- and high-benefit care), but that provide benefits worth less in
some sense than total social cost.

This problem is visible in most developed countries. It is
expressed in rapidly growing medical expenditures combined with
discontent over the trend and moves for medical cost
containment.[4] Under a system in which health care is provided free
to the patient and he is reimbursed for lost earnings, the financial
difference between supplying all care for which there is medical
need and all that is demanded is likely to be small. The difference
between these two quantities, on one hand, and the cost of supplying
all care that provides social benefits greater than social costs, on
the other, has become far larger than it was a generation ago
because of the technological revolution in health care. The cost in
resource misallocation of attempting to meet medical need has risen.

The situation just described does not exist in all countries, for
all groups within other countries, or for all services. In France,
some patients face cost sharing for some services. In Great
Britain, providers face tightly limited budgets and must ration services in various ways; the waiting lists for care for chronic
illnesses have received much attention. In the United States, private insurance coverage is incomplete. Many nations do not fully
reimburse wages lost because of illness, and some do not reimburse
them at all. A variety of limits in most countries has prevented
the purchase of all the modern equipment necessary to meet medical
"need," i.e., all that would produce positive medical benefits.[5]
Canada has placed hospitals on fixed budgets and the United States
is contemplating limits on hospital expenditures. However, the
upward drift in medical expenditures is large and pervasive (OECD,
1977). Whether this increase will continue depends, in part, on the
character of technological advances in medicine.

The increase in the proportion of the population that is aged,
already a problem in the United Kingdom and Germany and a future
problem in other European countries and the United States, makes
some increase in expenditures on medical care likely. This
demographic trend, together with the medical advances already mentioned, raises complex issues about the role of government in the
provision of long-term care. The auspices under which long-term
care is provided, the agency of government charged with respon-

sibility, and the relative importance of private and collective provision of care all differ widely. Because long-term care involves
not only medical care, but also numerous social services, I shall
not attempt to explore it here. It is important to recognize that
the application of the traditional ideology of medical care to long-
term care, including social services, involves very large and
increasing costs for a country with an aging population.

If the difference between efficient medical expenditures and those
that would be necessary to meet medical need remain large or
increase, the incentives from collective assumption of financial risk
(i.e., third-party reimbursement) for the excessive provision of
health care, and the resulting large and (possibly) growing medical expenditures, will place the ideology of health care, developed
when health technology was quite different, under increasing strain.

Alternative Roles of Government Under Modern Health Care Technology

As Uwe Reinhardt has pointed out (1975a), under various payment
systems it is possible, in principle, for patients to gain financially, to lose financially, or to be unaffected by additional
demands for medical care; the same three possibilities exist for
providers from increasing the supply of additional care. The result
is a nine-cell matrix based on policy with respect to cost sharing
and reimbursement. Three of the cells are seldom observed because
patients always incur time costs and seldom gain financially from
illness unless they are overinsured, a situation that can arise
under private insurance if people buy two or more indemnity policies, or under a national health plan if reimbursement for lost
wages is excessively generous (for example, if wage replacement
payments are nontaxable and exceed previous earnings).[6]

No health care system fits neatly in any one of the cells. Some
services in all countries are free to patients, while others
must be purchased. Some providers are reimbursed fee-for-service,
others are salaried, and some are at financial risk to provide all
services. Broadly speaking, however, the traditional ideology of
health care requires that patients directly bear little or none of
the marginal cost of health care and that providers either gain or
remain financially indifferent to the provision of additional care.
The British and Swedish systems approximate financial indifference
for both patients and providers. The German, Dutch, and American
systems approximate indifference for the patient (though in the U.S.
this is only true of hospital care for insured persons) and financial gain for the provider.

This section explores briefly the regulatory responses governments
can make to the changes in health technology if health systems
remain within these cells, and the quite different problems that
arise if a decision is made to place either patients or providers at
financial risk.

Marginal Cost for Patients: Negligible; Marginal Net Revenue for
Providers: Positive. This system, approximated in Germany and the
United States, contains incentives for patients to seek all care

that promises positive benefits and for providers to supply it. The
potential for economic waste within this system is at a maximum. For
that reason, the regulatory burden on the government, acting through
official instrumentalities or through private organizations, to
control the provision of excessive care and to encourage the selection of efficient methods is also at a maximum.

The regulatory devices available to governments are well known and
their use is general. First, governments can act to control the
number and type of trained health personnel and the nature of the
training they receive. Traditionally, governments have actively
subsidized, rationed, or otherwise controlled the training of health
personnel. Most developed countries attempted to increase the ratio
of physicians to the population during the three decades following
World War II. These policies were successful. Now a perception of
the opposite problem--that physicians, who have considerable if not
perfectly elastic control over the demand for their own services,
may be too numerous--is triggering widespread reconsideration of
policies to increase the ratio of health care providers to the
population.

Second, governments can act to control investment in medical capital. Usually, such controls focus on costly items--new hospitals or
major alterations, and expensive equipment. Such controls are the
instrument for supervising the introduction of new health technologies. Because technologies that do not depend on costly capital
slip through this screen, they are inherently more difficult to
control under this financing regime. It is important to note that
the regulator is hindered in his efforts to decide rationally
whether capital goods are scarce or overcrowded by the health care
provider's flexible capacity to determine the use of existing capital. High bed occupancy rates can mean either that space is unavailable to patients badly in need of hospitalization, or that
doctors have permitted excessive lengths of stay, or both. The
great differences in average lengths of hospital stay among (and
even within) developed countries for similar illnesses are compatible with supply-caused differences in medical practice.

Third, by regulating the reimbursement of physicians and health care
providers for various services, governments can influence the short-
run supply of various services by existing physicians, the location
of physicians, the flow of new physicians into various specialties
(and hence the long-run supply of various services), and the use of
ancillary health personnel. In many countries specialists receive
higher fees for the same service than do general practitioners, and
fees tend to be higher in areas where the ratio of physicians to the
general population is relatively high. Fees for certain standard
services are often lower for allied health personnel than those for
physicians. The causes of geographical imbalances in the density of
physicians are numerous and the consequences for health status are
unclear; the proper relationship among fees for various kinds of
service by individual providers, and for the same services by different providers, is subject to much debate. What is clear is that
regulation of the absolute and relative level of fees is one of the
few devices available to governments under "zero-marginal-cost,
positive-marginal-revenue" regimes to limit rents earned by providers, to influence physician location, or to alter the incentives to

provide various kinds of services. The effectiveness of control
over fees is open to dispute, but it is one of the few available
instruments of control.

Fourth, governments can promote utilization review. The United
States, the United Kingdom, and Germany all have such systems, as do
other nations. The purpose is to ferret out improper or excessive
care. Such reviews are carried out by physicians. I know of no
system that has had a significant measurable effect on practice or
cost. So long as the traditional ideology of care is dominant among
physicians and the incentives they and patients face encourage the
provision of all care with positive benefits at any cost, such
programs are unlikely to achieve more than marginal status.

Fifth, governments can attempt to impose expenditure caps on hospitals or other health care providers. Germany has imposed such
limits. After a period during which the growth of expenditures
slowed, these limits appear now to have been breached. President
Carter has sought such limits from the U.S. Congress, so far without
success. Such limits, if effective, remove covered providers from
the system of open-ended reimbursement. The tension that such
controls are bound to generate within a system otherwise predicated
on open-ended reimbursement is obvious: there is a continuing temptation to move services from the limited sector to the unlimited
sector and for providers in the limited sector to plead special circumstances as justification for exceptional treatment. For such
limits to succeed more than briefly, a complex and legitimized set
of institutions must arise for determining which of those patients
who would have received care in the absence of limits should be
denied care, and for enforcing and making acceptable such denial.
In short, effective limits and the traditional ideology of medical
care are flatly inconsistent.

Marginal Cost for Patients: Negligible; Marginal Net Revenue for
Providers: Nil. Under such a system, in its pure form, providers
are salaried and hospitals and other medical institutions must
operate on a fixed budget. Other combinations are possible; providers may be paid on a fee-for-service basis by organizations such as
hospitals which operate on a fixed budget. (Such a system is
equivalent to the effectively capped system mentioned above.)

British hospitals operate under such a system. The Swedish system
requires limited cost sharing, but most providers are salaried and
most hospitals budgeted. Many of the same regulatory problems faced
under fee-for-service continue. Policies to regulate the number and
type of health personnel may still be necessary, as there is no more
reason to think that existing institutions will train the "proper"
number under this system than under fee-for-service. Similar issues
will arise with regard to investment, except that the government
role is likely to be greater than under fee-for-service (as it is in
Great Britain and Sweden). The possible regulation of fee schedules
is replaced by the necessary regulation of salaries. Utilization
review becomes an ongoing element implicit in setting budgets, personnel targets, and capital planning.

The important difference between fee-for-service (positive marginal
revenue) and salary-fixed budget (zero marginal revenue) regimes is

that the latter creates an institutional setting for political
consideration of whether or not the nation wishes to adhere to the
traditional ideology of medical care, while the former does not.
There is no guarantee that the political process operating in such
an institutional setting will produce decisions to keep costs below
those generated with open-ended reimbursement. The pressures for
meeting "medical need" that tend to be satisfied automatically by
the mutual self-interest of patients and providers when marginal
cost is zero and marginal revenue is positive may be satisfied in
the political arena. But the opportunity for limits exists when
marginal revenue is zero, and it is hard to avoid in the face of
contemporary developments in medical technology and practice. The
political process quite clearly has been used to set limits in Great
Britain; the degree to which it has been so used in other countries
is less obvious.

Positive Marginal Cost. All health systems impose some charges on
some patients for some services. The issue is not whether such
charges should exist, but whether a policy of substantially
increasing the marginal cost patients face when they demand health
care is likely to be an equitable or efficient way of reducing the
demand for care that is worth less to society than it costs.
Increasing the cost of medical care at the margin will have some
effect on the demand for health care, as Newhouse's chapter in this
volume underscores. While some forms of cost sharing are costly to
administer--for example, copayments or coinsurance--others, such as
deductibles, are not. If cost sharing were required only of people
whose incomes exceed certain thresholds, the added cost of income
tests would result. On balance, it appears that cost sharing can
play a modest role in deterring care of which the social value is
less than cost.

Negative Marginal Net Revenue. The final device for encouraging the
explicit balancing of medical costs and benefits is to impose a
marginal net cost on providers for the provision of health care.
For a variety of obvious reasons this approach is viable only for a
group of providers capable of meeting and obliged to provide a
broad, predefined list of health care services. The group must
include sufficient providers to supply all services competently.
But the group must not be so large (e.g., the entire nation) that
the financial risk to individual providers from providing excessive
care becomes vanishingly small. Furthermore, patients who feel that
they are denied care worth more in their judgment than its cost must
have alternative groups or forms of care to which they can switch.

Several writers have advocated that the financing of health care in
the United States be organized to encourage patients to select prepaid group health plans under which providers are placed at risk to
provide all of a stipulated list of services to a closed panel of
patients. Under this system, patients could buy supplemental care
on a fee-for-service basis, but they would get no encouragement from
favorable tax treatment for medical outlays. Advocates of this
approach have pointed to several studies that indicate lower rates
of hospitalization and lower medical costs under closed-panel, prepaid group health plans. Part of this reduction in hospitalization
may be attributable to the tendency of people with lower prior rates
of hospitalization differentially to select prepaid group plans.

The fraction of savings that is genuine remains in dispute. Even
where freely available, prepaid group plans have not secured the
membership of more than one-third of the eligible population. The
practical question, therefore, is whether a health care subsystem
serving a fraction of the population can alter practice in the
remainder, either through competitive pressure or in some other way,
and thereby cut significantly into the excess of actual over efficient health care provision.

The incentives of prepaid group plans encourage providers newly
enrolling members to weigh the value of various kinds of medical
care against their costs, but once enrolled, members face the same
incentives as under full reimbursement by third parties. Newly
enrolling patients and providers exercise this choice through
various market decisions. These decisions, however, are conditioned
by government regulations. If public subsidies (directly or through
the tax system) are to be offered to encourage the purchase of care
up to a stipulated level (range of care, cost sharing, and so on),
or if the poor are to be provided free care, what should these
levels be? A political decision must be made expressing what those
levels of care should be, a decision that should embody a collective
judgment about what kinds of care yield social benefits at least as
great as cost. Other forms of regulation would continue, e.g., over
the number and kinds of health care providers who are trained. And
a new form of utilization review would probably come into existence,
to assure that providers did not stint on care. In short, the
growth of prepaid health plans would necessitate new forms of regulation in addition to some that would remain in effect for traditional forms of care. Advocates promise that this mode of
delivering care will reduce costs, both directly and through competition, and that it will permit government to assume a less intru-
sive role in the provision of health care. The first promise has
economic logic on its side; the second does not.

CONCLUSION

Health care is not and never has been a commodity whose production
and distribution satisfied the conditions for optimal allocation
through competitive markets. Many of its special characteristics
explain the special features of the market for health care: the
importance of insurance (private or governmental) and the pervasive
role of government. Until recently, however, the available technology made it relatively inexpensive to regard health care as a
right, not as an ordinary economic commodity. Little economic waste
attended this approach. The recent and continuing revolution in the
technology of medical care has inflated the cost of that right. If
all health care that provides medical benefit to the patient at zero
price is treated as a right, the scope for waste is large and
getting larger. Nations can deal with this situation (a) by
accepting waste as a price of sustaining a valued approach to human
life and of maintaining an institution that contributes to social
solidarity, (b) by imposing regulations to curb the natural tendency
of a zero-marginal-cost, positive-marginal-revenue system to
generate waste, (c) by imposing budget limits on providers, (d) by

increasing cost sharing for patients, (e) by putting providers at
financial risk, or by some combination of all of the above. Unless
countries choose option (a), the role of governments as guarantors
of the right to health care must end. They will be forced
increasingly to make ethically painful decisions about what care
shall not be provided.

                              NOTES

[1]Other hard-to-define services, such as those of lawyers, must normally pass
the market test (except in government where, many would argue, excessive supply is
a problem). Services of educators are normally purchased through fixed budgets.

[2]An unabashed expression of this ideology, contained in a recent letter to
The New England Journal of Medicine, may dramatize it for economists to whom
equating marginal costs and benefits is second nature.

Of late an increasing number of papers in this and other journals have (sic)
been concerned with "cost effectiveness" of diagnostic and therapeutic
procedures. Inherent in these articles is the view that choices will be predicated not only on the basis of strictly clinical considerations but also on the
basis of economic considerations as they may affect the patient, the hospital,
and society. It is my consideration that such considerations are not germane
to ethical medical practice, that they occupy space in journals that would be
better occupied by substantive matter, and that they serve to orient physicians
toward consideration of economics, which is not their legitimate problem. It
is dangerous to introduce extraneous factors into medical decisions, since consideration of such factors may eventually lead to considerations of age, social
usefulness, and other matters irrelevant to ethical practice. The example of
medicine in Nazi Germany is too close to need further elucidation.

....Optimization of survival and not optimization of cost effectiveness is the
only ethical imperative...Ethical physicians do not base their practices on
the patients' ability to pay or choose diagnostic and therapeutic procedures
on the basis of their cost..." (Loewy, 1980).

[3]For a similar point, see Newhouse and Taylor (1971): "We are used to
thinking about the traditional situation in which medical care was not very costly
and in which giving unlimited medical care to everyone who needed it did not mean
making much of a sacrifice elsewhere. In such circumstances, many came to view
medical care as an absolute 'right' and not simply as another service."

[4]The contrast between attitudes toward the rising proportion of GNP devoted to
medical care and the rising fraction devoted in the past to automobiles or
recently to computers is worthy of note. The fact that the ratio of consumer
expenditures on user operated transportation to GNP in the United States rose from
5.1% in 1930 to 8.1% in 1955, for example, elicited no calls for automobile cost
containment. The difference, of course, is that automobiles must meet a market
test. Medical care does not.

[5]The Office of Technology Assessment has gathered reports on the availability
of newly developed equipment and the frequency with which certain forms of high

technology care are provided in ten developed countries. The variations are considerable, suggesting that unless services producing no medical benefit are being
provided in some countries, some medical need (as defined above) is not being met
in others.

[6]This risk is realized with respect to people who are adjudged to be disabled.

HEALTH, ECONOMICS, AND HEALTH ECONOMICS
J. van der Gaag and M. Perlman (editors)
© *North-Holland Publishing Company, 1981*

AN INTERPRETATION OF GOVERNMENT INTERVENTION IN HEALTH:
THE ITALIAN CASE

Domenicantonio Fausto
Mario Leccisotti

INTRODUCTION

An extraordinary growth of medical expenditure has taken place in
most countries (OECD, 1977, p. 28). Such growth has mainly been
caused by government intervention in all aspects of health.
Compulsory and government-supported health insurance schemes or
national health services exist in almost all countries. Private
insurance and religious and other nonprofit hospitals enjoy considerable tax benefits and/or government subsidies. Not many people
in the western world nowadays bear the full cost of the drugs they
consume. Detailed regulation and control are enforced on many products and activities.

This growth of public expenditure on health care is not consistent
with the results of the empirical studies on the effects of medical
care. "The most important, and perhaps the most surprising, finding
of health economics is this: Holding constant the state of medical
technology and other health-determining variables, the marginal
contribution of medical care to health is very small in modern-
nations" (Fuchs, 1979).

We are, then, faced with an apparent paradox: resources and government intervention in health care are constantly increasing, but
health is not. How can we explain such a paradox? In this paper we
attempt to offer an explanation of government intervention by
referring to the motives which inspire the actions of politicians.

The behavior of the members of the party (or parties) in power is
constrained by the presence of an opposition in a parliamentary
system and by the independent behavior of bureaucrats and judges.
However, in the field of health there is no evidence of a serious
conflict of interest and opinion between the different parties or
bodies of government, so that, as a first approximation, we may
treat them as a single subject, whom we shall call the politician.

A Survey of Approaches

Government intervention in health is usually explained by recourse
to various social arguments. A number of authors stress the humanitarian motive of securing a certain level of medical care for

everyone, or the egalitarian motive of equal consumption of the
health commodity by all members of the community. The main core
of the literature is concerned with efficiency considerations:
the market fails to achieve the social optimum because of the
existence of externalities, public goods elements, ignorance on the
part of the consumer, etc.[1]

This "social approach" is really a normative theory that indicates
why government intervention in health can be justified. It can be
employed as an explanation of real-life events only if we make the
further assumption of a benevolent and perfectly operating
government, which is willing and able fully to implement the normative provisions.

Such an assumption is contradicted by everyday experience concerning
the motivations and behavior of people in government. Moreover, the
"social approach" is not able to explain the existing evidence of
the small contribution made by medical care to health. Indeed, it
points out that people want better health for themselves and for
their fellow citizens, whereas government expenditure only provides
more medical care. The "social approach" cannot explain why a benevolent and perfectly operating government or rational citizens
behave in such a way. An explanation must be found elsewhere.

Downs's pioneering book on representative democracy (1957) seems to
offer an explanation of government behavior. Downs assumes that
parties seek to maximize political support--"The fundamental
hypothesis of our model is that parties formulate policies in order
to win elections, rather than win elections in order to formulate
policies" (Downs, 1957, p. 28.). As long as voters support government expenditure on health, vote-maximizing politicians will be
induced to increase such expenditure. Downs's model, however, is
not able to explain voters' behavior in the light of the existing
difference between medical care and health. Downs's own thinking on
voter-taxpayers' behavior is inconsistent with the dramatic expansion of government expenditure. He suggests that voters' information is asymmetrical, in that they are more aware of the costs
than of the benefits of government programs.

Buchanan and Wagner (1977, pp. 129-30), referring to Puviani's
fiscal illusion, present the opposite view. For a variety of
reasons, voters underestimate the tax cost of government services,
thus favoring an excessively large government sector.

The fiscal illusion argument, by itself, is not able to explain the
relative growth of the government sector and of health expenditure
within it. It is only concerned with the efficiency problem of
government size relative to some optimum.

Buchanan and Tullock (1962) have also argued for overinvestment in
the public sector. Their explanation is that members of the winning
coalition approve those investments from which they expect benefits
and whose cost is shared with all taxpayers.

In this respect, Riker (1962), considering politics as a zero-sum game, holds that under majority rule, individuals will form a minimum winning coalition. People sharing the benefits will tend to be the minimum number required to ensure the victory. Such a hypothesis is unable to explain government intervention in health, which benefits a large and ever-expanding group of people.

A different explanation of government intervention, which seems consistent with the latter evidence, refers to the redistributional effect of government. A pure wealth-transfer model was suggested by Meltzer and Richard (1978), under the assumption that candidates seek voters and that voters choose the candidate who promises to act in their interests, which are represented by the difference between the expected benefits and costs of government programs. The majority will thus force a wealth distribution from the minority.

Brunner (1978) has extended the pure wealth-transfer model by considering "the entrepreneurial behavior of politicians and bureaus." He says, "The pure transfer model cannot explain, by itself alone, the relative growth of employment in the public sector or the increasing ramifications of the government apparatus. Neither can it explain the observable fact that wealth transfers do not occur in the form of a single uniform and huge system shifting money from the richer to the poorer." Brunner assumes that "Costs and benefits associated with general programs are more evenly distributed than the costs and benefits of specific programs... Information costs about costs and benefits of general programs are large relative to benefits... Information costs about costs and benefits of specific programs are relatively small to 'positively affected group' and comparatively large to 'negatively affected group.'" Therefore, "specific programs dominate general programs" (Brunner, 1978, pp. 670-73). Such a statement, however, is contradicted by the dramatic increase in the "general" health care program.

None of the existing theories seems able to offer a satisfactory explanation for the evidence of continuously increasing government intervention in health and for the above-mentioned paradox. On a theoretical level, such theories can be criticized for the incomplete specification of politicians' and voters' behavior. As far as the "social approach" is concerned, a politician's only role is to assure a perfect implementation of the preferences of the members of the community. Other authors restrict the role of politician to that of vote-getter and consider citizens as pure wealth-maximizers. A more satisfactory and consistent theory must explain the behavior of both politicians and voters according to the traditional postulate of utility maximization that is accepted by standard economic theory.

The "social approach," while assuming that members of the community have a complex utility function, including such "social" objectives as equality in consumption of some commodity, public goods, etc., limits the politician's utility to the pursuit of society's welfare. Other authors, in contrast, consider the politician and voters as merely concerned with their own material interests, which, for the former, are exclusively represented by the desire to be elected to office, and, for the latter, by their own wealth.

A GENERAL APPROACH TO GOVERNMENT INTERVENTION

Our hypothesis, therefore, is that the utility function of the politician and of individual voters is a complex one. In the first
place, such a utility function includes the "social" elements of
equality, wealth distribution, externalities, public goods, etc.,
which for analytical simplicity we shall indicate with the composite
variable $\underline{S}$. We shall not distinguish the different elements contained in $\underline{S}$, and, for the time being, rule out any contrast among
such elements, so that we may safely assume that an increase in $\underline{S}$
will increase an individual's utility. Ceteris paribus, if voters
are willing to support parties and candidates whose program promises
an increase in "social" expenditure, the politician is well disposed
to include such an expenditure in his program, both because it has
popular support and because he himself thinks it good.

However, individuals' actions are also motivated by their own personal wealth, $\underline{W}$. The wealth-transfer model has stressed how voters
behave accordingly, while the politician's interests are limited to
being elected. Such an assumption imposes an unnecessary constraint
on the analysis and renders it incapable of explaining much of the
politician's behavior. Undoubtedly his wealth is strictly connected
with the holding of office. He must promise a program which appeals
to voters, either by satisfying their "social" objectives or by
increasing their wealth. Any rational individual will, however,
have some trade-off between election and other forms of wealth.

Finally, individuals are also motivated by nonpecuniary goods, such
as social prestige and influence, etc., and are willing to sacrifice some of their own wealth or social objectives in order to
achieve more of them. We shall indicate such nonpecuniary goods
with the composite variable $\underline{X}$, without distinguishing among the elements contained in it and assuming that there are no contradictions
among them.

We can thus write the utility function of the members of a
community, either as politicians or as voters, in the following way:

$$U = U(S, W, X)$$

where U_S, U_W, $U_X > 0$.

In order to focus attention on the main strands of the argument, we
summarize our analysis by some postulates from which we will derive
propositions concerning the behavior of the politician and of
the voters. In the first place, since government action is determined by the politician, we assume that:

    1. Government intervention is determined by the utility function
of the politician.

The politician's behavior is subject to several technological and institutional constraints. However, since we are only interested in evaluating the direction of government intervention and not in determining an equilibrium or an optimum, we will consider only the constraints imposed by the voters or by possible contrasts arising in the realization of the different elements in the utility function of the politician.

Such a utility function includes the three variables we have previously indicated. A good proxy for the nonpecuniary goods of the politician can be found in the extent and degree of his control over resources that cannot be directly exchanged into money on the market, which we shall henceforth label as "power." In one way or another, power will probably increase the politician's wealth, but we prefer to keep it distinct both because it may also assume other connotations and because it entails a different kind of property right. Power is usually tied up with a particular office and cannot be freely disposed of. Consequently, the behavior of a person interested in acquiring, maintaining and increasing power may differ considerably from that of a wealth-maximizing individual.

A series of further postulates encapsulates various points in our argument:

   2. The politician's utility is a function both of the community's social objectives and of his own wealth and power.

   3. Voters support parties and candidates who promise to satisfy their own utility, as determined by their social objectives and by their own wealth and nonpecuniary goods.

We shall ignore all constraints on voters' behavior, with the exception of that depending by possible contrasts in the different elements in the utility function and of that relating to the cost of government expenditure. In this regard, however, because of the fiscal illusion, we assume that:

   4. Voters tend to underestimate the cost of government intervention.

In order to derive some meaningful and testable propositions, we need to specify how the attributes of government intervention affect the politician's interests and voters' behavior:

   5. The politician's discretionary power is greater in the sectors in which voters' control is weaker.

   6. Voters' control is weaker whenever well-established bounds and rules of government intervention do not exist; but when the sector is "long established," rules of government intervention and bounds become effective.

   7. Visible attributes of the output produced by government improve the politician's image more than invisible attributes.

From our seven postulates we derive four propositions concerning the behavior of voters and of the politician.

As far as voters are concerned, a contrast may arise between $\underline{S}$ and $\underline{W}$ or $\underline{X}$. A typical example from the area of health is the doctor, whose wealth may suffer from government intervention. However, "social" expenditure is likely to be favored by the majority of voters, both because they consider it good and/or because they tend to believe that it positively affects their wealth or nonpecuniary goods, given, also, the fiscal illusion indicated by Postulate 4. Next, the minority may find it more profitable to protect its own interests by affecting the shaping and implementing of social programs rather than by a strong, direct opposition, which has a great chance of being defeated.[2] As a consequence, in spite of a possible contrast between some voters' social objectives and their own wealth and/or nonpecuniary goods, we may formulate Proposition I.

I.   The majority of voters support government "social" intervention.

The politician is also motivated by social objectives and by his own wealth and power. First, personal interests of the politician can best be satisfied whenever he enjoys great discretionary power, because voters cannot adequately control his actions. Therefore, given the constraints imposed by his social objectives, we may formulate Proposition II:

II.   The politician prefers intervention in those sectors in which he can enjoy a greater discretionary power.

Next, as far as the politician is concerned, no contrast is likely to exist between the social objectives and his wealth and/or power. In the first place, since the majority of voters support government intervention in the "social" sector, by pursuing the community's social objectives the politician can gain popular support, thus increasing his power and wealth. Next, the characteristics of the social sectors tend to conform to Postulates 5 and 6, so that government intervention in the area leaves ample room for the satisfaction of the politician's power and wealth. Therefore, we may easily conclude that:

III.   The politician will propose large "social" programs.

One last proposition derives directly from our Postulate 7, and from the observation that often the production of visible attributes of output permits a greater increase in the politician's wealth and power:

IV.   The politician prefers visible attributes of government expenditure.

THE CHARACTERISTICS OF THE COMMODITY HEALTH

We attempt to find the explanation for government intervention in health as a commodity in the extent to which its characteristics satisfy our four propositions.

In the first place, as we have pointed out, health expenditure is usually regarded as a "social" good, because people want more equal consumption of such a commodity, because they want each person to have at his or her disposal a certain amount of medical care, because they fear infectious diseases and enjoy being surrounded by healthy people, etc. The "social approach" has specified in great detail the different ways in which health can affect individuals' utility functions. Both the politician and voters consider health as an economic good. Labor unions, intellectuals, and the man-in-the-street all praise politicians who support large and ever-increasing government intervention in the field. The politician is thus induced to promote such intervention, confident that he is doing the right thing, and the thing which will bring him votes.

Next, health expenditure satisfies Postulates 5 and 6, so that, according to Proposition III, it is to be preferred to other equally valued social objectives.

Health as a commodity does not possess precisely defined features and cannot be rigorously measured, in spite of attempts in literature to develop more or less sophisticated health indicators (see Culyer, Lavers and Williams, 1971). Government intervention is not valued in terms of its output, but according to the inputs employed,[3] thus leaving ample room for the politician's discretion in determining what to produce and how.

The measurement of government benefits by means of the inputs employed is common to most of government expenditures, such as justice, defense, instruction, etc. Why then has government expenditure in health increased more than in these other sectors?

An answer can be found both in the greater demand expressed by the voters and in Postulate 6. Health is a relatively new sector of government intervention, which does not exhibit well-established bounds and rules. The institutional framework is not yet solidly determined and is constantly changing with respect both to the services provided and to the population covered. In such a situation, the politician enjoys great discretionary power and can easily pursue his own interests, while officially attending to a widely accepted social good.

The politician's decisions will be motivated both by his desire to provide voters with clear evidence of his activity and by the possibility of increasing his own wealth and power. As Proposition IV says, both motivations lead to a preference for "visible" attributes of the output produced by government.[4] Moreover, the production of "visible" attributes of the output, such as the number of hospital beds, usually permits a greater increase of the politician's wealth and power than does production of invisible attributes, such as higher-quality services.

Why will voters accept such behavior from the politician? A general explanation can be found in Proposition I, derived from Postulate 4, which concerns the fiscal illusion relating to the cost of "social" programs. Medical care is usually financed by payroll taxes on employers and/or employees and by general taxation or budget deficits. The cost of health care tends to be underestimated by the voter-

taxpayer, who has, however, a clear perception of the benefits
offered. In particular, the demand for health services never seems
to be satisfied. People tend, or are induced to believe, that they
are frequently in need of medical care. Therefore, given the
voters' asymmetric awareness of benefits and costs they can easily
be convinced to support increased government expenditure on health.

The health commodity, therefore, closely satisfies our propositions,
so that we might predict a large and increasing government intervention in the field. The evidence presented in the introduction of
our paper is fully consistent with this prediction.

In the next section we will present some additional evidence
relating to the Italian case, which is consistent with the hypothesis that government intervention in health has constantly been molded
by the interests of politicians.

THE ITALIAN CASE OF GOVERNMENT INTERVENTION IN HEALTH

In our opinion, the financing, the hospitals, and the general organizational structure of the Italian system of health care are compatible
with such a hypothesis.

The Financing

Italy has had comprehensive national health insurance in recent
years. The Italian Parliament has made health care practically a
free commodity by passing new and increasingly comprehensive
legislation every few years.

The existing government agencies that financed and administered
national health insurance were officially terminated on December 23,
1978, when Parliament passed a bill which led to their replacement
by a new, governmentally administered structure, the National Health
Service (Servizio Sanitario Nazionale).

Payroll taxes were and are the most important source of financing,
together with budget deficits; so the politician is allowed to
exploit the phenomenon of fiscal illusion. In fact, since payroll
taxes are withheld at the income source, employees are unaware of
the fiscal burden of their contributions; whereas, for contributions imposed on employers, the burden is shifted wholly, either to
consumers by a rise in the price of products, or to workers, when
wages are adjusted (Brittain, 1972).

As for budget deficits, "elected politicians enjoy spending public
monies on projects that yield some demonstrable benefits to their
constituents" but "they do not enjoy imposing taxes on these same
constituents ... by creating budget deficits as a normal course of
events ... [So], as the public output enters positively into the utility functions of citizens, the expenditure by itself will secure support for the politicians" (Buchanan and Wagner, 1977, pp. 93-98).

The Hospitals

An Act of Parliament, on February 12, 1968, made profound changes in
the ways hospitals functioned. The old idea of hospitals as
nonprofit welfare institutions, often administered by private
boards, was replaced by the new view of hospitals as institutions
that provide a service to all citizens through national and regional
planning. The operation of hospitals passed under the control of
public boards, whose members are mainly appointed by local authorities. The control of political or governmental power over the
operation of hospitals is strengthened by the National Health
Service Act, which puts hospitals at the service of the Local Health
Care Branches.

The Act of Parliament, on February 12, 1968, also fixed a new method
for the financing of hospitals. The hospital cost per patient-day
is established by taking into account the real costs of various
hospitals. In this way a vicious circle is produced: expenditure
decision and payment decision are separated. On the one hand,
government agencies must pay hospital costs per patient-day and cannot check amounts expended,[5] since 80% of hospitalization concerns
persons insured by them; on the other hand, there is no incentive
for concern about efficiency on the part of medical-care personnel.
Consequently, hospital boards increased the number of hospital beds
and satisfied personnel demands both for increased salaries and more
costly forms of health care (Morcaldo and Salvemini, 1978).
Furthermore, the strong increase in hospital cost per patient-day
was augmented by specific regulations that set personnel standards
according to a minimum amount of time for health care per
patient.[6] Only with the Act of Parliament of August 17, 1974, was
the expansion of hospital staff prohibited until the establishment
of the National Health Service.

The same Act of Parliament that provided for the regionalization of
hospital health care also modified the method of hospital financing.
The new method is based on the National Hospital Care Fund (Fondo
Nazionale per l'Assistenza Ospedaliera), fixed annually in the
Ministry of Health budget and shared among the regions according to
prearranged parameters. As a matter of fact, during the years that
followed the act there was no rigid control of hospital expenses,
for many reasons: insufficient allocation of funds; the poten-
tiality or ability of hospital boards to run into debt with banks
and suppliers, the certainty of government intervention to pay off
any debts.

We have seen that, in the health care field, production of visible
attributes (such as number of hospital beds) allows an increase in
the politician's power. Italy is in second place among the European
Economic Community countries in number of hospital beds per 1000
people (Eurostat, 1977).

While hospital care has expanded greatly, at least from a quantitative point of view, other health facilities, such as
outpatients' departments, day-hospitals, and long-term hospitals,
which are less costly forms of health care, have been expanded
less, if at all. The reasons for such a policy are the following:

hospitals are a center of power for politicians and an opportunity
to increase the production of visible attributes and employment at
the local level.

The General Organizational Structure

Before the inception of the National Health Service in 1978, Italy
had comprehensive national health insurance with a government agency
for every category of employee. Government agencies were public
institutions charged by government to pursue public interests. On
their boards of directors were employees and employers, representing
their respective categories, and government bureaucrats. Therefore,
since the beginning, governmental intervention in the health care
system has been very strong. Such intervention was further increased
with the establishment of the National Health Service.

Since the inception of the National Health Service, all functions of
health and hospital care not reserved for central and regional
governments are assigned to town councils, which exercise them
through the Local Health Care Branches. These local branches--which
include from a minimum of 50,000 to a maximum of 200,000 citizens,
with certain exceptions for particular cases--are administrative
bodies of the town councils, with an assembly, a board of directors
and a chairman. The assembly has mainly political tasks: passing
budgets, programs, regulations and conventions. In some regions
there is the tendency to appoint as members of the board of directors, not only those politicians who have been elected at the local
level but also those who have not been reelected.

An Italian left-wing political leader has noted that with the inception of the National Health Service "the substantial change is that
health and sickness break into politics. Until now they had been
kept in a private circle, or in the field of social activities delegated to government agencies. From now on Government, parties,
local authorities, trade-unions, professional organizations and
mass associations will have to take care of the health of the
population" (Berlinguer, 1979, p. 65).

The power of politicians is increased by the structure that establishes goals for and controls health care institutions. The legislation allocates to government and Parliament, through the
National Health Plan, which is for a period of three years, the function of general guidance and coordination; to the regions, the function of planning and verification of the objectives of the National
Health Plan at the regional level; and to the town councils, the
delivery of services at the local level. As we can see, it is
a coordinate system, strictly ruled over by the politician.

We also want to underline that the legislation concentrates power in
the hands of the Minister of Health, who has the task of watching
over the expenditure and the effectiveness of the National Health
Service. The law has, however, left wide scope for discretion in
this, because there are no performance indicators or targets against
which progress can be monitored.

CONCLUSIONS

In this paper we have offered an explanation of government intervention in health according to the traditional postulate of utility
maximization by voters and by politicians. Both are motivated by
social objectives and by their own desires for wealth and nonpecuniary goods.

Our approach, we believe, is consistent with the observed facts; in
particular, we have attempted to explain government intervention
in health in the Italian case. In that case, increases in health
care spending programs were supported by the great pressure placed
on the health care sector by the rising demand for a more egalitarian society; that is, government did not operate independently
of the people and, therefore, produced results bearing some relation
to the wishes of citizens.

We have not been able to provide evidence that the rationale for
such a system can be found in the politician's interests and not in
his desire to fulfill a social objective in such a way. However, we
believe that we have been able at least to establish in the reader's
mind doubt for believing that such a concentration of absolute
power in the hands of politicians has been caused purely by their
interest in the general good.

                              NOTES

[1]This literature includes Lees (1961, 1967), Arrow (1963), Klarman (1965),
Titmuss (1968), Culyer (1971b).

[2]This is precisely what doctors have always done! See Glaser (1970).

[3]On the problems of defining, measuring and valuing the output and inputs of
health, see Hurst (1977) and Wright (1978).

[4]Lindsay (1976, pp. 1065-66) holds that such a preference for "visible" attributes is determined by the Congress's desire directly to monitor government
enterprises.

[5]Before 1968, hospital services were regulated by agreements among hospitals
and government agencies, with strict control over the kind and length of stay.

[6]It is estimated that personnel expenses are roughly 70% of hospital cost per
patient-day. See Iuele (1976, pp. 512-13).

HEALTH, ECONOMICS, AND HEALTH ECONOMICS
J. van der Gaag and M. Perlman (editors)
© *North-Holland Publishing Company, 1981*

THIRTY YEARS OF FRUITLESS ENDEAVOR? AN ANALYSIS OF GOVERNMENT
INTERVENTION IN THE HEALTH CARE MARKET

Alan Maynard
Anne Ludbrook

INTRODUCTION

This paper seeks to review the economic literature on the nature of
health care market "failure," to describe the current structures of
the health care systems of Britain, France and the Netherlands, and
to indicate how these health care systems have not effectively rec-
tified the defective outcomes of the market.* The conclusion of the
paper is that a different sort of policy of government intervention
is required: one which develops a system of micro-economic incentives which change the behavior of decision-makers (mainly doctors)
in such a way that they achieve policy outcomes which are both efficient and compatible with distributional targets aimed at specific
geographical areas and social groups.

In the first section, the economic rationale of government intervention is examined. Insurance markets seem to be inefficient, in part
because of moral hazard. Externalities, despite their ambiguity,
seem to indicate a need for government subsidies or nationalization
of health care. Market "failure" on the supply side, licensure, the
agency relationship, and the peculiarities of the pharmaceutical
market are sustained by government and make efficient resource allocation unlikely.

In the second section, the health care systems of Britain, France
and the Netherlands are described in general terms. The third section examines the distributional and allocation outcomes of these
three health care systems. It is shown that little analysis of the
efficiency of the health care delivery system has been undertaken:
perhaps 70-80% of current therapies have not been evaluated in a
scientific fashion. The distributional outcomes of these health
care systems show that both from the geographical and social-class
viewpoints, inequality is considerable and may have increased in the
last few decades.

The concluding section argues that the meager macro-controls of
government have to be augmented by a rigorous system of micro-

*The authors would like to acknowledge the Social Science Research Council (U.K.)
for a program grant in Public Sector Studies at the Department of Economics and
the Institute of Social and Economic Research, University of York, England.

incentives which oblige the doctor decision-maker to allocate
resources efficiently and to pursue, with rigor, the distributional
goals of society.

THE ECONOMIC RATIONALE OF GOVERNMENT INTERVENTION

The health economics literature is replete with references to the
"failures" of the price mechanism in the case of the health care
market. In this section we seek briefly to summarize this literature, starting with demand-side problems and then moving on to the
supply side of the market.

Demand-side "Failure"

In a world with no externalities, it is argued that the rational
risk-averse individual will insure himself against the costs of
health care if he is offered an actuarially fair premium. Arrow
(1963) argued that the insurance market was inadequate because it
failed to insure certain high-risk groups. Pauly (1968) pointed out
that such outcomes may not be market "failures" but may arise from
the fact that such high-risk groups fail to purchase coverage simply
because their premiums are so high. Arrow's advocacy of compulsory
insurance was criticized by Lees and Rice (1965), who first argued
that he had ignored transaction costs, and then went on to discuss
sellers' costs in particular. Arrow (1965) rebutted their arguments
by arguing that with compulsory insurance administrative costs would
be reduced, essentially an empirically refutable position.

Generally the problem of insurance markets may be that premiums bear
little relation to actuarial risk. It is likely that because of a
variety of factors, the price of insurance to the purchaser will be
less than its opportunity cost, and that, as a consequence, citizens
will over-insure themselves. Premium splitting (with the employer
paying an insurance contribution), tax offsets, group schemes (risk
pooling and adverse selection) and the inefficiency of the insurance
industry due to possible cartel effects may result in the premiums
being paid by citizens bearing little relation to the cost of
actuarial risk.

If the price of insurance coverage is lowered by these factors, two
outcomes may be over-insurance and welfare losses. The over-
insurance problem is compounded by the effects of moral hazard on
consumption: insurance, like a National Health Service, may remove
the price barrier to consumption. The little work which has been
done to evaluate the resultant welfare losses, by Pauly (1969) and
M.S. Feldstein (1973), for example, indicates that the magnitude of
these losses may be very great. However, these estimates may be of
limited utility: one criticism is that gains in efficiency arising
from the use of coinsurance may be outweighed to some degree by the
losses to individuals resulting from the increased risk bearing they
face. An interesting question in this area is whether the demand
curve can be identified: the agency relationship implies that the

market demand curve may reflect doctors' preferences rather than
patients' preferences. Whose demand curve is being identified in
these studies, and whose reaction to coinsurance is being evaluated?

The traditional textbook coverage of insurance tends to present an
incomplete discussion. The majority of people with insurance
coverage in the U.K. and the U.S.A. are members of group schemes.
The purchase of insurance is likely to be determined by the preferences of the marginal worker (Goldstein and Pauly, 1976), or by
the preferences of the median member of the trade union. It is
unlikely that premiums will bear much relation to actuarial risks.
Furthermore, it is to be remembered that certain attributes of the
insurance system, coinsurance and deductibles, may have effects
which frustrate the attainment of distributional goals (see Cairns
and Snell, 1978; Maynard, 1979a and 1979b; Barer, Evans and
Stoddart, 1979; and Maynard, 1980). The merits of this form of
health care finance seem quite limited, and the administrative costs
may be reduced by the use of tax finance, as in the U.K.

The problems associated with the insurance industry are compounded
if there are externality problems. Pauly (1971) argued that externalities arise from the absolute level of health care consumption
of one (e.g. poor) person affecting the utility of another (e.g.
rich) person. The implication was that in certain cases consumption
would have to be subsidized if efficiency was to be achieved.
Lindsay (1969) argued that the externality arises from inequalities
of absolute health care consumption and that the optimal form of
government intervention was a combination of subsidy and abstention,
the latter having inevitable "free rider" problems associated with
it. Culyer (1971a) examined an externality argument related to the
underconsumption of health care by poor individuals and concluded
that, given the slopes of the poor group's indifference curves, the
efficient policy would be collective provision of health care,
financed by progressive taxation.

These models related the externality arguments to inputs or consumption of health care. An alternative view would be that the
externalities arise from inequalities in outcomes or health status,
as Culyer (1979) and Maynard (1979b) have argued. This type of
argument emphasizes that increases in inputs (health care) may or
may not increase outputs (improvements in health).

Clearly there are problems involved in identifying and quantifying
the relevant externalities. However, the competing models
"explain" varying degrees of government intervention in the health
care market: subsidies, abstention, collective provision and
finance. All the analysis is set in terms of the traditional economic paradigm of consumer sovereignty. The agency relationship is
ignored and the demand/indifference curves used are assumed to be
those of the patient.

Supply-side "Failures"

Many of the imperfections on the supply side of the health care
market have been created and are sustained by government. We will

discuss two examples: occupational licensure and the regulation of
the pharmaceutical industry.

The licensing of doctors tends to be discussed in terms of two competing hypotheses, that of self-interest and that of the public
interest. The public interest hypothesis was well articulated by
Arrow (1963):

> The general uncertainty about the prospects of medical treatment
> is socially handled by rigid entry requirements. These are
> designed to reduce the uncertainty in the mind of the consumer
> as to the quality insofar as this is possible.

Thus society demands licensure because it is ignorant of the merits
of alternative therapies and is unpracticed in the arts of diagnosis. This argument can be extended to include the familiar
rationale of the agency relationship. Thus, it is argued, because
patients are ignorant of diagnostic techniques and the efficacy of
alternative therapies, they delegate their demand decision-making
powers to the cognoscenti (the doctors). This delegation of power
requires that the recipient is competent and ethical: that is, he
must be able to diagnose and treat patients efficiently, and he must
be trained to follow a strict ethical code which prevents his using
his agency powers in the interests of anyone other than his patient.

The self-interest argument is that the doctor-demander uses his
agency relationship powers to pursue ends other than those which are
in the interests of his patients: maximization of his income, and
the full employment of his staff and other parts of his "empire".
Thus licensure and the agency relationship may permit the profession
to control the quantity, quality and remuneration of doctors, and
regulation may benefit the regulated. This view sees the profession
as able to determine both the supply of and the demand for health
care. There are a variety of ways in which it is possible to test
the agency relationship and the income-maximization arguments associated with the self-interested explanation of licensure. If doctors can create demand for their services via the agency
relationship, we might expect increases in the supply of doctors in
any particular area to be associated with no reduction in the activities of doctors already at work in that area. While this type of
hypothesis has not been tested often and rigorously, the results
available seem to indicate that supply increases are associated with
activity reductions for previously active doctors. Increased
supplies of doctors tend to generate increased net activity levels,
but some of the new entrants' workload comes from previously active
doctors. This result is hardly surprising: we would not expect
doctors to get utility from income alone, and we might expect work
activity to decline over the life-cycle.

The incomplete nature of the tests of the agency relationship is
similar to the tests of the self-interest and public-interest explanations of licensure. The early rate of return results showed evidence of economic rents accruing to doctors (e.g., Friedman and
Kuznets, 1945). However, the use of different discount rates such
as those proposed by Lewis (1963), and the recognition that U.S.
doctors worked longer hours--the Lindsay bias--led to the results of
Friedman and Kuznets (1945), Sloan (1970), and Fein and Weber (1971)

being deflated considerably (Lindsay, 1973). Mennemeyer (1976) found for the U.S. that the rate of return earned by doctors was similar to that earned by lawyers and dentists but in excess of the earnings of other professions. Leffler (1978) showed the rates of return to be not very large, but to swell after Medicare and Medicaid. The results for the U.K. (Lindsay, 1980, and Walker, 1980) show that the rates of return have fluctuated and have been generally below 15% since 1955 (Lindsay, 1980, p. 59). These low U.K. rates have to be compared with even lower rates of return for other types of higher education: a perhaps inevitable result of the rapid expansion in the output of the higher education sector.

The result of government-inspired and supported licensure of the medical profession is that its members seem to have a powerful influence on both the supply and demand sides of the health care market. It is unfortunate that the exercise of this power takes place in an environment where the patient's agent, the doctor, is ignorant of the effects of many therapies and generally practices in an unscientific manner. (See Cochrane, 1972. This point is discussed further in the third section of this paper.) Clearly medicine is a technical subject and the consumer is likely to remain ignorant of many of its attributes. If these problems of uncertainty are met with licensure, careful monitoring and strong financial incentives are necessary if licensure is not to result in the inefficient and unethical use of resources.

The pharmaceutical industry is characterized by complex state regulation. Patents generate monopoly property rights in chemical substances, the power of the monopoly depending on the characteristics of the molecules, especially whether they are unique, and the size of the relevant market for these molecules. Safety and efficacy regulation reduces the effective length of the patent in an attempt to prevent the introduction of dangerous new drugs. The state often regulates prices (e.g., the U.K.'s Prices and Profits Regulation Scheme), and via its health care agencies (often monopolies like the NHS) it seeks to affect the consumption of drugs: these are two other effective means of reducing the rate of return to patents and to R & D.

The objective of these regulations, it is alleged by government officials, is to supplement the workings of the market. However, like so much regulation, it is very much concerned with means and not much concerned with evaluation of performance in relation to ends. Empirical evidence about the effect of patents on research and development is scant and it is not evident how the R & D process would be affected by the removal of patents. Safety and efficacy legislation is another area in which there are disputes about the cost-effectiveness of alternative institutions.

The government has chosen to change the market allocation of resources in the pharmaceutical market, and in doing so it ought to demonstrate that the effects of its intervention improve the market's allocative efficiency. Unfortunately, the little evidence that government agencies have produced (e.g., U.S. Department of Health, Education and Welfare, 1979) indicates that the performance of the industry during the last five years, as defined by the production of new, efficacious chemotherapies, has been quite unspectacular.

The nature of the market "failures" necessitating government intervention in the pharmaceutical market have not been clearly defined
by decision-makers and the performance of the appropriate (if any)
market "correction" policies is generally asserted to be good rather
than scientifically demonstrated to be efficient.

One argument put forward for state intervention in this market is
that property rights in inventions must be protected if rewards for
invention and innovation are to be such that these activities continue to thrive. Another argument is that safety and efficacy
legislation avoids (but does it?) defective drugs being marketed,
and that this generates benefits which are apparently absent from
voluntary (industry-run) testing codes. The latter, of course,
reduces the gains of the former, and from even casual analysis of
this market it is clear that policies are not clearly thought out or
monitored. Neither hypothesis has been rigorously evaluated.

There is a need for economists to analyze this market much more
carefully, and to demonstrate when, if ever, government regulation
is required. Perhaps a large number of the drug innovations of the
last decades could have been acquired at a lower cost and without
recourse to patents and other legislations.

Conclusion

The market for health care has some unusual characteristics. The
insurance mechanism exhibits severe defects; revenue gathering by
taxation may have no more defects and lower collection costs. A
variety of externality relationships have been postulated and these
indicate policies varying from government subsidization (Pauly,
1971, and Lindsay, 1969), to government provision and finance
(Culyer, 1971a). It seems that for demand-side reasons alone, the
health care market will, unless it is supplemented, fail to allocate
resources efficiently.

On the supply side, the problems of licensure and the agency relationship very imperfectly rectify the market deficiencies arising
from uncertainty regarding the evaluation of health care.
Furthermore in attempting to improve resource allocation, the state
has given increased market power to doctors, who may use it to
increase their pecuniary and non-pecuniary rewards from trading in
the health care market. Similarly, in the market for phar-
maceuticals it is not clear that state intervention has resulted in
marked improvements in resource allocation.

It is evident that there are serious defects in the efficiency of
the health care market's workings. The insurance mechanism is
likely to lead to overinsurance and demand-side inflation in expenditure. It is doubtful whether this mechanism can correct the
market failure arising from externalities in a more cost-effective
manner than an NHS. On the supply side, there are few incentives
available to induce efficiency, and the state has created severe
market imperfections which it has failed to monitor.

From this literature, we would expect to find institutions which are tax-financed and do not allocate care on an ability-to-pay basis. We might expect these institutions to fortify the market power of doctors, in part to overcome the problems of uncertainty, although given the state's unwillingness to monitor the efficiency of its interventions, we might not be surprised to discover that outcomes fail to meet government policy targets.

THREE WEST EUROPEAN HEALTH CARE SYSTEMS

The objective of this section is to outline the characteristics of the health care systems of Britain, France and the Netherlands. Of necessity each of these outlines will be terse and can be supplemented by other material (Maynard, 1975; Abel-Smith and Maynard, 1979).

Health Care in England

The National Health Service was created in 1948 with the objective of removing price barriers to consumption, reducing geographical inequalities in the distribution of health care resources, and improving the efficiency with which care was delivered (see Eckstein, 1964, and Stevens, 1966). The 1944 Government White Paper establishing the NHS stated:

> The Government ... want to ensure that in the future every man
> and woman and child can rely on getting ... the best medical and
> other facilities available; that their getting them shall not
> depend on whether they can pay for them or on any other factor
> irrelevant to real need. [Great Britain, Ministry of Health,
> 1944]

To achieve these objectives, the NHS is financed largely (95%) out of general taxation, and services are provided in public hospitals and by a labor force of nearly one million who, with the exception of general practitioners (less than half the doctor stock), are public employees. The Department of Health is small (around 5000 employees) and does not seek to determine day-to-day management decisions. The Health Department sets general policy objectives (Great Britain, Department of Health and Social Security, 1976a) and has allocated the health care budget to the 14 Regions by formula since 1970 (Great Britain, Department of Health and Social Security, 1976b; and Maynard and Ludbrook, 1980b). The Regions, and their constituent Areas and Districts, are obliged by law to provide a comprehensive health service in their localities. Thus the Department of Health sets general targets and distributes resources, and the Regions, Areas and Districts are responsible for the day to day management of the Service.

The NHS consumes about 5.5% of Gross National Product (£ 7711 million in 1979-80). The private sector is very small. The private

insurance companies hold policies, most of them group schemes,
covering about three million workers. The total activity of the
insurers and the private.health care providers adds up to little
more than 2% of the NHS budget (see Lee, 1978).

The nature of the British arrangements is that the health care
system is centrally financed, but provided by decentralized bodies
whose activities are loosely monitored by the center. It is not
surprising that inequality and geographical diversity have thrived
and that clinical freedom has been rarely circumscribed in this
structure.

Health Care in France

In France, a series of legislative developments since the last war
has created a health care system which is practically comprehensive. Workers and the insured (pensioners and the unemployed) are
obliged by law to be members of sickness funds. These autonomous
public bodies are responsible for the finance of the health care of
their members (the insured and their dependants). Public health
care benefits are supplemented by private sector schemes which
enable the purchase of "superior care" (e.g., private rooms in
hospital, etc.).

In effect, the state fixes the financial flows. The funds are by
law required to break even (i.e. income must equal expenditure) and
no cross-subsidization is permitted between the health funds and
other social security funds, such as that for pensioners or family
income support. However, the funds generally overspend and are
cross-subsidized. Furthermore, their contribution rates are carefully regulated by a state anxious to make the health care sector
financially viable and independent. Most of the membership contribution is paid by the employer. In 1976 6.8% of GNP was spent on
health care in France.

However, financial independence is unattainable merely by determining contribution rates (i.e. fixing the budget). The state has
become involved in fixing rates for the remuneration of doctors and
hospitals, and in attempts to control the quantity of health care
provided. Since 1970, the hospital sector has been regulated
through the control of capital investment in public and private
hospitals. There is some medical audit of doctors by means of a
comparison between the activities of doctors of the same type in the
same region. Coinsurance (the ticket modérateur), at a rate of 20%,
with exemptions, is also used to limit demands for care outside the
hospital and for short term hospitalization.

Thus while health care in France is provided by a system with more
private hospitals and more privately employed doctors than in
Britain, the degree of government involvement is considerable. As
in the NHS, the effect of the system is to reduce, incompletely in
the case of those with the ticket modérateur, the price barrier to
consumption. The use of planning policies, such as the "health map"
exercise, seeks to affect the spatial distribution of health care
facilities. However, as in the case of Britain, most of these poli-

cies have been evolved only in the last decade. They are weak and
have had little impact on the distributional or allocative outcomes
of the French health care market.

Health Care in the Netherlands

In the Netherlands, the lowest seven deciles of the income distribution are covered by the general medical scheme which requires compulsory membership in a sickness fund. This social insurance
coverage gives these people comprehensive health care which is provided by public and private institutions. The top 30% of the income
distribution buy private insurance coverage. All groups are covered
by the "heavy risks" program, which, in return for contributions,
gives benefits for long-stay hospitalization, chronic illness and
similar categories.

Contributions, usually split equally between the employer and the
employee, are paid to sickness funds (about 70 in total), and benefits are comprehensive and generally free of charge. In fact, the
sickness funds are obliged by law to guarantee benefits to their
insured. In 1976 about 8.1% of the GNP of the Netherlands was spent
on health care.

The Dutch health care sector is regulated by the government in a
variety of ways. The output of medical schools is controlled,
hospital investment is regulated, and all provinces have to plan
their hospital system. As in Britain and France, these developments
are quite recent; the latter began in 1971. Also, as in Britain
and France, there are significant geographical inequalities in the
distribution of health care facilities, little evidence of reduced
socio-economic disparities in consumption, and poor evidence as to
the efficacy of health care.

Health care policy in Great Britain, France and the Netherlands has
been characterized by a reluctance to set explicit policy targets,
and by a willingness to believe that the extension of public coverage
and the reduction or removal of the price barrier to consumption
would by itself improve the distributional and allocational characteristics of health care services. During the last ten years, there
has been a growing realization that policy targets, when they were
finally made explicit, were not being met. This has given rise to a
slow growth in the development of cautious remedial policies, mostly
of a macro-nature.

THE EFFECTIVENESS OF GOVERNMENT INTERVENTION IN BRITAIN,
FRANCE AND THE NETHERLANDS

In this section our objective is to analyze the effectiveness of
government intervention in relation to efficiency and distributional
objectives. In considering efficiency, we examine the allocation of
resources, first, to the health care sector and then, within the
health care sector. In the second part of this section, the distri-

bution of resources among different socio-economic groups and
regions will be analyzed.

Efficiency: Allocating Resources to Health Care

In all three countries, the process by which resources are allocated
to health care programs in the public sector is one of incremen-
talism. There is no explicit discussion about the appropriate level
of funding, based on the productivity of health care inputs and the
value of health care outcomes. The extent to which the government
is involved in this process does, however, vary.

In Britain, public sector funds are allocated centrally among different service areas. While the level of resources allocated to the
health care sector will be affected to some extent by the size of
the total budget, the allocation process can be characterized as
last year's allocation to maintain existing services, plus an
allowance for growth. The outcome is more the result of political
lobbying than of economic decision-making.

In France, funds for the social security schemes are raised from
contributions paid by employees and employers. The level of these
contributions and the share of total funds allocated to health care
are determined by the government, in consultation with the sickness
funds. The sickness funds have the difficult task of trying to
balance income and expenditures ex ante, through the contribution
levels and the tariff for health services. In fact, expenditure
will only be known ex post, as the funds have no effective control
on the quantity of services demanded or supplied. The final level
of expenditure is, therefore, determined to a large extent by supply
factors.

The Dutch system is similar to that of the French. The sickness
funds negotiate tariffs with the producers and also set the contribution levels, both of which must be approved by the government and
must conform with the government prices and incomes policy. As in
the French case, the sickness funds cannot effectively control the
quantity of fee-per-item services that are produced. If the funds
are operating with a deficit at the end of the year, they will
either seek direct government assistance or try to cover the deficit
by increased contributions for the following year.

This general scheme covers about 70% of the population, excluding
higher-income groups and their dependants. There is also a special
sickness expenses scheme, mainly for long term care, which has universal coverage. Again, the government exercises control over the
raising of revenue, but there is no effective control on expenditure. The insurance funds both public and private, which administer the scheme, must meet all demands that comply with the
medical conditions for admission.

In all three countries, the government's primary concern is to
guarantee the provision of adequate health care services at a politically acceptable level of tax or insurance contributions. There
is neither much discussion of the objectives, such as improving

health, nor much consideration of the relative productivity of different kinds of government and private activity in achieving them.
Even allowing for the inherent difficulties, there is little
apparent interest in measuring and valuing outcomes from health care
expenditure.

The importance of this point is illustrated by the data presented in
Table 1. The share of Gross Domestic Product (GDP) allocated to
health care has increased over the period 1960-1976 in all three
countries. The Netherlands has had the largest increase, and the
United Kingdom the smallest. With this increase in funding,
variations in the level of service have widened, proxied here by the
doctor/population ratio. However, this variation is not entirely
reflected by broad indicators of health status, such as the infant
mortality rate and the standardized mortality ratio (SMR). The
infant mortality rate has declined less in the Netherlands than in
the United Kingdom and France, and its SMR has increased relative to
the two other countries.

Efficiency: Resource Allocation Within the Health Services Sector

In Britain, the government is directly involved in the provision of
services, owning and employing the resources used. While the government retains a close control of total cost, there are few incentives
within the system to encourage efficient practices. Staff are paid
either by capitation fee or by salary. We would predict that own-
time saving practices will be adopted regardless of economic efficiency. Hospitals have to work within set budgets, and competition
for funds may produce some increase in efficiency, such as the·
substitution of brand name drugs by cheaper generic equivalents.
However, there is no incentive for decision-makers to adopt efficient practices if the savings accrue elsewhere. Indeed, hospital
decision-makers have an incentive to shift costs onto other budgets
whenever possible.

In France, the government is less involved in the provision of services. There are some public hospitals, administered by local
government. The main system of reimbursement is fee-for-item-of-
service, and this may encourage both an overproduction of services
and the allocation of physicians' time and hospital facilities
towards services which produce the maximum net income. The tariff
for physicians' services reflects the cost of inputs and the technical difficulty of the service. There is no evidence to suggest
that the sickness funds or the government attempt to use this tariff
system to encourage cost-effective or efficient practices. The
hospitals make per diem charges in the public hospitals based on the
average cost for broad specialties. Some attempts are being made to
improve efficiency by introducing different budgeting systems for
the public hospitals (e.g. global budgets), but there is considerable opposition to this, as it is seen to place public hospitals at a disadvantage vis à vis private hospitals, which would
continue to charge on a fee-for-item-of-service basis. (The average
cost-pricing in public hospitals already creates an incentive for
individuals to be treated in private hospitals for the relatively
minor complaints that are subject to copayment.)

Table 1.　Health Status and Share of GDP Allocated to Health Care

Country	Expenditure on Health as a Percentage of GDP		Doctors per 100,000 Population		Infant Mortality Rate		Standardized Mortality Ratio	
	1960	1976	1960	1976	1960	1976	1960	1976
France	4.0	6.8	108	163	23.5	12.7	99	95
Netherlands	4.5a	8.1	112	166	16.7	10.6	84	89
United Kingdomb	3.8	5.7	108	118	23.8	14.4	104	107

Sources:　For health care expenditure, see CREDOC, Comptes nationales de la santé: Méthodologie, résultats (1950-77) (Paris, 1979); Great Britain, Report of the Royal Commission on the National Health Service, Command Paper 7615 (London: HMSO, 1979); OECD, Public Expenditure on Health (Paris, 1977); Netherlands, Ministry of Health and Environmental Protection, Health Care in the Netherlands, Vol. 1 (Leidschendam, 1977).　For doctor ratio, see United Nations, Statistical Yearbook, 1962, 1963 and 1978; France, Ministère de la Santé et de la Famille, Annuaire statistique de la santé et de l'action sociale (Paris, 1978); Great Britain, Central Statistical Office, Annual Abstract of Statistics, 1977 (London: HMSO, 1977). For population and mortality statistics, see United Nations, Demographic Yearbook, 1961 and 1977; INSEE, Annuaire statistique de la France (Paris, 1978); Great Britain, Central Statistical Office, Annual Abstract of Statistics, 1961 and 1977.

a1963.

bFigures relate to the National Health Service only.　Other expenditure figures include both public and private sectors.

In the Netherlands, there is very little public provision of services. General practitioners are paid a per capita fee for publicly
insured patients, and specialists receive mainly fee-per-item-of-
service payments. This payment structure provides an incentive for
the referral of patients from primary care, where the doctor is not
paid any extra for his services, to more expensive secondary care.
The hospitals are paid a per diem fee which includes medical costs
if the hospital doctors are salaried. There is some attempt to
control the level of hospital charges by establishing norms for
inputs used by the hospitals, such as the number of nurses per bed.
However, the hospital has an incentive to lengthen patient stay,
since the cost of providing additional days of care declines.
Certain specialists also receive a fee per day of hospital care provided for their patients and so have an incentive to cooperate with
the hospital.

A crude indicator of hospital efficiency is length of stay. There
are obvious comparability problems. However, in 1977, the average
length of stay for patients in general and university hospitals in
the Netherlands was 15.2 days. By comparison, the average length of
stay for acute cases in Britain was 9.8 days in 1976, and in France
was 11 days.

Given the lack of incentives, it is not surprising that there is
relatively little evaluation of work practices in the health care
sector. In many cases, the scientific evaluation of clinical procedures has been tardy and incomplete (e.g., see Cochrane, 1972, and
Bunker, Barnes and Mosteller, 1977). There is little interest in
evaluating the cost-effectiveness of alternative treatments, but the
studies carried out have shown that the potential exists for more
efficient use of available resources (e.g., see Mather et al.,
1976, for a study of intensive care and home care for coronary
patients, and for a comparison of day-case treatment with longer
hospital stays for hernia cases see Russell et al., 1977). The
results of these and other similar studies have had limited effects
on medical practice because there are no incentives for other clinicians to adopt cost-effective procedures.

Distribution: Social-Class Equity

The first aspect of the distribution of health care resources with
which we are concerned is the division of resources between different social classes. The public health care programs in all three
countries remove or reduce the money cost-price barrier to the consumption of health care services, to some extent promoting greater
equality of access to health care. In Britain, the commitment to
equal access is embodied in the legislation setting up the National
Health Service. There are no charges to the patient for medical
services, and while there are small charges for items such as pharmaceutical products, all low-income groups are exempt. In France, a
system of copayment operates for everything except major illnesses,
maternity care and industrial injuries. Patients must pay 20% of
the cost of services, but the poor sections of the community are
exempted from these charges. The Dutch system is the least comprehensive in its coverage of the population, but the approximately 30%

A. Maynard and A. Ludbrook

Table 2.   Infant Mortality Rates (Per 1000 Legitimate Live Births)*

	Neonatal			Postneonatal			Total		
	1949–50	1970–72	% Decline	1949–50	1970–72	% Decline	1949–50	1970–72	% Decline
1. England and Wales									
Professional	13.5	8.7	35	4.9	2.9	41	18.4	11.6	37
Unskilled manual	21.9	17.6	20	17.9	5.8	68	39.8	23.4	41
2. France	1956–60	1966–70		1956–60	1966–70		1956–60	1966–70	
Liberal professions	12.7	8.8	31	4.1	3.0	27	16.8	11.7	30
Unskilled manual	23.1	18.4	20	21.7	12.0	45	44.8	30.4	32

Sources: V. Walters, Class Inequality and Health Care (London: Croom Helm, 1980); Great Britain, Office of Population Censuses and Surveys, Occupational Mortality: Registrar General's Decennial Supplement for England and Wales, 1970–72 (London: HMSO, 1978); INSEE, Tableaux démographiques et sociaux (Paris, 1976).

*As usual, the analysis is restricted to legitimate births in order to improve the comparability between classes. Infant mortality is higher for illegitimate births, which also show a social class bias.

of the population who are excluded from the general public program are generally affluent and have private insurance coverage. Those covered by public insurance pay virtually no charges, as in the United Kingdom.

If the performance of the Dutch health care system is judged by a comparison of public and private utilization rates, it appears to meet its objectives. Age-specific hospital utilization rates are higher for publicly insured patients (the lowest 70% of the income distribution) than for the population as a whole. Two studies of one group practice showed that, when other factors are controlled, publicly insured patients also have a higher utilization rate for primary care services (van der Gaag, 1978, and Rutten, 1978).

However, these outcomes may be related to a variety of factors, and it is to be noted that more detailed socio-economic utilization data are not available. An examination of more detailed evidence from France and Britain suggests that the lowering of financial barriers to health care consumption has not been particularly successful in achieving greater social equality. It seems that on crude measures of outcome (e.g. mortality) and of input (expenditure, doctors, etc.) significant inequality continues to exist and may have increased over the last 20 years.

In both France and Britain the social class gradient in mortality and morbidity rates has survived the "socialization" of health care services. In 1970-72, the standardized mortality ratio for males in England and Wales was 77 for social class I (professional) as against 137 for social class V (unskilled manual). This is a greater variation than that which existed in 1949-53, when the National Health Service was established (Royal Commission on the National Health Service, 1979). In France, the mortality rates for working-class males at age 55 and at age 75 have been increasing relative to those for the professional and upper classes (INSEE, 1976, 1979).

An analysis of infant mortality rates is also very revealing. Table 2 shows the infant mortality rates for the highest and lowest social classes and the percentage decline that has occurred. In both countries the improvement in the total infant mortality rate has been relatively greater in the lowest social class. However, this relative improvement has occurred only in the post-neonatal mortality rate. The percentage decline in the neonatal mortality rate is lower for the lowest social class.

Morbidity rates are reported annually for Great Britain in the General Household Survey. These show a strong social-class gradient, mainly with respect to chronic illness. In France, one health survey produced a weighted index showing that the working classes were affected by ill-health more than twice as often as the upper social classes (Santé Securité Sociale, 1977).

This evident variation in mortality and morbidity rates does not necessarily imply an inadequate provision of health services to the lower social classes. Firstly, improving access to health care may not have a significant impact on the health status of a population group, because health care may be ineffective and other factors such

Table 3. Regional Variations in Health Care Facilities, 1977

Services (per 100,000 population)	Highest Region	Lowest Region	National Average	Coeff. Variation
Doctors				
France	244	108	164	0.257
Netherlands	254	109	171	0.282
England	145	104	121	0.092
Beds				
France: Total	1170	570	840	0.179
Acute specialties	859	468	631	0.144
Netherlands[a]	670	370	540	0.153
England: All specialties	950	630	810	0.109
Acute specialties	350	240	290	0.141

Sources: Great Britain, Department of Health and Social Security, Health and Personal Social Security Statistics 1978 (London: HMSO, 1980); France, Ministère de la Santé et de la Famille, Santé securité sociale nos. 3A, 5, 6B (Paris, 1978); Netherlands, Centraal Bureau voor de Statistiek, Vademecum gezondheidsstatistiek Nederland (The Hague, 1978).

aUniversity and general hospitals only.

as education, housing and nutrition may be important. Secondly, an
individual with poor health may have a tendency to move into a lower
social class; these categories are based on occupation. The cause
for concern is that studies of the utilization of health services
show a tendency for under-utilization by the lower social classes,
relative to their need for health care (Ashford and Pearson, 1970;
LeGrand, 1978; Mizrahi, 1978).

It seems that the use of low or zero money prices may not be sufficient to achieve more equal access to health services. There are
other significant costs, such as time costs, involved in obtaining
health services, and institutional factors may be important. It may
be necessary to offer positive inducements to disadvantaged groups.
In France, policymakers are attempting to alter infant mortality
rates by encouraging the use of pre-natal services. Social
security benefits are linked to attendance at pre-natal clinics.
This policy effectively pays mothers to attend. However, it may be
that the lower classes regard the services provided by a health
system which is currently dominated by middle class professionals as
largely irrelevant to their needs.

Distribution: Geographic Equity

Finally, we turn to the problem of geographical inequalities in the
distribution of health care resources. This has been of particular
concern in the United Kingdom since the creation of the National
Health Service. The most recent attempt at equalization has been
through the use of the Resource Allocation Working Party (RAWP) formula in England (Great Britain, Department of Health and Social
Security, 1976b), and similar formulae in Scotland, Wales and
Northern Ireland. Essentially, the RAWP formula allocates capital
and revenue funds among the English regions on the basis of population weighted by "need." The weighting factors are expected utilization of services determined with respect to national utilization
rates, and standardized mortality ratios. (For a detailed
discussion, see Maynard and Ludbrook, 1980b.) The implementation of
this formula has produced a significant shift in resources away from
London and the south-east, with the northern regions being the most
significant "gainers." However, there has been no attempt to apply
the same allocation procedure to the total United Kingdom health
budget. At present, the expenditure level for each constituent
country is determined separately. This results in a higher level of
spending in Scotland and Northern Ireland, relative to need (Maynard
and Ludbrook, 1980a).

General practitioner services are excluded from the scope of the
RAWP formula, but the government is also concerned to improve their
distribution. Newly qualified doctors can be excluded from areas
that are considered to be well-endowed. In areas that are under-
provided, additional payments are made to encourage doctors to set
up practice.

The problem of regional disparities in health services is also being
faced in France and the Netherlands. Table 3 indicates the extent
of the variation in crude indicators of health service provision,

Table 4. Variations from Targets for Geographic Redistribution

Country	Distance from Target (as % actual allocation)	
	Highest Endowed Region	Lowest Endowed Region
England (1979-80)[a]	+12.98	- 8.76
France (1976)[b]	+31.23	-57.33
Netherlands (1977)[b]	+13.56	-22.70

Sources: For England, see Hospital and Health Services Review, 98 (1979); for France and the Netherlands, see F. Tonnellier, Etude régionale de la consommation de soins médicaux, (Paris, 1979); CREDOC, Comptes nationales de la santé; Méthodologie, résultats (1950-77) (Paris, 1979); and Centraal Bureau voor de Statistiek, Vademecum gezondheidsstatistiek Nederland (The Hague, 1978).

[a]Target figures are for the redistribution of hospital and community services budgets.

[b]Target figures are for hospital inpatient services (see appendix).

such as the doctor/population and bed/population ratios. The distribution of doctors is particularly uneven in both France and the Netherlands, having a coefficient of variation in excess of 25%, while that for England is less than 10% (the coefficient of variation is the ratio of the standard deviation to the mean). The governments of France and the Netherlands are unable to affect the distribution of resources as directly as the United Kingdom government, and there are no incentives for doctors to relocate in either the French or the Dutch system.

There is also considerable variation in hospital care, and both the French and Dutch governments are attempting to equalize provision by controlling capital developments. Targets are established for the number of beds in any area and no new developments are permitted if an area is over-provided. This approach has two main problems. In the first place, it is a very slow process, even if capital funds are being allocated centrally by the government. The second problem is that there are no positive incentives for the relocation of non-government capital. This is a particular problem for the Netherlands, where most of the capital funds are raised outside the public sector. There may be no incentive for anyone to provide new beds in a poorly endowed area and there are no incentives to force hospitals to rationalize their services in over-provided areas.

In order to illustrate the scale of the problem that exists in France and the Netherlands, a RAWP-type formula has been applied to calculate target allocations for hospital service provision (see Appendix).

Table 4 shows the position for the best and worst endowed regions in each country. The greatest degree of geographic inequality in access to health care is shown in France. The worst region is under-provided by over 50%, i.e., it uses less than two-thirds of the hospital services that would be allocated to the region if services were distributed according to "need." The Netherlands is a much smaller country and the degree of inequality is rather less than in France, comparing fairly well with the situation in England after four years of redistribution under the RAWP formula.

The problem of regional disparities in health care resources in France and the Netherlands might be tackled more effectively if the formula approach used in England were to be applied to geographical allocations of the total health care budgets. At this level, the sickness funds could then create incentives to attract physical and human resources into relatively under-endowed regions. Although the RAWP approach has met with some opposition in England, especially from losing regions, it has two distinct advantages. Firstly, the basis on which allocations are made is explicit and open to debate. Secondly, the inclusion of revenue as well as capital funds in the redistribution makes the process faster and more flexible. The rate at which progress is made towards equalization can be varied if necessary, and changes in the revenue expenditure program are rather easier to absorb than changes in the capital program.

CONCLUSIONS

The evidence reviewed in the previous section suggests that government intervention has been relatively ineffective in achieving
efficiency and distributional objectives, whether it takes the form
of public insurance or tax finance and direct provision. The health
care systems are characterized by much inefficiency, with little or
no evaluation, and there are no incentives for the adoption of more
efficient practices. Social inequality persists, both in health
status outcomes and health care consumption, and only in the United
Kingdom has there been significant direct intervention to reduce
geographic inequalities.

However, we reject a "nirvana" approach which would reject any
system that performs less than perfectly. Therefore, our conclusions should not be seen as an indictment of government intervention
per se. The rationale for government intervention is sound, and
there is no evidence to suggest that efficiency and distributional
goals can be pursued more effectively in its absence. Supply-side
defects, in particular, such as the agency relationship, the
monopoly power of the providers and the division between decision-
making and the financial consequences of decisions, imply that efficiency conditions will not automatically be met in a private market.
Distributional objectives will also require some form of government
intervention. The "failure" of the "private" market in the United
States has led to piecemeal government intervention (Medicare and
Medicaid) that has resulted in outcomes similar to those found in
Western Europe (perhaps in a more severe form). All systems,
whether public or private, face the same basic problem, in that
there are few incentives for the effective decision-makers--the
doctors--to trade off the costs and benefits of health care in a way
which uses resources efficiently.

In the absence of such incentives, we should anticipate that health
care resources will be used less than efficiently. The removal of
financial barriers will not create equal access for disadvantaged
groups unless there are also incentives for doctors to pursue such
objectives. As can be seen from the United Kingdom, more than 30
years of "equal access" have failed to achieve either greater
geographic or greater social equality. Direct intervention in the
distribution of resources has been necessary in order to move
towards a more equitable geographical solution.

Government intervention has been ineffective because of a failure to
specify objectives clearly and to monitor outcomes carefully.
Attention has been focused on macroeconomic issues, such as the size
of the health care budget or the length of waiting lists.
Microeconomic evaluation of medical practices and the creation of
incentives have been ignored in both the private and the public
systems. We would conclude, therefore, that the health care markets
in Britain, France and the Netherlands are suffering from too little
government intervention rather than too much, and that a different
type of government intervention is required.

Appendix

Target Allocations for Hospital Services in France
and the Netherlands

The procedure used was the same for both countries. The regional populations
were weighted for expected bed use, using national hospital utilization rates by
age and sex, and by the standardized mortality ratio as a proxy for morbidity.
The regional target share of hospital service provision was in proportion to its
weighted population share.

Variations in the extent to which medical costs were included in hospital costs
created problems in using total hospital expenditure as the basis for distributional targets. Because of this, the national total of hospital days provided
was used. The target share of hospital days provided was compared to actual consumption for each region, and the difference was expressed as a percentage of the
total allocation.

It should be noted that figures for the consumption of hospital services by
region for France were only available for the Régime Générale, which covered
about 70% of the population. The size of each weighted population was adjusted
to take account of variations in the percentage of the regional population
covered by the Régime Générale but, to the extent that the age/sex distribution
of these insured persons varied from the age/sex distribution of the total
regional population, some small degree of bias may have been introduced.

HEALTH, ECONOMICS, AND HEALTH ECONOMICS
J. van der Gaag and M. Perlman (editors)
© *North-Holland Publishing Company, 1981*

THE COST OF NURSING HOME CARE IN THE UNITED STATES:
GOVERNMENT FINANCING, OWNERSHIP, AND EFFICIENCY

H. E. Frech III
Paul B. Ginsburg

INTRODUCTION

The U.S. nursing home industry has undergone extremely rapid growth
and dramatic changes in the recent past.* In 1950, total expenditures for nursing homes amounted to only $190 million, of which
only 10% was financed by government (Gibson, 1979). By 1960, the
expenditures were $530 million, with government financing 22%. In
1966, the Medicare and Medicaid programs began, and by 1970, expenditures had increased to $4.3 billion, with government financing
43%. The latest data for 1979 show expenditures of $17.8 billion
and a public share of 57%. This extraordinary growth in nursing
home expenditures averaged 17% per year over the entire period,
substantially more rapid than the 10% annual growth in total personal health care expenditures over the same period.

The large size of the industry and its extensive government
financing make it an important object of study. Departures from
efficient production have major implications for resource
allocation.

Further, the nursing home industry is a natural testing ground for
theories about incentives and financing in the health care industry
as a whole. First, nursing homes provide much more homogeneous services than either hospitals or physicians. This makes it much
easier to measure relative costs and efficiency. Second, the large
number of nursing homes tends to permit more precise statistical
results. Perhaps most important, however, is the extensive
variation in ownership and reimbursement methods throughout the
industry.

Policymakers have shown considerable interest in the desirability of
having profit-seeking firms play a role in the provision of health
care. In contrast to the hospital industry, the nursing home
industry contains large numbers of profit-seeking firms, as well as
private nonprofit and government-owned firms. With none of these
ownership categories merely on the fringes of the industry, the

---

*This ongoing research has been supported by the National Center for Health
Services Research, U.S. Department of Health and Human Services, under Grant No.
1 R01 HS 02674.

nursing home industry provides a useful laboratory for the study of differences in efficiency among these various types of ownership.

The second area of policy interest is comparing the virtues of alternative types of reimbursement systems used to finance medical care for the poor and the aged. Here, again, the nursing home industry is a desirable one to study. Most public financing of nursing homes is associated with the Medicaid program, administered by the states with matching grants from the federal government. The states have used a great variety of methods of reimbursing nursing home care for Medicaid recipients, ranging from a flat rate per day to reimbursement of audited costs.

Our work to date indicates that both the ownership or property rights structure of the firm and the reimbursement system have important effects on efficiency. Either nonprofit legal status or a cost based reimbursement system may raise costs substantially. Further, some of these estimates are quite precise and reliable, especially for the ownership or property-rights variables.

Past Research

Christine Bishop has ably reviewed the literature on nursing home costs (1980). Of the nine studies reviewed that examined the effects of ownership on costs, all found nonprofit nursing homes to have higher costs. Some of the studies adjusted for patient characteristics and others adjusted for quality. In no case did these adjustments reverse the result that nonprofit homes are more costly.

Less work has been done on the effects of reimbursement systems. A number of studies examined the effect of the percentage of public patients, but the results have been mixed. A study not included in the Bishop review (Meiners, undated) found flat-rate reimbursement systems to be associated with lower costs. For the most part, reimbursement has not been treated in detail, so that many questions concerning the effects of reimbursements on costs remain unanswered.

Institutional Background

Traditionally, the nursing home industry in the U.S. has been dominated by private nonprofit firms. Most of the recent growth, however, has been in the for-profit sector. By 1977, 77% of the firms and 69% of the beds were in the for-profit sector of the industry (National Center for Health Statistics, 1979).

Nursing homes tend to be small. The average bed size is 74, with only 5% of the homes larger than 200 beds. Until recently, entry into the industry was essentially free in almost all states. However, beginning in the early 1970s, many states made entry a regulatory matter by passing certificate-of-need laws and applying them to nursing homes as well as to hospitals. Researchers suspect that some of these laws have restricted entry, but data quality problems and difficulties in separating the effects of certificate-of-need from restrictive capital reimbursement policies is at least

Table 1.   State Nursing Home Reimbursement Systems Under
Medicaid, 1972 (Skilled Nursing Homes)

Type of System	Number of States
Flat rate	7
Varies by level of care	2
Prospective rate setting	
No ceiling	4
With ceiling	2
Based on Group Performance	6
Cost Reimbursement	
With ceiling	11
No ceiling	18

SOURCE: Classified by authors on basis of an unpublished Medicaid
survey.

partly responsible for inconclusive results (Scanlon and Feder, 1980).

Medicaid plays a major role in the industry. In 1977, 53% of all residents in Medicaid certified homes were financed by Medicaid.[1] Until recently, the method (and to a large extent the level) of Medicaid reimbursement was a state prerogative.[2] In practice, the variation across states has been substantial. Some states had flat-rate systems, where a set amount is paid per patient day. At the opposite extreme is cost reimbursement, where each home is paid its audited costs. In between are cost reimbursement systems with limitations on the amount per day that is reimbursable and prospective reimbursement systems which set rates in advance, often based on a facility's costs in a prior year. Table 1 shows the array of reimbursement systems in effect in 1972, the year from which this study's cost data were drawn. Since that time, partly in response to new federal regulations, flat-rate systems have declined and prospective reimbursement systems have increased.

THEORY

The theoretical basis of this work is the property rights theory of the firm (Alchian, 1961; Williamson, 1969; Alchian and Kessel, 1962; Alchian and Demsetz, 1972; Furubøtn and Pejovich, 1972; Frech, 1980). Consider the top decision-maker of a single proprietorship firm under private property rights. In this situation, the owner will maximize utility by choosing the optimal combination of the nonpecuniary benefits of the firm (pleasant offices and colleagues, leisure, etc.) and the wealth of the firm. The top decision-maker will choose an optimum like the point Op in Figure 1.

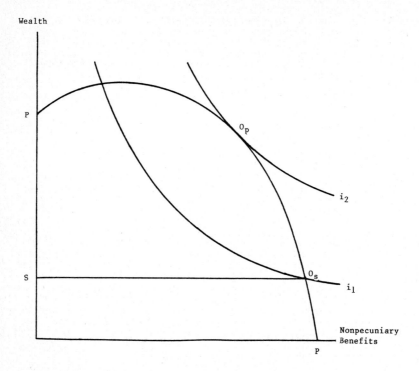

Figure 1. Property rights and choice.

Now impose a nonprofit constraint on the firm, which limits the
amount of the firm's wealth that the owner can keep to the present
value of a predetermined "reasonable" salary, S in Figure 1. The
addition of this new constraint leads the decision-maker to choose a
new optimum, a point like OS in Figure 1. In choosing to increase
the nonpecuniary goods, the decision-maker, of course, lowers the
efficiency of the firm. This theory has been examined empirically
in many industries and found to be a powerful explanatory tool.[3]

How can nonprofit firms survive in competition with profit-seeking
firms, given the results of the theory and the empirical evidence?
There are two answers to this question.

First, there are substantial tax and regulatory advantages for
nonprofit firms in most industries where they are found. This is
particularly true of the U.S. health care and health insurance
industries.

Second, the nonprofit legal form has important advantages for firms
whose output is subsidized by charitable donors (private or

governmental). The decision-makers of legally nonprofit firms cannot retain the residual. Thus, any contributions to the firm must
be spent within the firm. Since the donors desire to subsidize the
work of the firm, not the private wealth of the top decision-maker,
the private nonprofit firm is a natural vehicle for charitable
contributions, even at the cost of some loss in operating
efficiency.

The Case of Nursing Homes

The application of the theory to nursing homes includes both of the
main objects of this study: the property rights or ownership structure of the firm, and the state Medicaid reimbursement system.
Since the decision-makers of nonprofit and government nursing homes
cannot keep the residual, the theory predicts that these homes will
be less efficient.

Somewhat less direct is the application of the theory to the effects
of the reimbursement system. The reimbursement systems vary in the
extent to which the decision-maker (even of a profit-seeking firm)
can keep the increased residual resulting from improvements in efficiency. At one extreme is the pure cost reimbursement system.
Here, all of the increased residual which results from efficiency
improvements are taken by the government, since reimbursement declines with costs reductions. Such a reimbursement system converts the
natural strong incentives of the private property firm into
something like those of the nonprofit firm. At the other extreme is
the flat rate reimbursement system. Under this plan, the nursing
home is paid a flat rate per patient day, regardless of costs. In
this situation, the decision-maker of a profit-seeking firm can
retain all cost savings, so will have undiluted incentives to pursue
efficiency.

Thus, the theory predicts that nonprofit and government nursing
homes will be less efficient than profit-seeking ones where flat
rate reimbursement systems prevail, and that cost reimbursement and
similar systems will lead to higher costs. Further, the theory predicts some sort of interaction between the reimbursement system and
the property rights structure. Dulling the incentives for efficiency by means of the reimbursement system could not be expected to
have the same effects on a profit-seeking firm as it would on a
nonprofit firm with already poor internal incentives. The theory is
not powerful enough to tell us the exact nature of this interaction,
so the empirical results will have to stand on their own.

EMPIRICAL ANALYSIS

The data base for this analysis is the 1973-74 National Nursing Home
Survey.[4]   Reimbursement and regulatory data are from unpublished
Medicaid documents and an Urban Institute survey respectively.[5]

For this study, the sample was limited to

-- Firms providing nursing (as opposed to purely custodial) services to at least one-half of their residents;

-- Nursing homes certified for Medicaid;

-- Nursing homes located in a Standard Metropolitan Statistical Area (SMSA);

-- Nursing homes with complete reporting of the variables used.

These deletions reduced the sample of firms from about 2,100 to about 600.

The dependent variable was total operating or noncapital expenses. We used this rather than total expenses because of problems with the capital expense data. Nonprofit homes underreport capital costs associated with donated capital. Government operated homes underreport costs of government provided capital. Also, reported capital is endogenous to the reimbursement system. Cost reimbursement gives firms incentives to refinance frequently and to sell properties to increase depreciation reimbursements, incentives not found under flat rates. The results were not especially sensitive to the cost variable used (see below).

Independent variables include firm ownership, type of Medicaid reimbursement system, input prices, output, and variables to standardize for patient debility and for services provided and available (proxies for quality of care).

The property rights structure was measured by dummy variables for private nonprofit and government firms and interaction terms for nonprofit firms in flat-rate states and for government firms in flat-rate states. An additional variable for chain ownership of profit-seeking homes did not improve the equation and was dropped.

Reimbursement was modeled in detail. The type of reimbursement system and the recent history of the system were modeled with dummies. All reimbursement dummies were deflated by the proportion of the residents supported primarily by Medicaid, since the influence of the reimbursement system on the decision-maker must be strongly related to this proportion. In some states, different reimbursement systems were used for patients classified as requiring intermediate care and those requiring the higher level skilled nursing care. For homes with some residents of each type, we used the system and limits relevant for the majority. Variables for state regulations pertaining to fire safety and staffing ratios were also entered.

Input price variables included an index of SMSA construction prices, area-wide (SMSA) earnings for three levels of nurses and cleaning personnel. Area-wide earnings were preferred to firm-specific earnings, as the latter may be affected by reimbursement and/or ownership. Since the capital market is national in scope, interest rates were excluded.

Output was measured by the number of patient days, and standardized for occupancy rate, average length of stay, and a host of other dimensions. The data allowed us to control better than past studies for output type and quality. Standardizing variables included dummies for the types of rehabilitation therapies offered by the home and the proportion of patients receiving various routine services. The needs of patients were measured by an index which closely followed the one developed by Katz, called an Activities of Daily Living Index (Katz et al., 1970), but which was tailored to the data available from the survey used. We experimented with the scale gradient debility index pioneered by Skinner and Yett (1973) and an alternative version, but the results were not sensitive to the choice of index. The standardization for patient debility and routine service provision was incomplete because these variables were obtained from a sample of residents in each facility, the size of which averaged only 10 residents per facility. Appendix 1 lists all of the variables used.

The functional form was a hybrid of translog and log-linear. It is translog in the usual cost-function variables (input prices and output), while the property-rights, reimbursement and output-standardizing variables are entered in linear form.

$$\ln C = \alpha_o + \alpha_1 \ln Y + \Sigma_i \alpha_i \ln P_i + \frac{1}{2} \Sigma_i \Sigma_j \alpha_{ij} \ln P_i \ln P_j + \Sigma_i \alpha_{i\gamma} \ln P_i \ln Y$$

$$+ \Sigma_i \beta_i Pr_i + \Sigma_i \theta_i R_i + \Sigma_i \delta_i Rg_i + \Sigma_i n_i S_i$$

where:

C   = total operating expenses,

Y   = output, in-patient days,

P_i = the ith output price,

Pr_i = the ith property right structure variable,

R_i = the ith reimbursement variable,

Rg_i = the ith state regulatory variable,

S_i = the ith output standardizing variable.

The translog function is far more flexible than the more commonly used Cobb-Douglas form. Further, it can be usefully viewed as a natural second-order approximation to an arbitrary cost function (Christensen and Greene, 1976). The value of the greater flexibility was shown in sensitivity testing where the simpler Cobb-Douglas functional form was rejected.

Ordinary least squares was used to estimate the regressions. The treatment of ownership type and reimbursement scheme as exogeneous is straightforward, as is similar treatment of input prices (since they are taken from the market area of the nursing home). However, assuming that output is exogeneous is more complicated (Nerlove, 1965).

Nursing homes are not perfect substitutes, due to locational, amenity and medical differences, so that each nursing home is a price searcher. That is, each home has a (probably very small) degree of market power. Thus, the exact market conditions determine an optimal planned or ex ante size for the home, which we then take as exogenous for purposes of cost function estimation. In the regression we enter patient days for output. But since we hold occupancy rate constant, patient days are equivalent to planned output.

A potentially more serious problem occurs in taking the occupancy rate as exogeneous to costs. Clearly, occupancy rate and costs are both related to the way in which the firm is operated. However, the work of Greenlees, Marshall and Yett (1975) indicates that each nursing home faces random arrivals and departures. Thus, even if planned occupancy rate interacts with the error term of the regression, the actual occupancy rate observed contains a large random exogenous component. In any case, a regression was run with occupancy rate excluded, without upsetting the findings.

The assumptions necessary to avoid bias when estimating a production function with ordinary least squares are very different (Zellner, Kmenta and Dreze, 1966). As a form of sensitivity analysis, we are pursuing that approach as well, although we have more confidence in the cost-function approach. Preliminary results indicate that the production-function results are consistent with the cost-function results.

Heteroscedasticity may be a problem if the errors are strongly related to size. However, ordinary least squares is unbiased and consistent in any case. We have examined the residuals and determined that weighted least squares would not improve efficiency. The squared residuals were only weakly related to size. Although the sample was stratified, the cells were not oversampled, so weighting related to sampling would have no benefit.

Results

The cost function explained about 91% of the variation in total operating expenses. Table 2 gives the results for the ownership and reimbursement variables.[6]

Ownership. Nonprofit firms generally have higher costs than for-profit firms. The most expensive are government-owned nursing homes. Ownership differences are greatest in states using flat-rate methods of reimbursement. These cost differences appear at least partly to reflect differences in efficiency, although some uncertainty must be attached to this inference.

Table 2. Nursing Home Cost Function: The Effects of
Ownership and Reimbursement Method on Log
Total Operating Expenses

	Independent Variable	B Value	Standard Deviation
Ownership Variables	NONPROF	0.05	0.04
	GOVT	0.34	0.07
Reimbursement	TPMED2	-0.02	0.09
	TPMED3	0.56	0.32
	TPMED4	0.06	0.13
	TPMED5	0.03	0.12
	TPMED6	0.04	0.10
	TPMED7	0.41	0.14
Ownership/Reimbursement Interactions[a]	NPMED	0.24	0.12
	GMED	0.27	0.16

[a]Reimbursement variables and ownership/reimbursement interactions
are all interacted with PCAID, the percentage of patients supported
primarily by Medicaid. To obtain the effect of any of these
variables for homes with the mean Medicaid percentage for homes
included in the regression, multiply the coefficient by 0.615.

Private nonprofit homes appear to be more costly than for-profit
homes, but only in states with flat-rate reimbursement. In states
having other reimbursement systems, private nonprofit homes are estimated to have costs that are 5% higher, but this difference is not
statistically significant. In states with flat-rate reimbursement,
the difference at the mean Medicaid percentage of patients is estimated at 19%,[7] and this difference is statistically significant.

Government-owned homes are the most costly. In states without flat-
rate reimbursement systems, they have costs 34% higher than for-
profit homes. The difference increases to 51% in flat-rate states.
The magnitude of this difference appears somewhat unrealistic to us,
but the fact that there is a substantial difference is clear.

Our model did not distinguish between government-owned and private
non-profit firms, but the data show a substantial difference. One
explanation is that government-owned homes have more opportunities
to obtain subsidies from local governments than private nonprofit
homes have to obtain private donations to cover operating deficits.
Also, government homes may be required to pay wages according to
government salary scales.

To what extent do these cost differences imply indifferences in
efficiency? Two possible counter-hypotheses must be considered.
One is that the cost differences reflect unmeasured differences in
patient needs or quality of care. This possibility cannot be ruled

out. Nevertheless, the extent of the output standardization
variables employed and the size of the estimated cost difference, at
least for government-owned homes, implies that some of the cost differences are likely to reflect efficiency differences. Indeed,
while the patient and output standardizing variables improved the
equation, they did not have a major effect on the coefficients of the
ownership variables.

The other counter-hypothesis is that higher wages account for the
difference. Martin Feldstein has raised the possibility that
nonprofit organizations pay their employees more than their market
wage--philanthropic wage setting (M. S. Feldstein, 1971a). Our preliminary analysis of wage setting in nursing homes indicates that
private nonprofit and government-owned homes pay their employees
higher wages than for-profit homes, but the difference explains only
a small part of the difference in overall costs.

Reimbursement System. Pure cost reimbursement systems (those
without ceilings) are associated with the highest costs. Compared
to simple flat-rate systems (TPMED1), pure cost reimbursement
(TPMED7) has costs 21% higher in the typical home.[8] This result is
estimated with reasonable precision.

Note that cost reimbursement systems with ceilings (TPMED6) have
much lower costs than those without ceilings. Indeed, costs under
systems with ceilings are not much higher than those under flat-
rate systems. This implies that the ceilings are a binding
constraint for many nursing homes in these states.

Mixed results are shown for prospective reimbursement systems. Two
of the three types (TPMED4 and TPMED5) have costs comparable to
flat-rate systems and substantially lower than pure cost reimbursement. The third (TPMED3) has costs closer to pure cost reimbursement. This discrepancy is probably due to state effects. If all
prospective system categories were combined, costs would be
somewhere between pure cost reimbursement and flat-rate systems, but
the differences would not be statistically significant.

Flat-rate systems with rates varying by type of patient (TPMED2)
have costs similar to simple flat-rate systems. This is not
surprising since incentives are similar.

Sensitivity Testing. The major results were not especially sensitive to particular specifications of the model. A number of different versions were estimated.

First, total expenses was substituted for operating expenses as the
dependent variable. As expected, ownership differences have smaller
effects on total expenses than on operating expenses, but the qualitative patterns were unchanged. Private nonprofit firms had higher
expenses than for-profit firms, and government-owned firms had the
highest expenses. The ownership differences continued to be largest
under flat-rate reimbursement. Reimbursement differences followed
the same pattern, although pure cost reimbursement was somewhat more
costly relative to flat rates.

Second, various blocks of variables were excluded. When the
ownership variables were excluded, the results for the reimbursement

variables were virtually unchanged. When the reimbursement
variables were excluded, the ownership effects were estimated with
slightly less precision and showed slightly smaller effects.
Dropping the occupancy rates slightly enhanced the relative performance of the private nonprofit firms, but had no effect on the
government homes. Surprisingly, dropping the output standardization
variables, both a block at a time and all at once, had little effect
on either the ownership or the reimbursement coefficients. This
indicates that the various types of firms, operating under various
reimbursement systems provide roughly comparable care to roughly
comparable patients.

Discussion

The empirical results are consistent with the model. Within the
nursing home industry, nonprofit firms have higher costs than for-
profit firms, with a substantial part of the differences probably
related to efficiency. Within the nonprofit sector, government-
owned firms have higher costs than private firms.

Reimbursement systems make a difference. Pure cost reimbursement is
associated with substantially higher costs than flat-rate reimbursement. When ceilings are placed on cost reimbursement, the results
are closer to flat rates than to pure cost reimbursement. This
implies that the ceilings tend to be binding for a substantial proportion of nursing homes in these states.

Prospective systems give mixed results, though on average costs in
those states appear to be between flat-rate reimbursement and pure
cost reimbursement. The immaturity of most of the prospective reimbursement systems in the year for which the study's data were
collected (1972) and their heterogeneity (some are quite close to
flat-rate systems while others are closer to cost reimbursement)
prevents reliable inferences about the merits of prospective reimbursement. Prospective reimbursement should be seen as a continuum
between flat rates and cost reimbursement. When prospective rates
are established on the basis of statewide experience adjusted for
each home's characteristics other than actual costs, incentives are
comparable to flat rates. When prospective rates are based on a
home's cost experience in the previous year, these incentives are
diluted, and resemble cost reimbursement more closely.

Our results on the simple effects of ownership are consistent with
the previous literature. We were able to use a more extensive list
of output-standardizing variables and a more appropriate functional
form than many of the previous studies, but the qualitative conclusions are the same. Interestingly, while most of our blocks of
output-standardizing variables improved the equation, they did not
alter the basic results for ownership and reimbursement. Similarly,
our modified translog specification was a substantial improvement
over a simple Cobb-Douglas formulation, but did not alter the
results for ownership and reimbursement. While further refinements
are possible, the robustness of the results to data and specification implies that they are unlikely to be due simply to omitted
patient mix and quality of care variables.

Appendix 1

Variables

LTOTEXP = natural log of total costs

Ownership Variables

NONPROF = a dummy variable, taking on a value of one for a nonprofit firm

GOVT   = a dummy variable, taking on a value of one for government-owned firms

Type of Reimbursement System

TPMEDi = variable taking on the value of the proportion of the residents under Medicaid if the home is located in a state with the ith Medicaid reimbursement scheme. The index runs:

   1) = flat-rate,

   2) = flat-rate, varies by level of care,

   3) = prospective-rate, with a ceiling,

   4) = prospective-rate, without a ceiling,

   5) = prospective-rate, based on group performance,

   6) = cost-reimbursement, with a ceiling,

   7) = cost-reimbursement, with no ceiling.

Ownership-Reimbursement System Interaction

NPMED   = a variable taking on the value of the proportion of the residents supported by Medicaid if the home is nonprofit and also is located in a flat rate reimbursement state (NONPROF)(TPMED1 + TPMED2).

GMED   = analogous variable for government firms.

Other Reimbursement Variables

TRiC   = a variable taking on the value of the proportion of the residents supported by Medicaid if the reimbursement system was previously cost based (or flat rate) and has since changed.

Patient Debility

KATZi = percentage of residents in the ith Katz debility category. Debility
        increases with increasing i. The 0th category of no debility is excluded.

CSNF = the proportion of the residents classified by the state as requiring
        skilled nursing care, rather than intermediate care.

Services Received and Therapies Available

$ROUT_i$ = proportion of patients receiving the ith service during a seven day
        period. The index runs:

1) = nasal feeding,

2) = blood pressure reading,

3) = enema,

4) = catheterization,

5) = full bed-bath,

6) = bowel or bladder retraining,

7) = oxygen therapy,

8) = dressing or bandage,

9) = temperature-pulse-respiration reading.

$REHAB_i$ = a dummy variable, taking on a value of one if the home provides the ith
        rehabilitation therapy with a registered or licensed therapist on the
        premises. The index runs:

1) = physical therapy,

2) = occupational therapy,

3) = recreational therapy,

4) = speech and hearing therapy,

5) = counseling,

6) = other rehabilitation services.

Input Prices and Output

LDAYS = natural log of patient days.

LCONSDEX= natural log of an index of construction costs.

LRNEARN = natural log of registered nurses' earnings taken from the SMSA within which the home is located if possible, or nearest SMSA in other cases.

LLPEARN = natural log of licensed practical nurses' earnings.

LNAEARN = natural log of nurses' aides' earnings.

LCSEARN = natural log of cleaning service workers' earnings.

EPROXY = a dummy variable, for small SMSAs, taking on a value of one if the earnings variables are taken from a nearby SMSA.

CINTERi = interaction terms among the input prices and the output variable

1) = (LDAYS)(LRNEARN),	9) = (LRNEARN)(LCONSDEX),
2) = (LDAYS)(LLPEARN),	10) = (LLPEARN)(LNAEARN),
3) = (LDAYS)(LNAEARN),	11) = (LLPEARN)(LCSEARN),
4) = (LDAYS)(LCSEARN),	12) = (LLPEARN)(LCONSDEX),
5) = (LDAYS)(LCONSDEX),	13) = (LNAEARN)(LCSEARN),
6) = (LRNEARN)(LLPEARN),	14) = (LNEARN)(LCONSDEX),
7) = (LRNEARN)(LNAEARN),	15) = (LCSEARN)(LCONSDEX).
8) = (LRNEARN)(LCSEARN),	

Other Standardizations

OCC   = the occupancy rate.

LS   = average length of stay.

CONST = a dummy variable, taking on value of one if the home was originally constructed as a nursing home.

BED4 = proportion of beds in rooms with four or more beds.

STFO = a dummy variable, taking on a value of one for those states with a nursing staff requirement.

PCAID = proportion of residents supported by Medicaid.

NOTES

[1]This proportion is so high because of the age of nursing home residents and the fact that the high costs of care coupled with the long stays cause many residents to qualify for Medicaid under "medically needy" provisions.

[2]Section 249 of the Social Security Act of 1972 limits this freedom somewhat. Medicaid reimbursements to nursing homes must be "cost-related." The analysis in this paper uses data from a period (1972) before this law became effective.

[3]See Frech (1976) and the references therein, and the excellent survey of Louis DeAlessi (1980). The industries examined include savings and loan firms, insurers, hospitals and many others.

[4]Approximately 2,000 facilities were sampled. Within each facility, residents and employees were sampled. Sampling techniques are described in National Center for Health Statistics (1975).

[5]Additional details on the data are included in Frech and Ginsburg (forthcoming). We are grateful to Barry Chiswick for allowing us to use his data file of published SMSA data relevant to nursing homes.

[6]Space constraints preclude reporting the complete equation and discussing the results for other variables. Both are available from the authors.

[7]This number is the sum of the coefficient on NONPROF and the coefficient on NPMED, the latter amplified by the mean proportion of Medicaid patients, 0.615.

[8]The typical home reflects a weighted average of ownership types and the mean proportion of patients supported by Medicaid.

DEMAND ANALYSES

HEALTH, ECONOMICS, AND HEALTH ECONOMICS
J. van der Gaag and M. Perlman (editors)
North-Holland Publishing Company, 1981

THE DEMAND FOR MEDICAL CARE SERVICES: A RETROSPECT AND PROSPECT

Joseph P. Newhouse

During the past decade empirical knowledge about the demand for medical care services, especially its price or insurance elasticity, has increased enormously.[*1] Most of the relevant research has taken place in North America, especially in the United States, and has used American data. This survey concentrates on those studies.[2]

The U.S. debate about the appropriate role, if any, of patient cost sharing in a national health insurance plan has helped stimulate American research into the magnitude of insurance elasticities. The elasticity plays an important role at two levels. The U.S. Department of Health and Human Services (formerly HEW) has developed a model to estimate the monetary costs of alternative insurance plans; the elasticity of demand is a necessary input. At the same time, economists have developed normative models of insurance in which the optimum depends upon the elasticity of demand (Zeckhauser, 1970; M.S. Feldstein, 1973; Arrow, 1973).

Analysis of price and insurance elasticities tends to be of less significance outside the United States because other countries have historically had little or no interest in patient cost sharing. Nonetheless, quantifying nonprice determinants of demand appears to be of universal value (although the determinants may differ in their importance from one country to the next). For example, it is useful to know how travel and queueing times affect demand when making location decisions about facilities or medical manpower, or how trends in demographic variables affect demand when planning the appropriate number of physicians to train.

Before we review empirical estimates of demand functions, some problems in quantifying demand require comment. Broadly speaking, the literature has measured demand in two ways--expenditures and physical units of utilization. Although expenditures provide a ready metric for aggregating disparate services, they suffer from two potential disadvantages. First, insofar as prices do not reflect marginal cost, variation in expenditures has ambiguous welfare implications. Second, if the gross price for a given

*The research reported herein was performed pursuant to Grant No. 016B-7501/2-P2021 from the U.S. Department of Health, Education, and Welfare, Washington, D.C. The opinions and conclusions expressed are solely those of the author, and should not be construed as representing the opinions or policy of The Rand Corporation or any agency of the United States Government.

medical service changes when insurance changes, induced variation in
expenditure need not closely correspond to induced variation in real
resource use.

Alternatively, one can measure demand in physical units such as
hospital days or physician visits. Although such variables appear
to measure real resource use, they suffer in practice from
incompleteness. In the case of inpatient services, the variables
typically employed are admission rates and length of stay (or their
product, hospital days), but neither measures the intensity of
service, the most rapidly rising component of hospital expenditures
in developed countries. The same criticism applies to the usual
measure of demand for outpatient services, physician visits. Visits
can differ markedly in their intensity (e.g., in the number of
diagnostic tests performed) and a simple count of visits clearly
does not capture such variation. These imperfections should be
borne in mind when assessing the literature; I return to the issue
of measuring demand below.

THE PRICE ELASTICITY OF DEMAND

In 1971 Rashi Fein testified before the United States Congress that
he knew of no evidence to indicate that deductibles and coinsurance
"lowered utilization" (U.S. Senate, 1971). Although one might cavil
at this claim, the studies of this matter cited below came almost
entirely at or after this time. Elsewhere (Newhouse, 1978) I have
reviewed many of these studies and have described their estimates of
price elasticity, service by service.[3] Rather than repeat that
material here, I focus instead on the methodologies various analysts
have employed to derive estimates. The nature of the data used in
each study has, to a large degree, dictated the methodology used. I
have therefore classified studies by the type of data used to estimate elasticities. Each type possesses certain strengths and
weaknesses.

Studies Based upon Insurance Claims or Premium Data

These studies use quite simple methods. Expenditure data on
insurance claims, when available, are analyzed as a function of
insurance plan. When individual claims are not available, premiums
for different insurance policies contain implied elasticities of
demand with respect to insurance. For example, suppose premiums are
quoted for policies with 10% and 25% coinsurance. If demand elasticity were zero (and if loadings were proportional to actuarial
value), the premium for the 10% coinsurance policy would be 20%
(100-10)/(100-25) higher than the premium for the 25% coinsurance
policy. If the difference in premiums between the two policies is
greater than 20%, one can infer the elasticity from a formula found
in Phelps and Newhouse (1974a).

This method has been applied to estimate the response of demand to
variation in coinsurance and deductible rates. The medical services

analyzed include hospital and physician services (combined), hospital services alone, and dental services alone. Phelps and Newhouse (1974b) found demand for hospital and physician services combined to be 6% higher at 10% coinsurance than at 25% coinsurance.[4] Newhouse, Rolph, et al. (1978) estimated that demand per person at a deductible of $1,000 per person per year was about two-thirds of demand at a deductible of $50 per person per year (1975 dollars). Most of the response occurred in the range near $50, as theory would suggest (Keeler, Newhouse, and Phelps, 1977). Freiberg and Scutchfield (1976) found that a decline in out-of-pocket cost per day of hospitalization from $44 to $2.50 (which approximates a change in the coinsurance rate from 50% to zero) was associated with a 50% increase in hospital admissions. Phelps and Newhouse (1974b) found that demand for dental services was 30% higher at zero coinsurance than at 20% coinsurance.

This method has a number of strengths. It is usually straightforward to specify the variation in price, because one is examining a well-defined change in coinsurance or deductible rates. Premiums for policies with varying scopes of services, however, must be adjusted so they are comparable, and that is not always straightforward. Second, because the data usually pertain to large employer groups, one can reasonably presume that insurance is exogenous or that any self-selection is minimal. (One cannot, of course, generalize to those not covered by group insurance plans.) Third, the variation in utilization occurs for a small group in the market; thus, these estimates can be fairly taken to represent demand elasticities.

On the other hand, very little information is available about the characteristics of the insured, making it difficult to appraise the distributional effects of cost sharing. One could, in principle, examine how premiums vary for groups of individuals with differing characteristics, but in practice it is unlikely that the variation in group characteristics will suffice to permit many inferences. Nor will one collect any information about services that are not covered--for example, outpatient mental health services. Variation in coverage presents another difficulty: some services may be covered in certain policies but not in others (again, say, outpatient mental health). If such services have nonzero cross-price elasticities with other covered services, one must sometimes make untestable assumptions about the joint probability density function of demand for covered and noncovered services to obtain unbiased estimates of own-price elasticities.

To use this method to estimate the effects of a deductible (in contrast to coinsurance), one must know the probability density function of demand, something that may be difficult to obtain in practice. For example, policies that have a deductible will typically not generate information on demand by those who spend less than the deductible. At levels of deductibles that most individuals exceed, this is not a serious problem, but for larger deductibles it forces one to make unverifiable assumptions about the shape of the probability density function of demand in the region below the deductible. Furthermore, there exists a grey area. Individuals (or providers) may not claim reimbursement for all services actually used because of transaction costs incurred in filing a claim; again,

one must typically make unverifiable assumptions about the rate of
underfiling. The seriousness of this problem clearly depends upon
the magnitude of underfiling, but is of some importance when estimating the effects of variation in a deductible because underfiling
is concentrated in the region of total expenditure near the
deductible.

Studies Based upon Natural Experiments

These studies typically compare demand by a group of individuals
before and after their insurance policy changed. For example,
Scitovsky and Snyder (1972)and Scitovsky and McCall (1977) measured
how frequently Stanford University employees made physician visits
before and after the employee's coinsurance rate changed from zero
to 25%. Visits fell approximately 25% 1 year after the change: the
decline maintained itself 4 years later. The method has also been
applied to hospital services by Heaney and Riedel (1970) and by
Williams (1966), to dental services by Morehead, Donaldson, and
Zanes (1971) and by Grubb (1964), and to drugs by Smith and Garner
(1974). In the case of dental services and drugs, full insurance
caused demand roughly to double relative to situations in which services were not insured. In the case of hospital services the
response was, speaking very roughly, about half as great as for dental care.

Roemer et al. (1975) estimated that a $1 copayment for office
visits in the California Medicaid program decreased office visits,
but increased hospitalization to such a degree that total expenditure
increased (see also Brian and Gibbens, 1974). This finding caused
them to characterize the copayment as "penny-wise and pound-foolish."

For estimating price elasticities natural experiments share many of
the advantages of using premium or claims data. The price variation
is usually straightforward to specify, and because the same group of
individuals is compared before and after, self-selection problems do
not arise. On the other hand, this method confounds the effects of
the change in price with changes in any other variable affecting
demand (e.g., an influenza epidemic in one period and not another).
The more preferable design, a comparison with either an equivalent
control group or an equivalent alternative treatment group, is not
available.[5] Usually the change occurs for a relatively small group
in the overall market, but not always. For example, Beck (1974)
analyzed the natural experiment that occurred when Saskatchewan
implemented a province-wide copayment. The resulting fall in utilization could have reflected elements of both supply and demand, as
is also true with similar comparisons for the United States
Medicare program (Bombardier et al., 1977). Natural experiments,
too, may have the advantage of permitting us to determine whose
demands are more affected by the change (i.e., estimation of
interactions between price elasticities and demographic variables);
for example, in the Stanford data collected by Scitovsky and
Snyder, demands of female dependents were more responsive than those
of any other group (Phelps and Newhouse, 1972). Of course, the
group among whom the natural experiment occurred may not be
representative: Stanford University employees may differ from the

United States population. But insofar as the group is large enough
to study variation in response within it, this disadvantage may be
overcome by appropriate weighting.

Studies Based upon Comparison of Individuals with Different Insurance Policies

The economics literature has most commonly used this method. When
the unit of observation is the individual (or household), the method
utilizes data from surveys that ask the household about its
insurance and use of services. These data, together with the
covariates available in the survey, are then used to estimate a
demand curve (Colle and Grossman, 1978; Davis and Reynolds, 1976;
Holtmann and Olsen, 1976; Manning and Phelps, 1979; Newhouse and
Marquis, 1978; Newhouse and Phelps, 1976; Phelps, 1975; Rosenthal,
1970; Rosett and Huang, 1973). Alternatively, data on area averages
have been used in place of data upon individual households (Davis
and Russell, 1972; M. S. Feldstein, 1971b, 1977; P. J. Feldstein,
1973, 1971b; Fuchs and Kramer, 1972; Rosenthal, 1964).

These studies exhibit a wide variety of price elasticity estimates.
Some of the variation in the estimates may reflect true differences
in the populations sampled; some reflect differences in specification (Newhouse, Phelps, and Marquis, 1979). Other variation may
stem from a (true) nonconstant demand elasticity, with observations
coming from varying ranges of price or insurance. Newhouse and
Phelps (1976) give among the lowest values; they estimate elasticities around -0.1; studies of Martin Feldstein (1971, 1977) yield
somewhat higher estimates (around -0.5), as do those of Fuchs and
Kramer (1972) and Davis and Russell (1972). Perhaps the highest
elasticities reported in the literature are those of Rosett and
Huang (1973), who find an elasticity of around -0.35 at a coinsurance rate of 0.2, but an elasticity of -1.5 at a coinsurance rate
of 0.8. The estimates around -0.1 more closely resemble estimates
using other methods, but comparisons are difficult, for many
reasons. The estimates from the studies cited in this section come
from a wide range of insurance; some are true price elasticity estimates with no insurance present; in others, rather extensive
insurance is present. Thus, the interval within which insurance or
price varies may be quite different across studies. This difference
can make it difficult to compare these studies, one with another,
and also with studies based on other methodologies.

These studies have, nonetheless, a number of advantages. Data can
be collected from a representative sample (e.g., a national probability sample), and the ability to aggregate by geographic regions
allows for the possibility that physicians (or other health care
providers) gear their treatment advice to some average or modal
insurance coverage in a local market area, instead of, or in addition to, the coverage of the individual being treated (the so-called
"norms hypothesis"). Collection at the household level usually
allows us to gather enough information about other characteristics
of the household to allow one to estimate interactions of price
elasticities with demographic variables. One can also obtain information on the consumption of services that are not insured, either

because they fall outside the scope of coverage or below a
deductible.

This model does have drawbacks, however. Price or insurance is difficult to specify. Actual insurance policies can vary along so many
dimensions that simple parameterizations, such as the frequently
used average coinsurance rate, can cause inconsistent estimates
(Newhouse, Phelps, and Marquis, 1979). For example, if one computes
the average or marginal coinsurance rate for those facing a deductible, and uses that rate to estimate a price elasticity, the
resulting estimate will be biased away from zero, because the error
term will be negatively correlated with the average coinsurance
rate.[6]   Such problems are necessarily present when the data are
averages from a geographic entity such as a state, and the direction
of the inconsistency cannot always be signed a priori.

Another misspecification of the price variable occurs if no direct
information on price is available, and price is estimated by
dividing total expenditures by quantity consumed. In that case
measurement error in the quantity consumed variable can result in a
well-known bias away from zero in the estimate of the price elasticity. Fuchs and Kramer (1972) attempt to avoid this problem by
using an instrumental variables estimator, but asymptotic properties
of consistency may be of little solace with a small number of observations. Aggregation presents other problems. Use of aggregate
data raises the possibility of aggregation bias or instability. For
example, suppose one wishes to predict what will happen if a uniform
national plan is enacted. In such a case the change in insurance
across individuals will vary depending upon their prior coverage.
Unless that coverage is independent of the individuals' insurance
elasticities, or varies in a known way, aggregating across individuals will introduce bias.

Aggregating across services presents another kind of problem, if
services vary in the extent of coverage. In that case theory permits such aggregation only when relative prices are constant. This
problem is particularly dramatic in the Rosett and Huang (1973)
study; the authors examine expenditures at various average coinsurance rates, but the rate is computed as the average rate for all
observed expenditures. Those entering the hospital typically had
their hospital bills covered; those who did not go to the hospital
typically had much smaller expenditures that were not covered by
insurance. Hence, insurance appeared to induce a large increase in
total expenditure. If one knew the coinsurance rates for hospital
and outpatient services, of course, one could enter such rates in
the demand equation.

The theory of demand for insurance suggests that individuals with
high demands for medical care will seek relatively greater coverage
(Phelps, 1976). If so, insurance is endogenous, but unfortunately,
no instruments are known that strongly identify its effects. For
individual data, the best conceptual variable appears to be work
group size, because the size of the loading falls systematically as
work group size increases (Phelps, 1973), and work group size
arguably does not affect the demand for medical services directly.
Nonetheless, a two-stage least squares estimator, when applied to a
sample of several thousand observations, did not yield statistically

significant estimated price elasticities (Newhouse and Phelps, 1976). In light of the evidence of nonzero price elasticities that other methods show, it seems unlikely that this imprecision occurred because the true price elasticity is zero; rather, the difficulty seems to be weak identification. Whether household surveys will be sufficiently large to achieve reliable results is thus problematical.[7]

Both price and utilization variables may be subject to considerable measurement error. Households are asked to recall utilization over some past period; studies show that as high as 40% of total variance could represent errors in household-reported annual hospital and dental expenditure (Marquis, Marquis, and Newhouse, 1976; Marquis, 1979). Random error in measuring utilization, of course, only degrades precision. But random error in the price variable will bias the coefficient toward zero, and the household cannot necessarily be relied upon to furnish error-free information about insurance. The large American surveys (the National Medical Care Expenditure Survey; the Center for Health Administration Studies surveys) attempt to verify the household-supplied insurance information with employers or insurance companies, but verification efforts do not always succeed and can miss policies that the household respondent simply does not mention.

Designed Experiments

Two experiments (at least) have been designed to gather information about the price elasticity of medical care. One took place in Kansas during an 8-month period in the 1960s (Lewis and Keairnes, 1970; Hill and Veney, 1970). The other is the Health Insurance Study, a multi-year project that is still in progress. Some initial results from the Health Insurance Study are reported in another paper at this conference (Manning et al., 1980).

Designed experiments randomly assign individuals to an experimental treatment(s) and to a comparison group (or use related techniques). The treatments vary the price of care. The Kansas study tested the hypothesis that reducing the coinsurance rate for outpatient care would reduce total expenditure by reducing demand for hospital services; in contrast to the results of Roemer et al. (1975) described above, the hypothesis was not supported.

The Health Insurance Study (Newhouse, 1974) was designed to estimate the own-price elasticity for most medical services, the interactions, if any, of that elasticity with various demographic characteristics, and the cross-price elasticity between inpatient and outpatient care. Preliminary results suggest that demand for care is on the order of 50% higher when care is free than when it is subject to an income-related catastrophic insurance plan. Results for the cross-price elasticity between inpatient and outpatient care are consistent with those from the Kansas study.

In appropriately executed designed experiments, insurance is exogenous and readily parameterized, and it is approximately orthogonal with other covariates. The range of variation in price is high

relative to most natural experiments, yielding information on elasticities over a wider range of coinsurance, as well as increasing the
precision with which one can test the hypothesis that price affects
demand.

Artifacts of the experiment may, however, interfere with reliable
estimation. If the study in Kansas had run for more than 8 months,
results might have differed (although in this particular instance
the results from the Health Insurance Study suggest not). More
generally, there is the problem of Hawthorne effects and methods to
test whether behavior differs in an experimental situation do not
always exist.

Designed experiments are, moreover, relatively expensive; if they
are not properly executed, substantial resources may be wasted.

THE EFFECTS OF OTHER VARIABLES ON DEMAND

Empirical studies have found that a number of nonprice variables
importantly affect demand. These include health status, age (which
may reflect imperfect measurement of health status), sex, income,
time price, and race; the effect of education has been more difficult to isolate.[8]

Health status, when included, usually explains more variation than
any other single variable (Newhouse and Phelps, 1976). The observed
relationship between health status and utilization frequently,
however, represents reverse causality. The mechanism is as follows.
Household surveys typically measure health status at the time of the
interview or during the past twelve months, and utilization over the
past twelve months. But individuals who visit the physician at
higher rates are more likely to have health problems discovered and
may perceive their health to be poorer than those who do not visit
the physician very frequently. Manning, Newhouse, and Ware
(forthcoming) show that when self-rated health status is used to
"predict" past utilization the estimated coefficients of health status and all variables not orthogonal to it are inconsistent. The
empirical magnitude of the inconsistency varies from moderate to
small. Not surprisingly they also demonstrate that, other things
equal, those in poorer health will have a greater demand for medical
services.

Estimated income elasticities have varied from near zero to approximately 1.0. Grossman (1972a) has suggested that wage and nonwage
income will affect demand differently because an increased wage
raises both the value of time used in consuming medical services and
the value of any reduction in sick days. To date, the evidence is
consistent with this view, although the effect of nonwage income
upon demand has not been estimated with any precision.

The greater the distance one must travel to receive medical care,
the less the demand (Acton, 1975, 1976; Phelps and Newhouse, 1972;
Simon and Smith, 1973). Distance is one of several variables that
affect the time price of care; using Becker's general approach,

Phelps and Newhouse (1974a) and Acton (1975, 1976) have developed
the theory of how time price affects the demand for medical care.
If elasticity with respect to total price (time price plus money
price) is constant, observed time price elasticities should rise as
money prices fall and observed money price elasticities should rise
as time prices fall. The latter prediction is borne out by the
greater price elasticities (in absolute value) for home visits than
for office visits, and the former prediction is consistent with the
relatively high values for time price elasticities at zero or near-
zero money prices (Phelps and Newhouse, 1974b).

Of considerable interest is the interaction, if any, between income
and price elasticities; in particular, are the poor more sensitive
to price than the more well-to-do? Evidence from Canada (Beck,
1974) suggests that this is the case; U.S. data are inconclusive
(Phelps and Newhouse, 1972; Newhouse and Phelps, 1976; Manning et
al., 1980). The Canadian data have the considerable advantage of a
very large sample: on the other hand, they measure the effect of a
copayment that was implemented province-wide; if queues fell as a
result of the copayment, the resulting change in the time price
could have led to less of a decline in demand for those with high
prices of time (who would be disproportionately nonpoor). But
failure to find an effect in the smaller American data sets (where
time price presumptively did not change) could merely reflect a lack
of power.

DOES SUPPLIER-INDUCED DEMAND INVALIDATE THE DEMAND FUNCTIONS
IN THE LITERATURE?

There exists a serious challenge to the estimated demand functions
just described. Many argue that the important determinant of demand
is supply, especially the supply of physicians (Detsky, 1978; Evans,
1974; M.S. Feldstein, 1967; Roemer and Shain, 1959). In particular,
the physician is said to have sufficient discretion in advising the
patient (i.e., unexploited demand-creation ability) to offset exogenous changes in demand. But if the demand of only a small number of
individuals changes, the physician has little incentive to do so,
hence, the studies of demand cited above could greatly overestimate
the response of demand to changes in insurance or to changes in
demographic variables such as income and age.

Recent evidence, however, suggests that both the physician's
unexploited demand-creation ability, and his ability to offset exogenous changes, are limited.[9]

Newhouse, Williams et al. (1979) have shown that, as their numbers
have grown, specialists of a given type have systematically entered
smaller and smaller towns in the United States. These data directly
refute the hypothesis that specialists can gratify their supposed
preference for living in larger cities by creating ever more demand.
Rather the data are quite consistent with standard economic location
theory, which implies that as the number of physicians has grown,
the market area surrounding each has shrunk. As a result, small
towns that were previously part of larger market areas have now

become the focus of new market areas. Although some amount of
unexploited demand-creation ability could exist, physicians appear
to locate as if they are constrained by standard market forces. Of
course physicians' location preferences might have changed in favor
of smaller towns, but such direct evidence as exists does not
suggest it (U.S. GAO, 1978).

Between 1969 and 1977, controlling for specialty and location,
physicians' real incomes in the United States fell around 1.75% per
year (Newhouse, Williams et al., 1979). Data in Hadley, Holahan,
and Scanlon (1979) are consistent with these figures; these same
authors also show that Canadian physicians' real incomes fell after
the implementation of Medicare and the subsequent growth in the
number of Canadian physicians. If physicians have sufficient
demand-creation ability to fully offset adverse changes in the
external environment, one presumes they would not tolerate a fall in
real income. Fuchs (1978) has estimated that a 10% increase in
surgeons will induce a 3% increase in operations. The true elasticity figure may, however, be less, if an increased number of
surgeons is correlated with an increase in quality that in turn
increases demand.[10] Even if we accept Fuchs's estimate, unexploited
demand-creation ability is clearly limited.

These observations cast serious doubt on the extreme version of the
supply-creates-its-own-demand argument that physicians can or will
offset any changes in market demand that might be induced by changes
in insurance or other variables. Thus, demand analysis remains of
interest, but the way in which changes in demand at the market level
affect utilization is an important unknown.

FRONTIERS OF DEMAND ANALYSIS

In this section I speculate on the direction of demand research in
the next decade. Such speculation is hazardous, but the risk of
appearing foolish--either ex ante or ex post--will have been worth
taking if the discussion stimulates fruitful research.

Specification of the Price, Income, and Health Status Variables

Own price. Most empirical work has assumed the insurance policy
could be treated by one parameter, a nonvarying coinsurance rate,
and has analyzed demand per unit of time, typically 1 year. If the
coinsurance rate varies with total expenditure (e.g., it has a
deductible or upper limit), the appropriate theoretical price
variable is unobservable; moreover, it varies with the time left in
the accounting period and the amount of expenditure necessary to
change the coinsurance rate when decisions about treatment of a
given illness are made (Keeler, Newhouse, and Phelps, 1977). A more
appropriate unit of observation when insurance is of this form is
the illness episode rather than total demand per unit of time.
During the 1980s data from the Health Insurance Study should facilitate analysis on this basis: they provide enough information to

group expenditures into illness episodes and date them within the
accounting period.

Cross Price. Specification of relevant cross-price variables will
probably improve. For example, estimates will probably be made of
the cross-price elasticity between outpatient mental health services
and general medical services, and between prescription and
nonprescription drugs, about which little is known.

Income. Most empirical studies have measured income as current
income; Andersen and Benham (1970) are an exception. Yet current
income suffers from two well-known defects: it contains transitory
income, which will bias the estimated income elasticity toward zero
if demand in fact relates to permanent income; it also is presumptively endogenous because of the effect of sickness on both income
and demand for medical services. Both these problems could be
avoided by using a measure of permanent income, yet there is no
standard method for measuring it. That various instrumental
variables all provide consistent estimators provides rather little
comfort, given usual sample sizes. Measures that better approximate
permanent income (e.g., use of several years of income) should
improve the estimation of both income elasticities and the interaction of price elasticities with income. It may also make possible a
better test of Grossman's hypothesis that non-wage-related income
should affect demand differently from wage-related income.

Health Status. Measurement of health status variables seems likely
to improve in several ways. The comprehensiveness with which health
is measured will increase; for example, physical, mental, social,
and physiological dimensions rather than just self-assessed general
health perceptions can be included. (For a first step, see Manning,
Newhouse, and Ware, forthcoming.) Greater attention will probably
be paid to possible biases from random measurement error in the
health status variable, either through formal reliability measures
to adjust least squares estimates or the use of latent variable
techniques (van de Ven and van der Gaag, 1979). The endogeneity of
the frequently used measured health variables may also be addressed.

Specification of the Stochastic Term and Appropriate Estimators

Most demand modeling has used very simple stochastic assumptions,
typically assuming that the distribution of the error term is normal
or lognormal and that observations are independent. Because of the
Central Limit Theorem, the assumption of normality is appropriate
when using aggregate (area-wide) data. But for individual data, the
assumption of normality is not a good approximation. Lognormality
is better, but preliminary analysis of Health Insurance Study data
suggests that one can reject at the 1% level the hypothesis that
medical expenditures come from a lognormal distribution. The actual
distribution departs from lognormality in part because of a group
that spends nothing during a particular time period (typically about
20% of the people in any one year). Additionally, the conditional
distribution of annual expenditures (conditional upon spending some
positive amount) has systematic departures from lognormality in the
right-hand tail.

Typically, researchers using family level data have not accounted
for intrafamily correlation, yet such correlations appear pronounced
(Manning et al., 1980; van der Gaag and van de Ven, 1978). In
general, one can anticipate the use of more appropriate stochastic
specification, which should lead to more efficient estimators.

Specification of the Dependent Variable

Most analysts have measured demand either as expenditures per unit
of time or in physical units consumed per time period (e.g., visits
or hospital days per year). The relationship between physical units
and expenditures will probably be explored much more fully in the
next decade.

As pointed out above, measures such as visits and hospital days are
seriously incomplete, because they fail to analyze the intensity of
service. Ancillary services, for example, everywhere represent a
substantial component of expenditure on both outpatient and
inpatient services, but few analyses of demand for ancillary services
have been undertaken. (Scitovsky and Snyder, 1972, estimated that
the price elasticity for outpatient ancillary services was approximately half that of the elasticity with respect to visits.)

How one analyzes intensity of services depends in part upon the
meaning one attaches to prices. A quite conservative approach keeps
the estimation as much as possible in physical units. Such an
approach could extend beyond the demand for various types of medical
procedures to encompass choice of physician. It is important to
know the determinants of choice between, say, a specialist and a
general practitioner in those countries where choice is permitted
(e.g., United States, Canada), because governments there tend to see
the specialty distribution as a policy instrument, and their actions
may affect both the supply of and demand for different types of manpower. To study how individuals choose providers, one could place
providers into a discrete category (e.g., general practitioner,
board-certified family practitioner, board-certified pediatrician),
and analyze how variables such as insurance, income, and education
affect choice.

Unfortunately, the conservative approach just outlined tends to
break down when large numbers of categories must be analyzed, and
large numbers will be the rule, not the exception. For example,
providers differ in many ways other than specialty, and medical care
consists of hundreds--if not thousands--of different types of services or procedures.

The alternative approach uses price (or an analogue) to aggregate
across types of providers or services, but this approach is hardly
problem-free. First, different prices appear relevant to different
aspects of the expenditure decision, implying that expenditures
need to be disaggregated. Goldman and Grossman (1978), for example,
point out that fixed costs such as travel and waiting times apply to
units of service such as visits but do not necessarily apply to the
intensity of service, nor to what they define as quality, namely the
type of provider used. They have built upon the theoretical work of

Rosen (1974), who suggested that the analyst approach the demand for
different products by first estimating a hedonic price equation and
then using the implied prices of product characteristics to estimate
the demand for various types of characteristics.

Because of its current popularity with economists generally and its
promise for addressing the issue of variation in quality, it is
worthwhile emphasizing two practical difficulties that Rosen noted
for this method. In the usual case, the hedonic price equation (the
first stage) cannot be linear, or there will be no variance in the
price of quality in the sample. But to justify one nonlinear form
rather than another is typically a difficult task, and the estimated
marginal prices could be quite sensitive to the choice of functional
form.

Even assuming, however, that the nonlinear functional form of the
hedonic equation is correct, a serious identification problem can
arise. To identify a demand curve, one must have at least as many
variables that affect the supply price of quality and do not affect
demand as one has dimensions of quality. If quality takes several
dimensions to represent, the requirement for several excluded exogenous variables can be onerous.

One clearly exogenous variable (or set of variables) is the possible
differences among local areas in factor prices or regulations that
affect the cost or production. Whether the variation in factor
prices that exists will suffice to yield reliable estimates is, of
course, an empirical issue, but the matter seems problematical. At
a minimum, one would like data from several local markets.

Goldman and Grossman, who were working with data from one local
market, proposed different solutions to the problems of identification and variation in the price of product characteristics
across consumers. They postulated that consumers faced different
prices because of assumed differences in the cost of search. The
variables they used to measure the cost of search, however, arguably
affect demand directly: if so, identification has still not been
achieved.[11] Identification may be possible, however, by analyzing
choices of consumers who face varying prices because of varying
insurance coverage; such an approach also permits using a linear
hedonic price equation. Rosen's methods, or extensions of them, may
prove quite useful to the degree that meaningful prices can be used;
as discussed below, however, observed prices in heavily insured
markets may have little or no significance.

The Norms Argument and Technological Change

Further tests of the norms hypothesis seem likely; they will shed
light on the degree to which demand studies based upon individual-
level data yield meaningful elasticity estimates. The tests carried
out to date have examined whether variation in area-wide insurance
affects utilization of individuals, holding constant individual
insurance coverage. The tests have not supported the hypothesis,
but precision has been poor (Newhouse and Marquis, 1978). Similar
tests may well be repeated on other data sets.

Another variant of the norms hypothesis that focuses attention on
variation across time rather than space deserves testing. Theory
suggests that the rate of technological change in medical care
reflects the market willingness to pay for new products.[12] Suppose
ideas for new products or services are generated at a constant rate,
but that those actually meeting the market test reflect income and
insurance coverage generally. Specifically, more meet the test as
insurance and income grow. Expenditures on medical services over
time could then rise more rapidly than would be predicted from
cross-sectional variation in income and insurance (which holds technology constant). The markedly higher income elasticities in time-
series than in cross-sectional data are suggestive of such a
phenomenon, although other explanations for this difference can be
found. The straightforward approach to this issue requires
measuring technological change and analyzing its determinants, a
very difficult problem. Some progress may be possible in the next
decade, but it will not be easy.

How Do Price and Utilization Respond to Changes in Demand?

One of the major applications of demand analysis in most industries
is to predict how price and utilization (or quantity bought and
sold) will change if determinants of demand or supply change. The
use of estimated demand curves in forecasting future beef prices is
a well-known example. But the applicability of the beef market
paradigm to medical care is in dispute; both the stability of the
supply curve and the mechanisms used to clear the market are not
settled issues.

As insurance tends towards completeness, the consumer loses the usual
incentive to purchase from less costly, more efficient providers
(Evans, 1971; Newhouse, 1979). If insurance simply reimburses
costs or charges, the meaning and stability of the supply curve are
called into question. Inefficient producers are not necessarily
weeded out, and one cannot assume that an estimated supply curve
represents an aggregation of marginal cost functions, all representing efficient production.

How price is determined in markets with substantial insurance is not
a settled issue either. In many, if not most, countries price is
nominally determined or negotiated by a governmental or centralized
body; considerations of public finance and political economy will
clearly play a role in determining price.

In other instances, such as in some U.S. private insurance (as well
as the Medicare program), price determination is decentralized. The
literature typically assumes that the extent of insurance makes
little difference to the process by which price is determined, that
is, insurance simply shifts the demand curve in some fashion, and
that a standard supply curve exists and is stable.[13] Prices then
adjust to equate supply and demand. This usual tale appears applicable if insurance covers only a minor portion of the market;
insurers could reimburse at a market price, determined in the usual
fashion. But when most consumers are insured, the behavior of the
insurer as well as the consumer becomes presumptively relevant to

the reimbursement that the provider receives; although the standard partial equilibrium model could still apply, its usefulness is open to question. How prices and utilization behave in heavily insured markets looms as one of the most important frontiers to explore.

Three examples may clarify matters. Many believe that the United States has too many surgeons, and too few primary care physicians such as pediatricians. The study of Fuchs et al. (1972), for example, suggests underemployment among surgeons. Suppose these beliefs are true; what might explain them? The pattern is suggestive of markets with prices fixed at levels other than the price in competitive equilibrium. Could prices be fixed? Insurance coverage for physicians whose services are mostly rendered in the hospital, such as surgeons, has historically been quite extensive, whereas insurance for physicians whose services are primarily delivered on an outpatient basis, such as pediatricians, has been more scanty.[14]   Might extensive insurance coverage have fixed fees in a way that induced excessive entry into specialities such as surgery?[15]   The standard partial equilibrium model suggests not; if prices are flexible, surgeons should not be underemployed. Alas, we seem to have no theory other than the standard model to explain how prices are set in heavily insured markets and whether they might be set so as to induce an inappropriate distribution of physicians across specialties.

A second example pertains to hospital financing. Although the private hospital in the United States is doubtless subject to some ultimate product market constraint, the extent of reimbursement insurance makes it appear that the constraint may not now be binding.[16]   Over 90% of hospital expenditure is reimbursed by third parties, and for many hospitalized individuals the marginal dollar is fully reimbursed. Presumptively, there is little or no basis for price competition. This reasoning led the Carter administration to propose public regulation of hospital budgets while it was simultaneously proposing deregulating several other industries. Yet if the hospital is not subject to a binding product market constraint, what determines its production choices? And why do certain hospitals become bankrupt, while at others labor disputes and strikes occur? If the hospital does operate under some constraints, what exactly are the nature of those constraints? Until we have answers to such questions, the theory of how suppliers respond to changes in demand will be incomplete.

The final example concerns equilibrating or market clearing mechanisms. When complete insurance for outpatient services was introduced in Montreal in 1970, waiting times for an appointment increased from 6 to 11 days (Enterline et al., 1973). This increase presumptively cleared the market. But why were waiting times to an appointment used as an equilibration mechanism? What does theory predict about the dimensions along which equilibration will occur when price is controlled? (One can imagine other dimensions, such as longer waits in the office, shorter visits, fewer revisits, or more telephone visits.) How does the use of alternative equilibration mechanisms affect demands of various individuals? For example, do longer delays for appointments affect demand by children more than by adults because of a higher incidence of self-limiting diseases among children? The decline in the rate of visits by

children in Montreal is consistent with such a hypothesis. Some
beginning on this question have been made for inpatient services
(M. S. Feldstein, 1967; Rafferty, 1971; van der Gaag, Rutten, and
van Praag, 1975); almost nothing is known about outpatient services.
With answers to such questions, we will better understand the effect
of a change in demand upon who obtains what kind of medical service
for what type of medical problem.

CONCLUSION

To seriously entertain the notion that we do not have a convincing
explanation for the determination of price and utilization when
insurance is complete or nearly so seems heretical; if true, it
would tempt an observer to characterize health economics as among
the most backward of economic subfields. But however dismal the
current situation in health economics, it seems vastly better than
15 years ago, certainly with respect to demand analysis.

Fifteen years ago almost no theoretical work on insurance had been
done; reflecting this state of affairs, empirical analyses of demand
specified insurance in an ad hoc fashion. For example, they sometimes employed a dummy variable indicating that the person was
insured and at other times used its aggregate analogue, the percentage of an area's residents with any kind of insurance. In general,
empirical demand studies were more concerned with testing hypotheses
than seriously estimating elasticities.

Both conceptual and empirical knowledge are now much improved. The
availability of experimental data in the 1980s should ensure further
progress on many fronts. Indeed, we should have reasonably defini-
tive answers to many of the important questions that small-scale
demand studies can answer; that is, when one individual's circumstances change, how does that individual's demand change,
assuming the behavior of all other consumers is unchanged? Progress
will probably be slower in understanding the effects of changes in
demand at the market level, but even for that prickly set of issues
the progress of the past decade bodes well for the next.

NOTES

[1]Phelps and Newhouse (1974a) show that price and insurance elasticities differ
only by an empirically negligible income effect, provided the gross price is
invariant to variation in insurance.

[2]For reasons of space I do not take up analysis of demand for insurance or
demand for prepaid plans such as health maintenance organizations; see Phelps
(1973, 1976), Keeler, Morrow and Newhouse (1977), Roemer and Shonick (1973), and
Luft (forthcoming). Nor do I treat the demand for health; see Grossman (1972a).

[3]See also Freeburg et al. (1979) for an annotated bibliography of past studies. Other reviews of this literature include: M. S. Feldstein (1974), P. J. Feldstein (1966), Ginsburg and Manheim (1973), Hall (1974), Joseph (1971), Kimbell and Yett (no date), and Pauly (1974).

[4]Where possible I have reported percentage differences rather than elasticity estimates, so that one can clearly keep in mind the range of coinsurance under discussion.

[5]The Roemer et al. study (1975) may be an exception; in this study there was a nonequivalent control group which was exempted from the copayment before. Unfortunately those who were hospitalized before may have been disproportionately in the no-control (copayment) group. If so, hospitalization in the control group would have fallen spuriously; see Helms, Newhouse and Phelps (1978).

[6]Use of the average coinsurance rate if a deductible is present introduces error into the measurement of the own-price variable as well as correlation with the error term; this errors-in-the-variables problem causes an inconsistent estimate of the price elasticity, and the direction of this inconsistency cannot be signed a priori. See Newhouse, Phelps and Marquis (1979). In practice, the negative correlation of the price variable with the error term seems likely to dominate the direction of the overall inconsistency.

[7]The distribution of insurance in Newhouse and Phelps's data was also not favorable: few individuals had insurance for ambulatory care. A population with greater variance in the insurance variable would yield more precise estimates, although significant estimates were obtained using OLS.

[8]On occasion the estimated effect of education has been negative (Colle and Grossman, 1978); at other times it has not explained much variation (Manning et al., 1980).

[9]Sloan and Feldman (1978) reviewed the findings of earlier studies and found them consistent with both the standard, neoclassical view of negligible or no demand-creation ability as well as the alternative view that the physician has important unexploited demand-creation ability.

[10]Fuchs's estimates rely on a variable measuring per capita hotel and motel receipts in an area to identify the effect of supply on demand. The premise is that such receipts are higher in attractive areas and so will cause an increase in supply that is independent of demand. If, however, areas with many tourists also have more border-crossing by patients (e.g., both surgeons and hotels in very large metropolitan areas draw from larger market areas), then Fuchs's estimates are biased away from zero. A more captious objection is that areas with many tourists may have more accidents requiring surgery; a ski resort would be an unfair example.

[11]The variables used were race, length of residence, and location. Race may affect demand because of differences in culture (e.g., tolerance for pain; see Zola, 1966); those living longer in an area or living in a particular subarea may systematically differ in respects other than their knowledge of the local medical care system, and such unmeasured differences may affect demand.

[12]Willingness to pay in most instances should be measured at the level of the

J.P. Newhouse

world market. Temporal variation in insurance and income changes, therefore, must
be measured for the entire world, not just a single country.

[13]One exception is Holahan et al., 1979. See also Steinwald and Sloan (1974).

[14]There is a good economic explanation for this pattern; loading fees are much
higher for small outpatient expenditures than for large inpatient expenditures.

[15]Indeed, rents could still exist. One can show a significant correlation
between the percentage of revenue derived from third parties and average income in
a specialty.

[16]Insurance in the United States typically reimburses the hospital its costs
or a "price" quoted by the hospital.

HEALTH, ECONOMICS, AND HEALTH ECONOMICS
J. van der Gaag and M. Perlman (editors)
North-Holland Publishing Company, 1981

A TWO-PART MODEL OF THE DEMAND FOR MEDICAL CARE:
PRELIMINARY RESULTS FROM THE HEALTH INSURANCE STUDY

Willard G. Manning, Carl N. Morris, Joseph P. Newhouse,
Larry L. Orr, Naihua Duan, Emmett B. Keeler,
Arleen Leibowitz, Kent H. Marquis, M. Susan Marquis,
and Charles E. Phelps

How the extent of health insurance coverage affects the demand for
medical services has been a key issue in the American debate over
national health insurance.* Past studies of this issue have used
nonexperimental data that suffer from several flaws: insurance is
potentially endogenous; existing policies are difficult to describe
parametrically; utilization data are frequently based on recall and
are subject to reporting biases; and coinsurance rates and deductibles often vary little.

To overcome these problems, The Rand Corporation is conducting a
social experiment, The Health Insurance Study, or HIS, on behalf of
the United States Department of Health and Human Services
(previously Health, Education, and Welfare).

In late 1974 the HIS enrolled 389 families living in Dayton, Ohio,
and in 1976, 2367 additional families in five other sites were
enrolled. The families were given health insurance plans with differing coinsurance rates and upper limits on families' financial
exposure; in return they assigned to the experiment the benefits of
any nonexperimental plans for which they were eligible. If the
assignment could make the family worse off, the family was given a
lump-sum payment equal to the maximum it could lose from participating. Seventy percent of the families (60% in Dayton) were
enrolled for three years, the remainder for five years.

This paper reports the initial results of analyzing data from the
first two years of the experiment in Dayton;[1] subsequent papers will
report results from later years and other sites. These results
should be considered preliminary in two senses. Even if the models
estimated are correct, sampling error will decrease with additional
observations.[2] More importantly, the models estimated embody certain restrictions upon parameters and stochastic terms. Although

---

*We would like to thank Dan Relles and Dan Shapiro for their programming help.
William Rogers and John Rolph have provided us with helpful comments. Professor
Bradley Efron of Stanford has provided excellent advice throughout this analysis.
The research reported herein was performed pursuant to Grant No. 016B-7901-P02021
from the U.S. Department of Health and Human Services, Washington, D.C. The
opinions and conclusions expressed herein are solely those of the authors, and
should not be construed as representing the opinions or policies of any agency of
the United States Government.

the available data do not reject those restrictions, additional data
may, thereby forcing the estimation of more complex models.

The paper is organized as follows: The next section briefly
describes the design of the experiment, the data, and the sample.
Then we provide the rationale for a model which separates expenditures into a two-equation model--one for the decision to seek care
and one for the level of nonzero expenses. The fourth section
reviews the empirical results. The final section describes the
shortcomings in the model that we have discovered to date.

THE DESIGN OF THE EXPERIMENT, DATA, AND SAMPLE

The Design

The 389 families in Dayton were assigned to 11 different insurance
plans. About one-quarter of the sample received all services free
(their coinsurance rate was zero), and nearly one-quarter paid 25%
coinsurance subject to an upper limit on annual out-of-pocket family
expenditures of 5, 10, or 15% of the previous year's income, or
$1000, whichever was less. This limit was called the Maximum Dollar
Expenditure (MDE). Just under one-fifth of the sampled families had
a 50% coinsurance rate, also subject to three different MDEs, and
one-quarter had a 100% coinsurance rate, subject to the three MDEs.
In effect, this last group of families had an income-related family
deductible. (In Year II the 100% coinsurance rate was changed to
95% to increase the incentive to file a claim, although there was no
statistical evidence of underfiling. This change will be ignored in
the results that follow.) Finally, around one-tenth of the families
were enrolled in a 100% coinsurance plan that limited annual out-of-
pocket expenditures to $150 per person ($450 per family), providing
in effect an individual deductible. The coinsurance applied only to
outpatient services, while inpatient services were free to the
family. The coinsurance rate also changed to 95% in Year II in this
plan.

In all plans a wide variety of services were covered. The only
significant exclusions were outpatient mental health services in
excess of 52 visits per year, nonpreventive orthodontia, and cos-
metic surgery unrelated to accidents occurring after the start of
the experiment.[3] Dental services and outpatient mental health services were, however, treated somewhat differently in the first year
of operation in Dayton, and so analysis of those services will not
be considered here.[4] The same coinsurance rate applied to all
services, except for the individual deductible plan.

Our analysis controls for three artifacts of the experiment. First,
because the length of the enrollment period was varied to help
determine how the duration of the experiment may have affected
demand, we compare the behavior of families enrolled for varying
periods. Second, some families were given an initial screening
examination to improve the precision with which changes in physiological health could be measured at the end of the experiment. The

results of the examination were reported to a physician designated
by the family, with abnormal results noted. Because one could
expect followup of abnormal results, a random (within-plan) 38% of
the families were not examined (half in Dayton). We compare their
behavior with families who received the examination. Third, a diary
was mailed to the families periodically so they could report disability days and information about medical care utilization not contained on claims forms (e.g., time spent with the physician,
telephone visits). Because the diary may have stimulated both
better reporting of utilization and more true utilization, we compare a random half of the families that received it weekly with the
other half that received it biweekly in Dayton Year I.[5]

The sample was a random sample of the Dayton metropolitan area, but
the following groups were not eligible: 1) those 62 years of age
and over; 2) those with incomes in excess of $25,000 (1973 dollars);
3) those eligible for the disability Medicare program; 4) those in
institutions such as jails and the military; 5) veterans with
service-connected disabilities. Over 80% of the Dayton population
was eligible. The lower third of the income distribution was
(intentionally) mildly oversampled; the middle third undersampled.
The sample has not been reweighted to reflect the disproportionate
sampling, because we are not interested in generalizing to the
Dayton population.[6]

Families were enrolled as a unit with only eligible members participating. No choice of plan was offered; the family could either
accept the experimental plan offered or not participate. A family
was either an individual, or a group of related individuals living
together, some of whom were economically dependent on the others. A
self-supporting son living with his parents thus constituted his own
family unit.

Families were assigned to plans using the Finite Selection Model
(Morris, 1979). This model is designed to achieve as much balance
among plans as possible while retaining randomness; that is, it
makes the experimental plans approximately orthogonal to the
demographic covariates. The expected gain in precision from using
this model, rather than simple random assignment, is about 25%
(Morris, 1979). Random refusals of the enrollment offer, however,
degrade the expected gain in proportion to the refusal rate (Morris,
Newhouse and Archibald, 1979); fortunately, the refusal rate of the
enrollment offer in Dayton was only 7%. With this low a refusal
rate, no statistically significant unintended differences have been
found between the enrolled group and the Dayton population.

Dependent Variables

In this paper, we have confined our analysis to covered medical
expenditures other than dental or outpatient mental health care.
Thus, total medical expenses (MED) include all inpatient care, medical outpatient care, including services provided by nonphysicians
such as chiropractors and optometrists, and (largely prescription)
drugs and supplies.[7] Claims filed by participants, including those

for unreimbursed expenses, provide data on the amount and type of
expenses.

Insurance Plan Variables

We have employed two alternative specifications of the insurance
plans. One uses an analysis of variance (ANOVA) specification with
four dummy variables, one each for: a family medical coinsurance
rate of 25% (P25); a family medical coinsurance rate of 50% (P50); a
family medical coinsurance rate of 100% in Year I or 95% in Year II
(behaviorally the same as a family deductible--PFD); the individual
deductible of $150 per person or $450 per family for outpatient
care, with free inpatient care (IDP). The free care plan is the
omitted group. The second specification models the characteristics
of the insurance plan itself, using four variables: a logarithmic
coinsurance function (LC), a dummy for the individual deductible
plan (IDP), a maximum dollar-expenditure function (FMDE), and a
logarithmic participation-incentive payment function (LPI). The
FMDE measure is based on the gross dollars necessary to exceed the
maximum dollar expenditure (MDE). For example, a family with an MDE
of $1000 and a coinsurance rate of 25% requires $4000 of gross
expenditures to receive free care, whereas a family with an MDE of
$1000 and a coinsurance rate of 100% requires only $1000. The participation payment is the lump sum amount paid to families for participating in the experiment. The formal definitions of the
variables are:

LC   = ln [coinsurance + 1] where $0 < $ coinsurance $ < 100$
       (coinsurance is expressed as a percentage), and
       coinsurance for the Individual Deductible and the
       Free Plan is $0.$[8]

FMDE = 0 if Free or Individual Deductible Plan,

     = ln [max (1.0, MDE/(.01 coinsurance))], otherwise.

LPI = ln [max (1.0, annual participation incentive payment)].

Other Experimental Variables

Three other experimental treatment variables were described above,
namely: whether a household was given a pre-enrollment screening
examination (EXAM) or not; whether the family reported disability
days weekly (WEEKLY) rather than biweekly; and whether the family
was enrolled for three (YR3) or five years.

Other Covariates

The remaining variables control for variation in socio-economic factors. They include income, family size, prior contact with the
medical system, race, age, sex, self-reported health, pain and worry

about health.[9] Table 1 contains the formal definitions. We
selected a functional form for the continuous variables (e.g.,
income and pre-experimental utilization) that would yield homoscedastic residual plots. For example, the transformation for positive
pre-experimental physician visits is neither linear nor logarithmic
because those specifications overfit individuals with many pre-
experimental visits--in both cases, the residual variance decreases
markedly as visits increase.

Pre-enrollment interviews provided data on all of these characteristics.

The Sample

The sample consists of those enrolled individuals who participated
for a full year. Excluded are newborns, adoptees, suspended participants, participants who voluntarily attrited, and persons who
died or were involuntarily terminated for noncompliance during the
year.[10] These exclusions account for 52 of the 1160 Dayton Year I
enrollees and 50 of the 1148 Year II enrollees. The unit of analysis is the individual.

THE EXPENDITURE MODEL

The distribution of medical expenses has three characteristics that
require special attention to obtain reliable estimates of the demand
for medical care. First, part of the distribution is located at
zero. Second, the distribution of positive expenditures is very
skewed. Third, the error terms for different family members are
positively correlated. To treat the first two characteristics, we
have developed a two-equation (compound) model of expenses and
transformed positive expenses. An estimation technique for variance
components is appropriate given the intrafamily correlation.

Rationale for Compound Model

Given our sample size, the nature of health expenditure data causes
an ordinary least square (OLS) regression of raw dollar expenses on
the covariates to yield estimates with unsatisfactory precision.
Table 2 contains the results of an ANOVA regression of medical
expenses on plan indicator variables. A very few large expenses
lead to violation of the monotonicity that one expects in the
response to coinsurance.

We have developed a two-part model as an alternative to OLS with raw
dollar expenditures as the dependent variable. The first equation
of the model determines whether or not a consumer seeks medical care
during the year, and is estimated using logistic regression. This
equation resolves the problem of the large number of observations
located at zero dollars.

Table 1. Socio-Economic Variables

Indicator (0,1) Variables

BLACK   = 1 if race of head is black

FEMALE   = 1 if female

CHILD   = 1 if age < 18

FCHILD   = female child

AFDC   = 1 if someone in family received AFDC

NOMD   = 1 if no regular physician for any family member

NOMDVIS = 1 if no visits to physician in past year

HLTHG   = 1 if self-rated health is good ⎫

HLTHF   = 1 if self-rated health is fair ⎬ (excellent health
                                          ⎪   omitted)

HLTHP   = 1 if self-rated health is poor ⎭

PAING   = 1 if in great pain ⎫

PAINS   = 1 if in some pain   ⎬(no pain omitted)

PAINL   = 1 if in little pain ⎭

WORRG   = 1 if health is of great worry ⎫

WORRS   = 1 if health is of some worry   ⎬(no worry omitted)

WORRL   = 1 if health is of little worry ⎭

NEWMEM   = 1 if added to family after interviews (nonfamily
             variables zero)

Continuous Variables

LINC   = ln (average 1972, 1973 family income in 1972 dollars:
             income set at $1000 if reported to be less)

LFAM   = ln (family size)

INMDVIS = $[max (1, last years physician visits)]^{-1}$

MAGE, FAGE = a function relating utilization to age and sex (MAGE
             for males and FAGE for females), based on National
             Center for Health Statistics data on physician visits.

Table 2. Expenditures by Plan (ANOVA Regression)

Plan	Year I		Year II	
	β	S.D.[a]	β	S.D.[a]
Free	$310	40	$410	55
25%	340	43	350	60
50%	210	51	220	71
Family Deductible	180	42	310	59
Individual Deductible	270	70	170	98

Source: Data from Rand's Health Insurance Study.

[a]Lower bound. Estimates are not corrected for intrafamily correlation.

The second part estimates how the logarithm of positive expenses depends on explanatory variables. The logarithmic transformation removes the skewness in positive expenses.

This approach allows us to model the behavior of consumers with zero expenses differently from those with nonzero expenses; this is less restrictive than the tobit model. Consumers incur fixed costs in order to receive care. In contrast, for individuals undergoing treatment, these costs are sunk costs; their decisions about level of care are largely unaffected (Goldman and Grossman, 1978). Also, the decision to receive some care is largely the consumer's, while the physician influences the decision about the level of care.

The logarithmic transformation of nonzero expenses provides more robust and efficient estimates than the use of raw dollars. A normal plot of the logarithm of positive expenses indicates a close fit to normality. Because of the relatively low R^2, we should expect the residual error for the positive expense equation to be normally distributed. Minimizing the departures from normality makes the estimates more robust. The log transformation eliminates the possibility that a few large expenses will unduly influence the estimation, as they did in Table 2. Because the coefficient of variation is decreased, the estimates using the log transform are more precise than using the raw dollar scale if log normality holds.

The two equations of the model are estimated separately without bias or loss of efficiency. The log likelihood function is separable in the parameters of the decision to have nonzero expenses and in those of the decision about the level of nonzero expenses. Separability

results from the way conditional distributions are calculated, not
from any independence assumption in the model. Hence, a model of
the type suggested by Heckman (1974, 1976, 1979) is not appropriate,
if in fact positive expenditures are log-normally distributed.[11]

Variance Components Model

We have used a random effects variance components estimator to analyze the expenditure levels. This enables us to obtain efficient
estimates of regression coefficients and consistent estimates of
standard errors.[12] The intra-family correlation is nearly a positive constant across family roles and sizes.[13] Thus, the residual
correlations are similar to those of a variance components model
with a family-specific error component. The model is

$$y_{fi} = x_{fi}'\beta + \mu_f + \varepsilon_{fi} \tag{1}$$

where

$$y_{fi}, x_{fi} = \text{dependent and independent variables for person i in family f,}$$

$$\mu_f = \text{unmeasured family effect, and}$$

$$\varepsilon_{fi} = \text{unmeasured individual effect.}$$

Further, we assume

$$\mu \sim N(o,\sigma_\mu^2) \text{ i.i.d. across families,} \tag{2}$$

$$\varepsilon \sim N(o,\sigma_\varepsilon^2) \text{ i.i.d. across persons, and} \tag{3}$$

$$E(x\mu) = E(x\varepsilon) = E(\mu\varepsilon) = 0. \tag{4}$$

The variance of the error $(\mu + \varepsilon)$ is

$$V(\mu + \varepsilon) = \sigma^2(1 - \rho)I_n + \sigma^2\rho D \tag{5}$$

where $\rho = \sigma_\mu^2/(\sigma_\mu^2 + \sigma_\varepsilon^2)$ is the intrafamily correlation, D is a
block diagonal matrix with a block of 1's for each family, $i_{mj} i'_{mj}$,
where i is a column vector of 1's and m_j is the size of the
j^{th} family, and $\sigma^2 = \sigma_\mu^2 + \sigma_\varepsilon^2$.

Equation (1) is estimated by maximum likelihood, iterated on ρ and
β.[14] Taking account of intrafamily correlation is important for
variables that do not vary within the family, such as insurance
plan. In our sample, the OLS-estimated t-statistics for such coefficients are as much as 30% too large. For variables which vary as
much within as across families, the OLS t-statistics are about right.

Table 3. The Distribution of Medical Expenses

| | % with MED > 0 | Positive Expenses ln (MED \| > 0) | | | |
		mean	variance	skewness	kurtosis
Dayton I					
Free	91.6	4.949	1.673	.034	.540
25%	81.1	4.836	1.996	.428	.506
50%	81.9	4.656	1.740	.131	.296
Family Ded.	76.4	4.468	1.882	.082	.179
Individual Deductible	80.4	4.707	2.285	.247	-.531
Dayton II					
Free	88.5	5.100	1.958	.101	.429
25%	81.3	4.812	2.098	.448	.517
50%	77.2	4.563	1.909	.321	.641
Family Ded.	73.4	4.766	2.441	.138	.185
Individual Deductible	88.5	4.636	1.871	.004	-.241

Source: Data from Rand's Health Insurance Study.

Table 4. Effect of Insurance on Medical Expenses

Variable	Dayton I				Dayton II			
	Logit		$\ln(\text{MED} \mid > 0)$		Logit		$\ln(\text{MED} \mid > 0)$	
	β	|t|a	β	|t|a	β	|t|a	β	|t|a
ANOVA Specification								
Intercept	2.9983	---	4.9551	---	2.6199	---	5.0826	---
25%b	-1.1507	3.75	-.1946	1.42	-0.7820	2.76	-.3287	2.38
50%b	-1.3318	4.02	-.4518	3.00	-1.3365	4.49	-.6544	4.22
Family Deductibleb	-1.4256	4.83	-.5762	4.20	-1.2113	4.57	-.3988	2.86
Individual Ded.b	-0.9786	4.01	-.3765	2.00	-1.4126	4.00	-.5510	2.75
Insurance Function Specification								
LC	-.2189	2.37	-.1745	3.37	-.2977	2.58	-.1363	1.93
FMDE	-.0788	1.33	+.0429	1.35	-.0399	0.56	-.0028	0.07
LPI	+.0170	0.31	-.0094	0.34	+.0967	2.02	+.0365	1.30

Source: Data from Rand's Health Insurance Study.

at's are on the difference from the Free Plan.

bPlans are taken as deviations from the Free Plan (≡ intercept).

EMPIRICAL RESULTS

In reporting the empirical results, we will limit the discussion to total medical expenses, but our qualitative findings apply equally well to outpatient care, drugs, and supplies. Estimates for other covariates and dependent variables are omitted here because of space limitations.

Responses to Insurance Plan

Insurance influences the decision to seek care and the decision about the amount of care. Table 3 summarizes the medical expenditure distribution by plan--the probability of positive expenses and the mean, variance, skewness, and kurtosis of log-positive expenses. Table 4 contains the coefficients from both the ANOVA and the coinsurance function specification of insurance. Generally, higher coinsurance rates lower the probability of seeking care and the amount of medical care purchased. The reversal between the 50% and family deductible plans in Dayton Year II is statistically insignificant. In the coinsurance specifications, the effects of the MDE are not discernible, which is expected in a sample of this size because the MDE affects relatively few people.

The largest coinsurance response occurs if some out-of-pocket amount must be paid, that is, between the free and 25% coinsurance plans. This may reflect a greater proportion of families exceeding the MDE in plans with higher coinsurance rates; about one-third of the families exceeded the MDE in the Family Deductible plan, but only around one-tenth did so in the 25% coinsurance plan.

The overall elasticity of demand with respect to coinsurance depends on the elasticity of the probability of seeking care and the elasticity of the conditional (nonzero) demand. For the log coinsurance specification, the elasticity of the probability (prob) of seeking care is $(1 - \text{prob})\,\hat{\alpha}_{LC}$, where $\hat{\alpha}_{LC}$ is the logit coefficient. The conditional elasticity is $\hat{\beta}_{LC}$. The estimated overall elasticity is

$$\hat{\varepsilon}_{\text{compound}} = (1 - \text{prob})\hat{\alpha}_{LC} + \hat{\beta}_{LC}. \tag{6}$$

A substantial part of the overall elasticity is in the decision to seek care. Table 5 provides the two components and the overall elasticity, both evaluated at the sample mean probability. The overall elasticity is -0.2, a value which is consistent with non-experimental studies reported in Phelps and Newhouse (1974b). Averaged over the two years, about one-quarter of the coinsurance response is due to the response in the logit.

An alternative way of describing plan effects is to examine the predictions by plan. Table 6 contains the average predicted probability of seeking care, the average predicted positive expenditure, and the average predicted total expenditure for each of the plan subsamples. The bottom half of the table contains each plan's

W.G. Manning et al.

Table 5. Coinsurance Elasticities for Medical Expenses

Year	Probability of Seeking Care	ln (MED | > 0)	Total
I	-.038	-.175	-.212 $(\sigma = .089)$
II	-.060	-.136	-.196 $(\sigma = .117)$

relative--the value of the variable for that plan divided by the free plan value.

The response of expense to plan is more complex than the simple summary elasticity at the mean probability suggests. Most of the coinsurance response in the decision to seek care occurs between the free plan and the 25% plan. The probability falls at a decreasing rate as coinsurance increases; this is also true in Table 3. In the free-to-25% range, half of the plan response is in the decision to seek care. For higher coinsurance plans, the response is increasingly in the decision about the amount of care.[15]

To the extent that health is a durable good, one would expect that individuals moving to more generous plans (e.g., the free plan) would experience a transitory surge in demand while those moving to less generous insurance (e.g., the family deductible plan) would postpone medical expenses until they returned to their more generous coverage at the end of the experiment. The first year, however, exhibits only slightly more price responsiveness than the second year (a coinsurance elasticity of -.212 compared to -.197), and the difference (.015) is quite insignificant.[16]

Response to Other Experimental Treatments

We included indicators for other experimental treatments to detect possible Hawthorne effects in the experimental response. The results, presented in Table 7, are consistent with the hypothesis that these treatments have no effect on either the decision to seek care or the decision about the level of care. In Year I the signs of the coefficients are in the expected direction but are imprecisely measured. The results for the three year dummy, like the comparison of insurance elasticities in Year I and Year II, suggest that people do not behave as though medical services were a durable good.

Response to Other Socio-Economic Variables

A substantial amount of the response to some covariates is in the

Table 6. Predictions for Total Medical Expenses

	Dayton I			Dayton II		
	PROB (MED > 0) (1)	E(MED | MED>0) (2)	E(MED)[a] E((1) X (2))	PROB (MED > 0) (3)	E(MED | MED>0) (4)	E(MED)[a] E((3) X (4))
Actual Levels						
Free	.918	$357	$336	.885	$455	$414
25%	.803	306	261	.802	336	285
50%	.821	266	231	.803	311	266
Family Ded.	.767	210	174	.724	276	220
Individual Deductible	.804	279	240	.705	273	213
Relative to Free						
PDO	100	100	100	100	100	100
P25	87	86	78	91	74	69
P50	89	75	69	91	68	64
Family Ded.	84	59	52	82	61	53
Individual Deductible	88	78	71	80	60	51

Note: The mean of the product does not equal the product of the means, because the model is nonlinear.

[a] $E(MED \mid MED > 0) = e^{x\beta + \sigma^2/2}$

$E(MED) = prob\ (MED > 0)\ e^{x\beta + \sigma^2/2}$

Table 7. Effect of Other Experimental Treatments

Variable	Year I				Year II			
	Logit		$\ln(\text{MED} \mid > 0)$		Logit		$\ln(\text{MED} \mid > 0)$	
	β	t	β	t	β	t	β	t
Exam	+.2071	1.09	+.0226	0.23	-.1431	0.79	+.0198	0.19
Weekly Health Report	+.2479	1.31	+.0825	0.84	+.0675	0.38	-.1225	1.21
Three Year Enrollment	-.2653	1.41	-.0227	0.23	-.0535	0.30	+.1260	1.25

Source: Data from Rand's Health Insurance Study.

decision to seek care. As Table 8 indicates, most of the detectable
response to being black, receiving AFDC, or having no physician at
the outset of the experiment is in the decision to seek care.
Individuals with these characteristics have historically had poorer
access to the medical system. The inhibiting effect of being black
or being on AFDC diminishes in Year II but is still quite pronounced.

Caution is indicated when interpreting coefficients in the second
stage if the variable in question has an effect in the first stage.
For example, the true coefficient of being black may be zero in the
second stage either because the medical system ignores race when
treating patients, or because blacks who enter the system may on
average be sicker but receive less care for given symptoms.

Income has a strong effect on both the decision to seek care and on
the level of care. The income elasticity for the probability of
seeking care is .13 in Year I and .17 in Year II. The total income
elasticity is .38 in Year I and .36 in Year II at the mean
probability.[17] Thus about 40% of the response to income is in the
decision to seek care.

The magnitude and sign of income-plan interactions are not clear
from these data. Although individuals in lower-income families
appear to have larger (in absolute value) elasticities when the LC
variable is made to interact with income (i.e., free, 25%, 50%, and
family deductible plans are compared), the opposite pattern holds
when the IDP variable is made to interact with income (i.e., when
individuals on the free and individual deductible plans are
compared). To further complicate interpretations, the results
differ between Year I and Year II. Data from additional sites and
years will enhance the precision with which interactions between
plan and income can be estimated.

Larger families spend less per person for medical care. The total
family size elasticities are -.24 in Year I and -.17 in Year II.

Individuals with numerous pre-experimental physician visits have
high experimental consumption in both Year I and Year II. The
coefficients on INMDVIS imply elasticities for MD visits of 0.39 in
Year I and 0.37 in Year II. The impact of the INMDVIS variable is
strong in both the decision to seek care and the decision about
level of care.

Intrafamily Correlation

As we noted earlier, there is a significant positive correlation in
the error term among family members. The intrafamily correlations
for log-positive medical expenses are .173 and .081 in Years I and
II, with standard errors of .039 and .035 respectively. This
correlation decreases the effective sample size for making
inferences about family level variables. For medical expenses in
Year I, the 918 positive spenders actually contained the information
equivalent to 667 independent observations. Thus a seemingly "mild"
correlation of .17 is equivalent to a 27% drop in sample size. Most

Table 8. Effect of Socio-Economic Variables

Variable	Year I				Year II			
	Logit		ln (MED | > 0)		Logit		ln (MED | > 0)	
	β	t	β	t	β	t	β	t
LINC	+.7700	4.34	+.2474	2.63	+.8444	5.13	+.1918	1.91
LFAM	-.4094	1.85	-.1720	1.65	-.6097	3.02	-.0499	0.47
BLACK	-1.8072	3.67	-.0920	0.50	-.6328	2.13	+.0347	0.18
AFDC	-1.3464	2.75	+.2253	0.56	-.9593	1.98	+.0835	0.19
NOMD	-1.0233	2.74	+.2832	0.96	-1.1413	2.86	-.3307	0.98
NOMDVIS	-.2431	0.92	+.0554	0.37	-.5650	2.24	+.0788	0.44
INMDVIS	-1.5437	4.51	-.5153	3.37	-1.4080	4.46	-.4518	2.60
CHILD	-.1996	0.80	-.3787	3.48	+.1929	0.72	-.3806	2.81
FEMALE	+1.4258	1.16	-.5092	0.94	+.7511	0.60	-1.1437	1.77
CHILD·FEMALE	-.9780	2.14	-.1052	.53	-.2208	0.45	+.2881	1.17
MAGE	+.6870	1.09	+.5620	2.30	+2.0689	2.88	+.4831	1.58
FAGE	+.1469	0.24	+.9204	3.28	+1.5632	2.08	1.2699	3.40

Source: Data from Rand's Health Insurance Study.

of this cut in sample comes in large families. For $\rho = .17$, a
family with 5 positive spenders has the information content of 3
independent observations.

AN INTERIM CONCLUSION

The results presented here represent our first efforts to understand
and to estimate how the annual expenditures of individuals responded
to experimental variation in insurance coverage in the Health
Insurance Study. In modeling that response, our goal has been to
estimate inter-plan differences that are insensitive to or robust
regarding departures from the underlying model assumptions.

Specifically, we have introduced the following modifications to
ANOVA or regression on individual expenditures. The clustering of
expenditures at zero was explicitly treated by the introduction of a
logit equation to explain zero expenses. The influence of the long
tail for positive expenditures was diminished by the natural
logarithmic transform. Correlated errors among family members
required fitting a family variance-components model. Residual plots
and outlier analysis not reported here suggested that the specification of the independent variables is appropriate.

We see the following shortcomings in the present model: (1) the
assumption of no family effects in the logistic part of the compound
model; (2) the restriction that the intrafamily correlation and
other parameters, e.g., variances, be constant across plans; (3) the
difficulties in retransforming predictions from a log linear model
to obtain estimates of health expenditures (rather than of the log
of health expenditures) if the data are not perfectly log normal;
(4) the inability to determine the effect of plan, if any, on
catastrophic expenditures; and (5) the absence of efforts to pool
data across years. These problems will be addressed when more data
are available.

Intrafamily Correlations in the Logits

The present logistic model ignored intrafamily correlation.
Intuitively, we expect to find some residual family correlation in
the decision to receive any care because of similar tastes, parental
decision-making for children, etc. Preliminary estimates suggest
that as much as half of the unexplained logit variance is a family
effect. If so, the present standard errors in the logistic model
may substantially overstate the precision of the estimated coefficients. Major changes in the coefficients themselves are not
expected.

Constant Intrafamily Correlations Across Plans

The present model assumes that the intrafamily correlation ρ for

positive expenses is constant across plans. Although this assumption greatly simplifies the estimation, we know that the correlations in the positive expenditure equation tend to rise with
coinsurance, as theory would suggest, given the MDE. Thus, the t
and F statistics, but not the coefficients, may be biased.
Abandoning the OLS model in favor of one with constant ρ corrects
the major effect of intrafamily correlation on inferences by
reducing the bias in the t and F statistics. Some residual bias in
the present t and F statistics remains because ρ depends on plan.
In particular, the true precision of estimates of family variables
for the free plan would be slightly higher than reported, and those
for the family deductible plans slightly less.

The Retransformation Problem

One of the main HIS goals is to predict average expenditures or the
ratios of average expenditures on different treatments or plans.
The use of a logarithmic dependent variable raises certain problems
in estimating mean expenditure. If the error term ε in a regression
using the logarithm of positive expenditures is normally distributed, then the expectation of positive expenditures is

$$E(y) = e^{\mu+\sigma^2/2} \tag{7}$$

where

$$\mu = E(x\beta) \text{ and } \sigma^2 = Var(\varepsilon).$$

If, however, the error term has nonzero skewness s, and kurtosis k,
and other higher cumulants so that it is not exactly log normal,
then

$$E(y) = e^{\mu+\sigma^2/2!} + s\sigma^3/3! + k\sigma^4/4! + \dots. \tag{8}$$

Residual plots reveal some departure from log normality for total
medical expenses, so the higher order correction terms are important. For Dayton Year I, the retransformation based on assuming
log normality may understate the true value by as much as 5%.

If the plans differ only in the means of their log expenditures,
however, then the coefficients (exponentiated) for plan relatives in
the text do accurately reflect ratios of plan means. For example,
with equal variance, skewness, etc., the ratio of mean expenditures
of the family deductible plan to the free plan will not depend on
the departure from a homoscedastic normal error. On the other hand,
if there is plan-related heteroscedasticity, then plan coefficients
do not fully reflect differences in mean expenditures. For example,
in Dayton Year I the 12% higher variance in log expenditures on the

family deductible plan than that on the free plan implies a ratio of mean expenditures of .57 instead of .52.[18] This is a large change, but it is measured imprecisely. Although we have evidence that variances increase with coinsurance, we cannot yet accurately tell by how much. Comparison of plan means can also be affected by plan differences in higher order cumulants, as ratios of (6.2) for two plans would indicate.

Catastrophic Expenditures

The present version of the model assumes that individuals with catastrophic expenditures are drawn from the same distribution as the remaining 98% or so of the population. Theory suggests something very different. Individuals with very large expenditures will always exceed their maximum dollar expenditures (MDE), which are never more than $1000 out-of-pocket. After that, they should not be influenced by the size of the coinsurance rate because care is free.[19] Thus our estimates of plan differences in expenditures reflect a mixture of coinsurance-responsive individuals and a few very large but coinsurance-insensitive expenditures. About 6% of the population have gross expenditures over $1000 in a year. These individuals account for half of all medical expenses.

Misestimating the extreme right tail of the distribution can greatly affect estimates of the means for various insurance alternatives. If, as theory would predict for an insurance policy with an MDE, expenditures in the right tail are not as sensitive to plan as other expenditures, our estimates will overstate the true difference among plans. An intuitively more appealing method would model catastrophic expenditures separately, assuming little or no price sensitivity for them, and use the compound model for the remaining cases. Then expenditure estimates would involve the probability of no expenditure, the probability and cost of catastrophic illness, and the cost of noncatastrophic but coinsurance-sensitive care.

In any one site year there are insufficient catastrophic illnesses to analyze them separately, but we plan to do so when more data have accumulated. At that time the degree of overstatement in the estimates will be clearer.

Summary and Prospects

Although predicting medical expenses presents some problems, the qualitative inferences we have drawn should be insensitive to those difficulties. The out-of-pocket price of medical care does affect demand. The coinsurance elasticity at the sample mean is on the order of -0.2. We found the demand in Dayton to be income-inelastic. The demand for medical care can be decomposed into decisions to seek any care during the year and decisions about the amount of care. A substantial fraction of the overall coinsurance and income responses is in the decision to seek any care. Most of the detectable response to being black, to being on welfare, or having no regular MD is in the decision to seek care.

Further data and modeling should enhance our understanding of the
annual expenses. We also plan to disaggregate the data in order to
analyze episodes of illness according to whether they are chronic or
acute, and episodes of well care. The effects of insurance on
health status will be addressed later in the experiment (Brook
et al., 1979).

NOTES

[1]These two years, which correspond roughly to calendar 1975 and 1976, are
referred to below as Year I and Year II.

[2]The two site years analyzed below represent around 10% of all observations;
roughly speaking, therefore, one might anticipate a fall in standard errors by a
factor of three when all data are analyzed, provided the models estimated are
correct.

[3]In the case of each exclusion it is questionable whether anything could have
been learned about steady-state demand during the three to five year lifetime of
the experiment.

[4]Dental services for adults were only covered in the plan with a zero coinsurance rate; expenditures on outpatient mental health services did not count
toward satisfying the MDE. After Year I in Dayton and in all other sites, dental
services for adults and outpatient mental health services (up to 52 visits per
person annually) were covered like any other service in all plans.

[5]In Year II all families filed bi-weekly, and in all subsequent sites the bi-
weekly periodicity was followed. In some subsequent sites, however, the diary was
omitted entirely for part of the sample. Additionally, verification of utilization with physicians' offices has been pursued to distinguish more complete
reporting from additional utilization. For a more detailed discussion see
Newhouse, Marquis, et al. (1979).

[6]Given the absence of any strong interaction effects between plan and income,
our estimates of plan effects should be approximately unbiased.

[7]We have also analyzed medical outpatient care and drugs plus supplies
separately. The results are similar to those reported below for total medical
expenses.

[8]The functional form was chosen to fit the ANOVA plan coefficients as closely
as possible. The specification of the coinsurance function can explain in excess
of 90% of the between-plan variation in either the probability of seeking care or
the level of expenditures, given that it is nonzero.

[9]We did not include education because early analyses indicated that its coefficient was insignificant, once a good income specification was found.

[10]We expected these cases to behave differently from the full year population.
With the data available, there are not enough cases to analyze the differences
with precision. Inclusion of an indicator variable for the condition would essentially dummy the cases out. Instead, we delay their analysis until we have enough
data to analyze them properly.

[11]Another way to state this is that the parameter ρ in Heckman's model is identically zero in this model, but not because of any assumption about independence; Heckman's method could not gain because the plim of $\hat{\rho}$ is zero if log normality in the conditional distribution holds.

[12]See Balestra and Nerlove (1966), G. S. Maddala (1971), Searle (1971, Chap. 9-11), and Mundlak (1978) for a discussion of this model.

[13]The one exception was that in families of four or more members, there was a negligible father-child correlation.

[14]We are indebted to Dan Relles at Rand for providing us with a computationally efficient maximum-likelihood program that can handle the unbalanced design (e.g., unequal family sizes) of our data.

[15]Since rare characteristics (e.g., NOMD) are not perfectly balanced by plan, there are a couple of minor violations of monotonicity (e.g., 25 vs. 50% plan in Year I).

[16]If there is no correlation from year-to-year, the standard error on the difference is 0.147. Because there is positive correlation, this number understates the true standard error of the difference.

[17]This elasticity is somewhat higher than that found in the literature. See Phelps and Newhouse (1974b) and Newhouse, Phelps, and Marquis (1980).

[18]The underlying numbers for Dayton Year I are in Table 2.

[19]The coinsurance rate may affect the initial desire to seek care, which could affect the likelihood of diagnosis and treatment. For catastrophic expenditure, this seems unlikely, unless it is iatrogenic.

HEALTH, ECONOMICS, AND HEALTH ECONOMICS
J. van der Gaag and M. Perlman (editors)
© *North-Holland Publishing Company, 1981*

RISK AVERSION AND DEDUCTIBLES IN PRIVATE HEALTH INSURANCE:
APPLICATION OF AN ADJUSTED TOBIT MODEL TO
FAMILY HEALTH CARE EXPENDITURES

Wynand P. M. M. van de Ven
Bernard M. S. van Praag

INTRODUCTION

This chapter concerns the demand for deductibles in health insur-
ances, or more specifically the demand intentions of individuals who
are completely insured but have made up their mind as to whether
they would take a deductible if the option were available to them.*

Acceptance of a health insurance policy with a deductible and a
premium reduction obviously depends on the health status of the
respondents and the anticipated expenses for health care during the
period of insurance. A second factor determining attitude toward a
deductible is one's general attitude toward financial risk,
assessed, for example, by Pratt's (1964) measure of absolute risk
aversion. The purpose of this chapter is twofold: first, to estimate the parameters of the distribution function of family health
care expenditures; second, to shed light on the measure of risk
aversion insofar as it influences the demand for health insurance
policies with a deductible and a premium reduction.

In the next section we estimate from a data base of 6068 privately
insured families the distribution function of family health care
expenditures, the parameters of which are a function of relevant
explanatory variables. The model we use is an adjusted tobit model,
which removes some shortcomings of the classical tobit model. In
the following section a theoretical model is developed in order to
assess the expected utility gain from a health insurance policy with
a deductible and a premium reduction as compared to one with
complete coverage. Some preliminary estimates of risk aversion

---

*The authors wish to thank Jacques van der Gaag, Evelien Hooijmans, Theo van der
Star, and René van Vliet for their helpful comments and suggestions on a previous
draft. We thank the health insurance company "Het Zilveren Kruis" for making
available the data that were used.
This study forms a part of the Leiden Health Economics Project.
This research is financially supported by a grant from the Sick Fund Council of
the Netherlands.

are given. The advantage of estimating risk aversion (or propensity to insure) is that it provides a variable that may be of help in identifying the parameters of structural health care utilization models which specify a simultaneous relation between health care utilization and health insurance.

FAMILY HEALTH CARE EXPENDITURES

The Data

This section estimates the parameters of the distribution function for one year (1976) of family health care expenditures for hospitalization and treatment by specialists. The data base consists of about 8000 questionnaires with information on approximately 20,000 individuals. All families were privately insured by a health insurance company, Het Zilveren Kruis. The 8000 questionnaires which were returned were matched with health care expenditures data available in the company's records. A complicated procedure was used to retain anonymity for the respondents. Most of the families in the survey belong to the upper three deciles of income distribution because in The Netherlands all employees (and their families) whose annual income is below a certain amount, which in 1976 was 30,900 guilders (two guilders equal approximately one U.S. dollar), are compulsorily insured, a partial form of national health insurance. The original sample is fairly representative of those who are not in the national program.

We excluded from our data set about 2000 families who had no standard insurance policy or for which some variables are missing. We were left with observations on 6068 families who were completely insured against the cost of hospitalization and treatment by specialists.

Model

Defining y_i as annual health care expenditures (hospitalization and specialists' treatment) for family i,[1] our model is as follows:

$$\ln y_i = \begin{cases} -\infty & \text{if } y_i^* < 0 \\ \\ \mu_i + \varepsilon_{2i} & \text{if } y_i^* \geqslant 0, \end{cases} \qquad (1)$$

where

$$\mu_i = \sum_{j=1}^{\ell} \beta_j X_{2ij}, \qquad (2)$$

$$y_i^* = A_i + \varepsilon_{1i} \qquad \text{with } A_i = \sum_{j=1}^{k} \alpha_j X_{1ij}, \qquad (3)$$

and

$$
\begin{bmatrix} \varepsilon_{1i} \\ \\ \varepsilon_{2i} \end{bmatrix} \sim \text{Biv. N} \left(\begin{bmatrix} 0 \\ \\ 0 \end{bmatrix}, \begin{bmatrix} 1 & \rho\sigma \\ & \\ \rho\sigma & \sigma^2 \end{bmatrix} \right), |\rho| < 1. \tag{4}
$$

We interpret y_i^* as some unobserved index of demand for medical care, e.g., an index of <u>unhealthiness</u>. If $y_i^* < 0$, then the observed annual expenditures are zero; if $y_i^* > 0$, the observed expenditures are positive; we assume the nonzero health care expenditures for family i to be log-normally distributed with parameters μ_i and σ^2, where μ_i is a function of some explanatory variables. The assumption of log-normally distributed nonzero health care expenditures seems quite realistic and is often made (see, e.g., Keeler, Morrow, and Newhouse, 1977, p. 796; Keeler, Newhouse, and Phelps, 1977, p. 653).[2]

For the moment we will assume the parameter σ to be constant for all families. Abandoning this assumption would seriously complicate the rather simple estimation method we use (see below, "Estimation Results").

It seems realistic to assume that the error terms ε_{1i} and ε_{2i} contain some common omitted variables, so we assume them to be correlated with correlation coefficient ρ. We have fixed the variance of ε_{1i} at 1, which is the usual probit normalization. Looking now at the structure of our model and that of the well-known tobit model (Tobin, 1958), we see that the main differences (besides the logarithmic transformation of y_i) are that in the tobit model $\alpha \equiv \beta$, $X_1 \equiv X_2$, and $\varepsilon_1 \equiv \varepsilon_2$ (which implies $\rho = 1$). We will refer to our model in equations (1-4) as an <u>adjusted tobit model</u>. Three advantages of this adjusted tobit model (see also Cragg, 1971; Nelson, 1977; De Vos and Bikker, 1978) over the classical tobit model are as follows:

1. There may be explanatory variables which only influence the decision whether or not to go to the doctor, <u>or</u> only influence the nonzero expenditures.

2. The influence of an explanatory variable on the decision whether or not to go to the doctor <u>and</u> on the size of the nonzero expenditures need not to be the same (e.g., one influence may be positive and the other may be negative).

3. The error-term in the nonzero expenditures equation is no longer truncated as it is in the classical tobit model (and which in some cases may be quite restrictive).

Specifying the vectors X_1 and X_2, we start with family composition and morbidity, those being factors which influence both the probability and the extent of nonzero expenditures. We define 12 family-size variables, FSi, i = 1,2,...,12, each indicating the number of family members within some age-sex group (see Table 1 for a defi-

Table 1. List of Variables (in alphabetical order)

Variables	Mean	Standard Deviation	Definition
BED	1.630	0.207	Logarithm of the total number of beds (in general, university and categorical hospitals) per capita in the region.[a]
DIST	3.599	0.916	Logarithm of [distance (HM) to the nearest hospital + 1].
EDUC1	2.487	0.342	Logarithm of the number of years of education of the family head.
EDUC2	0.498	0.500	Dummy variable: equals 1 if the family head has received a vocational training; equals 0 in case of a generally educative schooling.
EMPL	0.637	0.481	Dummy variable: equals 1 if family head is employee; equals 0 if not.
EXPEND	b	b	Logarithm of family health care expenditures (1976).
FS1	0.101	0.334	Number male family members ages 0–4.
FS2	0.316	0.642	Number male family members ages 5–14.
FS3	0.254	0.499	Number male family members ages 15–29.
FS4	0.437	0.496	Number male family members ages 30–49.
FS5	0.226	0.418	Number male family members ages 50–64.
FS6	0.102	0.302	Number male family members age 65+.
FS7	0.094	0.326	Number female family members ages 0–4.
FS8	0.302	0.626	Number female family members ages 5–14.
FS9	0.243	0.471	Number female family members ages 15–29.
FS10	0.400	0.490	Number female family members ages 30–49.
FS11	0.218	0.413	Number female family members ages 50–64.
FS12	0.100	0.301	Number female family members ages 65+.
GP	-1.119	0.108	Logarithm of the number of general practitioners per capita in the region.[a]
ILL	1.105	1.381	Logarithm of (the maximum number of illness days during a half year, + 1) maximum taken over all family members.
INC	10.267	0.390	Logarithm of the annual after tax family income (1976).

Table 1 (continued)

Variables	Mean	Standard Deviation	Definition
INS1	0.439	0.496	Dummy variable: equals 1 if the family has bought an additional insurance for medical assistance by the general practitioner (GP) and for pre-scribed medicine; equals 0 if not.
INS2	0.243	0.429	Dummy variable: equals 1 if the family's hospital insurance is a so-called "class 2b" insurance, which in case of hospitalization provides more luxury facilities than a "normal" hospital insurance (e.g., a double room instead of a ward); equals 0 if not.
INS3	0.044	0.205	Dummy variable: equals 1 if the family's hospital insurance is a so-called "class 2a" insurance, which in case of hospitalization provides still more luxury facilities than a "class 2b" insurance (e.g., a single instead of a double room); equals 0 if not.
PINS	4.180	0.065	Logarithm of the percentage of publicly insured in the region.[a]
SPEC1	-0.805	0.272	Logarithm of the number of all specialists per capita in the region.[a]
SPEC2	2.143	0.182	Logarithm of the number of clinically working specialists per bed in the region.[a]
SELF	0.208	0.406	Dummy variable: equals 1 if the family head is self-employed; equals 0 if not.
URB	0.647	0.478	Dummy variable: equals 1 if the family lives in an urbanized region; equals 0 if in a rural region.

[a]In order to calculate the variables PINS, GP, SPEC1, SPEC2, and BED, The Netherlands were divided into 63 regions, and each family was assigned the relevant value of the region in which the family was living. For a detailed description of the calculation of these variables, see E.M. Hooijmans and W.P.M.M. van de Ven, "Implementing a Health Status Index in a Structural Health Care Model," Report No. 80.13, Center for Research in Public Economics, Leiden University, 1980.

[b]31.1% of all families had zero expenditures (1976). The mean value of EXPEND over the 4180 families with nonzero expenditures is 6.354 (st. dev. 1.647). The average expenditures over all 6068 families equals 1449.25 guilders (st. dev. 4471.73).

nition of all explanatory variables). As an indicator of morbidity
we use the number of days of illness, as reported by the
respondents. Because the partial nonresponse for this individual
question was relatively high, we took the maximum of illness days,
the maximum taken over all reported family members (ILL).

Generally speaking, a patient in The Netherlands has no direct
access to the specialist or the hospital (emergency cases excluded).
When a health problem arises, the patient first contacts his general
practitioner, who may refer the patient to a specialist; it is the
specialist who decides whether the patient is to be hospitalized.
Without a referral by the general practitioner the insurance company, as a rule, does not refund any claim. So if the expenditures
for hospitalization or specialists' treatment are nonzero, this
means that (a) the patient first contacted his general practitioner,
and (b) the general practitioner decided to refer the patient to a
specialist. In specifying the vector X_1 and in interpreting the
vector of estimated coefficients α, we should be aware of the fact
that there may be variables with a different or even opposite
influence on these two different decisions.

All families were completely insured against medical cost of hospitalization and specialists' treatment, but only 44% of them had
bought insurance covering medical assistance by the general practitioner (indicated by the dummy INS1). This additional insurance
lowers the (financial) threshold to contact the general practitioner. We may therefore expect a positive effect of being
insured for general practitioner's assistance on the probability of
nonzero expenditures for hospitalization and specialists' treatment.
A second reason to expect this positive effect might be that less
healthy families did buy the additional insurance. For this last
reason we may also expect a positive effect of INS1 on the extent of
the nonzero expenditures. Another aspect of the insurance mode is
that 29% of the families had bought an insurance policy which in
case of hospitalization provides more luxurious treatment in hospitals than the standard policy offers--e.g., single or double room
instead of ward (indicated by two dummies, INS2 and INS3). We expect
this to have some effect on the nonzero expenditures only, but not
on the probability of nonzero expenditures.

We also included characteristics of the region where the family was
living. With respect to the distance (DIST)[3] to the nearest hospital
(i.e., the place where the specialist works), we hypothesized that a
larger distance implies (a) smaller (probability of) nonzero expenditures (cf. Kruidenier, 1977). With respect to the degree of urbanization (indicated by the dummy URB) we expected that families
living in a rural area as a rule would enjoy a more healthy life
than those living in an urbanized area because of less environmental
pollution, fewer traffic accidents, more physical exercise on the
job, and other similar factors.

An important determinant of the use of health care facilities (and
consequently of medical expenditures) is their availability.
According to established experience, we expected that the probability of nonzero expenditures would increase with the number of specialists per capita in the region (SPEC1). We further hypothesized
a positive effect of the number of beds per capita (BED) and the

number of clinically working specialists per bed (SPEC2) on the extent of the nonzero expenditures.

The fewer patients a general practitioner has, the more attention he can give to each patient--by treating the patient himself instead of referring him to a specialist or, after having referred a patient to the specialist, by taking him over from the specialist as soon as possible. We therefore expected both a negative α and β coefficient for the number of general practitioners per capita in the region (GP).

A special characteristic of the region is the percentage of publicly insured people in that region (PINS). As already mentioned, all employees with an annual income below 30,900 guilders (in 1976) were compulsorily insured by the Sick Fund, a kind of public insurance. We included the variable PINS to control for differences in the remuneration system between the private and the public sector[4] (both groups of patients share the same services).

Finally, as socioeconomic family characteristics we took (a) the annual family income after taxes (INC); (b) the education of the family head--total years of education (EDUC1) and a dummy variable indicating whether the family head has received a vocational training (EDUC2); (c) two dummies indicating whether or not the family head works in a paid job, and if so, whether he or she is an employee (EMPL) or is self-employed (SELF). These two dummies may be interpreted as accounting for, first, differences in time prices (in the case of receiving medical assistance); second, if EMPL = SELF = 0 the family head is nonactive, e.g., a pensioner, unemployed, or chronically disabled.

Because we consider a constant elasticity of the extent of the non-zero expenditures with respect to BED, DIST, EDUC1, GP, ILL, INC, PINS, SPEC1, and SPEC2 to be more realistic than an elasticity which increases with increasing value of the explanatory variable, we applied a logarithmic transformation to these variables.[5] (The variables ILL and DIST were raised by 1 because they may take on the value 0.)

Summarizing the above discussion, we specify the two vectors of explanatory variables, X_1 and X_2, as follows:

$$X_1 = (\text{ILL, FS1, ..., FS12, INS1, DIST, URB, SPEC1, GP, PINS, INC, EDUC1, EDUC2, EMPL, SELF, constant term}); \quad (5)$$

$$X_2 = (\text{ILL, FS1, ..., FS12, INS1, INS2, INS3, DIST, URB, SPEC2, BED, GP, PINS, INC, EDUC1, EDUC2, EMPL, SELF, constant term}). \quad (6)$$

The next section discusses the estimation results of model (1-6).

Estimation Results

The parameters of the adjusted tobit model have been estimated by means of the simple estimator devised by Heckman (1976, 1979).[6] In

Table 2 the estimation results are presented for the probit equation
"yes or no expenditures" and the regression-equation explaining the
nonzero annual family health care expenditures both with and without
Heckman's correction term λ, i.e., estimating ρ freely and fixing ρ
at 0. The estimated value of ρ equals 0.345.

Inclusion of the correction term λ results in a considerable upward
shift of the absolute values of $\hat{\beta}$,[7] which could be expected if ρ is
wrongly assumed to be zero instead of positive (De Vos and Bikker,
1978, p. 7).

Our estimates do not, however, indicate that the coefficient of the
correction term λ is "significantly different from zero." This may
be due to the high multicollinearity between λ and the vector of
explanatory variables (X_2). Nevertheless, because of the theoretical advantages of the model without the a priori restriction of
uncorrelated errors (ρ = 0), we will further focus on the equation
with Heckman's correction term (ρ ≠ 0).

Table 3 gives the elasticities of the (probability of) nonzero
annual family health care expenditures. Main variables in
explaining health care expenditures are the variables which represent the family's morbidity (ILL) and the age-sex family composition. A 10% increase in ILL results in a 4.6% increase in
expected family expenditures.

As an illustration, the effect of a simultaneous change of the
variables ILL and FS1 through FS12, holding all other variables
fixed at the sample mean, is given in Figure 1. In this figure we
see that the expected expenditures at the age of 75 are about eight-
fold that at the age of 25.

In Table 3, the influence of the availability of health care facilities on the expected medical expenses is as expected. The number of
specialists per capita (SPEC1) has a small but positive influence on
the probability of nonzero expenditures. The elasticity of the nonzero expenditures with respect to the number of hospital beds per
capita (BED) equals 0.40. Increasing the number of general practitioners per capita lowers both the expected probability and the
expected nonzero expenditures (but the estimated coefficients are
not significantly different from zero). The distance to the nearest
hospital has a significantly negative influence on the probability
of nonzero expenditures; its influence on the extent of the nonzero
expenditures is negligibly small.

The expected family health care expenditures are, holding all other
variables constant at the sample mean, 37.1% higher for a family
that lives in a region with relatively few general practitioners and
many beds and specialists (6.25 beds per 1000 population, an average
of 1700 patients per specialist and 3300 patients per GP, and a 1-km
distance to the nearest hospital) than for a family living in a
region with relatively many general practitioners and few beds and
specialists (4.5 beds per 1000 population, an average of 3000
patients per specialist and 2600 patients per GP, and a 10-km
distance to the nearest hospital).[8]

Rutten (1978) analyzed aggregate medical consumption of the
publicly insured patients. Using his estimation results in order to

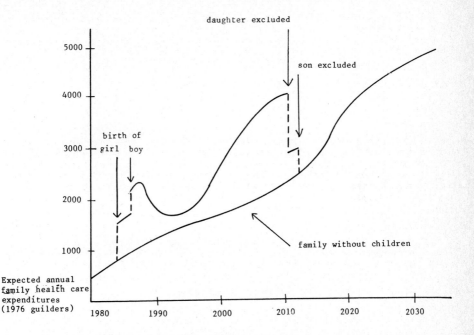

Figure 1. Annual family health care expenditures during 50 years for two fictive families.

Note: In 1980, two fictive families each consist of a 24-year-old woman and her 27-year-old husband; in 1984 and 1987 one of the two families is enlarged by the birth of a girl and then a boy; these children are later excluded from the family health insurance policy, the girl at age 26, in the year 2010, the boy at age 25 in 2012. For both families the variable ILL is set at two days in 1980, and every year ILL increases with 1/3 day (in 2030; ILL = 18.67).

The average (1976) premium for two adults is 1386,45 guilders; for two adults plus two children younger than 16 years old; 1950,93 guilders; and for two adults plus two children between 16 and 27 years old who are students, 2426,29 guilders. (These are all weighted averages, where the mean values of INS2, INS3, and 1-INS2-INS3 are used as weights.)

Table 2. Estimation Results of Probit Equation "Yes or No Expenditures" and OLS-Equation Explaining the Nonzero Annual Family Health Care Expenditures

Variable	Probit Equation		OLS Equation without Heckman's Correction Term λ		OLS Equation with Heckman's Correction Term λ	
	Coefficient	t-value	Coefficient	t-value	Coefficient	t-value[a]
ILL	0.246	16.30	0.416	25.99	0.468	9.61
FS1	0.173	3.02	0.190	2.65	0.240	2.85
FS2	0.166	4.79	0.064	1.58	0.101	1.94
FS3	0.175	4.28	0.156	3.14	0.194	3.23
FS4	0.447	7.55	0.355	4.19	0.474	3.50
FS5	0.492	7.63	0.433	4.86	0.557	3.94
FS6	0.561	7.18	0.786	7.27	0.931	5.55
FS7	0.266	4.45	0.280	3.92	0.348	3.72
FS8	0.174	5.01	-0.013	0.33	0.027	0.49
FS9	0.376	8.25	0.233	4.45	0.311	3.60
FS10	0.517	10.18	0.186	2.63	0.308	2.39
FS11	0.674	10.31	0.241	2.65	0.405	2.36
FS12	0.527	6.10	0.375	3.07	0.506	3.00
INS1	0.155	4.07	0.110	2.23	0.148	2.48
INS2			0.144	2.42	0.139	2.34
INS3			0.255	2.11	0.249	2.06
DIST	-0.057	2.16	0.0007	0.02	-0.012	0.32
URB	0.064	1.33	-0.0001	0.002	-0.017	0.26
SPEC1	0.149	1.71	0.053	0.36	0.085	0.57
SPEC2						
BED	-0.203	0.97	0.368	2.34	0.402	2.51
GP	-0.215	0.76	-0.293	1.07	-0.341	1.23
PINS			-0.177	0.43	-0.219	0.53
INC	0.126	2.38	-0.045	0.60	-0.011	0.14
EDUC1	0.072	1.05	0.057	0.62	0.072	0.78

	Model 1		Model 2		Model 3	
EDUC2	-0.045	1.08	-0.054	1.00	-0.064	1.16
EMPL	-0.196	2.50	0.067	0.66	0.027	0.25
SELF	-0.223	2.78	0.290	2.73	0.242	2.13
CONSTANT	-1.145		4.938		4.034	
λ					0.518	1.13
σ	1.0		1.4996		1.4995	
ρ			0.0		0.345	
Observations	6068		4180		4180	
R^2 b	0.1572		0.1708		0.1709	

a In the OLS equation with Heckman's correction term, the t-values are only approximate (see J.J. Heckman, "Sample Selection Bias as a Specification Error," Econometrica, 47 [1979], 158).

b In the probit equation, R^2 equals the squared correlation coefficient between the dependent variable and its predicted value.

Table 3. Elasticities of Nonzero Annual Family Health Care Expenditures at the Mean Value[a] and the Effects of Change of Some Variables

	Elasticity			Effect of a "Normal" Change[b]		
	of probability of nonzero expenditures	of expected expenditures conditional upon a positive value	of unconditional expected expenditures	on probability of nonzero expenditures[c]	on expected expenditures conditional upon a positive value[d]	on unconditional expected expenditures[e]
ILL	0.074	0.386	0.460	+29.9%[f]	+248.3%[f]	+352.3%[f]
DIST	-0.019	-0.002	-0.021	- 4.2%	- 0.5%	- 4.7%
SPEC1	0.050	-0.025[g]	0.024	+ 2.9%	- 1.5%	+ 1.4%
SPEC2	-	0.085	0.085	-	+ 3.6%	+ 3.6%
BED	-	0.402	0.402	-	+ 17.9%	+ 17.9%
GP	-0.068	-0.306	-0.374	- 1.5%	- 6.5%	- 7.9%
PINS	-0.072	-0.182	-0.254	- 0.9%	- 2.4%	- 3.3%
INC	0.042	-0.032	0.010	+ 3.8%	- 2.8%	+ 0.8%
EDUC1	0.024	0.060	0.084	+ 1.5%	+ 3.7%	+ 5.3%

[a]The elasticities of "the probability of a nonzero y-value" (η_{PROB}) and the conditional and unconditional expected value y (η_{COND} and η_{UNC}) with respect to the first explanatory variable of X_1 and X_2 after logarithmic transformation are

$$\eta_{PROB} = \alpha_1 \frac{\phi(A)}{\Phi(A)},$$

$$\eta_{COND} = \beta_1 + \alpha_1 \frac{\phi(A+\rho\sigma)}{\Phi(A+\rho\sigma)} - \frac{\phi(A)}{\Phi(A)},$$

$$\eta_{UNC} = \eta_{PROB} + \eta_{COND} = \beta_1 + \alpha_1 \frac{\phi(A+\rho\sigma)}{\Phi(A+\rho\sigma)},$$

where $A = \alpha_1 \log X_{1.1} + \sum_{j=2}^{k} \alpha_j X_{1.j}$, and $X_{1.j} = \frac{1}{N} \sum_{i=1}^{N} X_{1ij}$,

and with $\phi(\cdot)$ and $\Phi(\cdot)$ the density, respectively, the cumulative distribution of a standard normally distributed variable. For a derivation of these formulae, see W.P.M.M. van de Ven and B.M.J. van Praag, "Risk Aversion and Deductibles in Private Health Insurance," Report No. 80.12, Center for Research in Public Economics, Leiden University, 1980.

b A "normal" change of a variable is defined as a ceteris paribus change from the mean value of this variable <u>minus</u> its standard deviation (in the sample) to the mean value <u>plus</u> its standard deviation. The other variables are set at their mean values.

c $P(y_i^* > o) = \Phi(A_i)$.

d $E(y_i/y_i^* > o) = \exp(\mu_i + \frac{1}{2}\sigma^2) \times \Phi(A_i + \rho\sigma) \times [\Phi(A_i)]^{-1}$.

e $E(y_i) = \exp(\mu_i + \frac{1}{2}\sigma^2) \times \Phi(A_i + \rho\sigma)$.

f The reported effects are the effects of a change of ILL from 1 to 37 days. The effects of an ILL change from 1 to 8 days are +17.5%, +87.3%, and +120.0% respectively; the effects of an ILL change from 8 to 37 days are +10.6%, +85.9%, and +105.6% respectively.

g Although SPEC1 is not included in the OLS equation explaining the nonzero expenditures, it does influence $E(y_i/y_i^* > 0)$ because $E(\varepsilon_{2i}/y_i^* > 0)$ is a function of SPEC1.

Table 4. Effects of Ceteris Paribus Change in Some Exogenous Variables

Change in Exogenous Variable[a]	Effect on Probability of Nonzero Expenditures	Effect on Expected Expenditures Conditional Upon a Positive Value	Effect on Unconditional Expected Expenditures
INS1 = 0 → INS1=1	+5.2%	+12.9%	+18.8%
INS2=INS3=0 → INS2=1,INS3=0	-	+15.0%	+15.0%
INS2=INS3=0 → INS2=0,INS3=1	-	+28.3%	+28.3%
URB=0 → URB=1	+2.2%	+ 0.6%	+ 2.8%
EDUC2=0 → EDUC2=1	-1.5%	- 5.4%	- 6.9%
EMPL=SELF=0 → EMPL=1, SELF=0	-5.8%	+ 6.0%	+ 0.2%
EMPL=SELF=0 → EMPL=0,SELF=1	-6.7%	+32.1%	+23.3%

[a]Keeping all other explanatory variables at the sample mean.

calculate the effect of a comparable "normal" change of bed density, specialist density, GP density, and population density (as a proxy for distance) on the total cost of clinical and hospital outpatient care (in 1973) of publicly insured patients, we find a 34.7% difference,[9] which conforms fairly well with the above-mentioned difference of 37.1% for privately insured patients.

The influence of the insurance variables is as expected: for families with the additional insurance for general practitioner assistance the probability of nonzero expenses is, other things being equal, 5% higher than for families without that insurance; and their total expected expenditures are 19% higher (see Table 4). For families with the additional insurance for luxury hotel facilities in case of hospitalization (INS2 and INS3) the expected expenditures are respectively 15% and 28% higher than for families with the "normal" hospital insurance.

Looking at the family characteristics, we see that income has a significantly positive effect on the probability of nonzero expenditures. This might be an indication that high-income families have a high demand for good health which is reflected in more visits to the general practitioner or pressure to refer them to a specialist. After a referral to a specialist, however, income has no effect on the extent of the nonzero expenditures.

Finally, if the family head is an employee (EMPL) or self-employed (SELF), the probability of nonzero expenditures is lower than in the case of a family head not working in a paid job. The expenditures of a self-employed family, however, if there are any, are significantly larger than for a family that is not self-employed. The high time-price may be a reason that self-employed people do not consult their physician for relatively less severe cases.

In the next section, we develop a theoretical model of the relation between risk aversion, risk premium, and deductibles; we then use the estimated coefficients as presented in this section for the calculation of the truncated expected expenditures in case of a deductible and for making estimates of the measure of risk aversion.

RISK AVERSION AND DEDUCTIBLES

Risk Aversion and Risk Premium

One of the questions we asked in the questionnaire was "Would you like to have a health insurance policy with a deductible if you would get an appropriate premium reduction?"[10] To all policyholders who answered in the affirmative, we additionally asked "If you would get a premium reduction q, what maximum amount would you be prepared to take as a deductible?" Each policyholder was invited to consider five alternative values of q: q_{ij}, $j = 1,2,...,5$ (10%, 20%, 30%, 40%, and 50% reduction of p_i, the premium of family i for full insurance).[11]

For a policy with a deductible D, the health care expenditures that
family i has to pay in one year is $y_i(D)$, with

$$y_i(D) = \begin{cases} y_i \text{ if } y_i < D \\[2ex] D \text{ if } y_i > D, \end{cases} \tag{7}$$

where y_i is the total health care expenditures for family i in that
year.

For family i with income z_i and utility function of income $U_i(z)$, we
define the Expected Utility Gain (EUG) in case of a policy with
deductible D and premium q as compared with a complete insurance
with premium p_i as

$$EUG_i(q,D) = E_{y_i}\left[U_i\left[z_i - (p_i - q) - y_iD)\right]\right] - U_i(z_i - p_i). \tag{8}$$

If D_{ij} is the maximum deductible that family i is willing to accept
in exchange for the premium reduction q_{ij} (j = 1,2,...,5), we have
for each j

$$EUG_i(q_{ij},D) = \begin{cases} > 0 \text{ for } D < D_{ij} \\[1ex] = 0 \text{ for } D = D_{ij} \\[1ex] < 0 \text{ for } D > D_{ij}, \end{cases} \tag{9}$$

which implies

$$E_{y_i}\left[U_i\left[z_i - (p_i - q_{ij}) - y_i(D_{ij})\right]\right] = U_i(z_i - p_i), \tag{10}$$
$$j=1,2,...,5.$$

For a deductible D we define $v_i(D)$ and $\tau_i^2(D)$ as the expected value,
respectively the variance of $y_i(D)$:

$$v_i(D) = E_{y_i}\left[y_i(D)\right], \qquad \tau_i^2(D) = E_{y_i}\left[y_i(D) - v_i(D)\right]^2. \tag{11}$$

In Figure 2 we have sketched the relation between $v_i(D)$ and the
premium reduction q for family i. For instance, in exchange for a
premium reduction q_{i3} family i is prepared to take at most D_{i3} as
the deductible amount, which implies that all pairs of combination
$[v_i(D), q_{i3}]$ with $D < D_{i3}$ are "acceptable" to family i, while if

$D > D_{13}$ family i prefers the complete insurance without deductible.[12] In this way, all points in the shaded area of Figure 2 represent pairs $[\nu_i(D), q]$, and their corresponding pairs (D, q), which are acceptable to family i. For paying the uncertain amount $y_i(D_{13})$ instead of the certain amount q_{13}, family i wants to receive the extra amount $\pi_{13} = q_{13} - \nu_i(D_{13})$. In general we define the <u>risk premium</u> as

$$\pi_{ij} = q_{ij} - \nu_i(D_{ij}), \tag{12}$$

which is the <u>minimum</u> amount additional to the expected expenditures $\nu_i(D_{ij})$ belonging to deductible D_{ij}, that family i wants to receive for exchanging certainty for uncertainty. On the other hand, if family i has a policy with a deductible D_{ij}, π_{ij} is the <u>maximum</u> amount family i is prepared to pay in order to exchange uncertainty for certainty. Rewriting equation (10) as

$$E_{y_i}\left[U_i(z_{ij} - y_{ij})\right] = U_i(z_{ij} - \pi_{ij}), \quad j=1,2,\ldots,5, \tag{13a}$$

where

$$y_{ij} = y_i(D_{ij}) - \nu_i(D_{ij}) \text{ and } z_{ij} = z_i - (p_i - q_{ij}) - \nu_i(D_{ij}), \tag{13b}$$

we see that family i is indifferent between paying the risk premium π_{ij} (with certainty) and taking the actuarially neutral risk y_{ij} $[Ey_{ij} = 0$ and $Ey_{ij}^2 = \tau_i^2(D_{ij})]$.

Following Pratt (1964) we consider the behavior of π_{ij} as $\tau_i^2(D_{ij}) \to 0$, and we derive Pratt's measure of risk aversion r by expanding U_i around z_{ij} on both sides of (13a):

$$E_{y_i}[U_i(z_{ij}) - y_{ij}U_i'(z_{ij}) + \tfrac{1}{2}y_{ij}^2 U_i''(z_{ij}) + \mathcal{O}(y_{ij}^3)]$$

$$= U_i(z_{ij}) - \pi_{ij}U_i'(z_{ij}) + \mathcal{O}(\pi_{ij}^2). \tag{14}$$

Under the assumption that $\mathcal{O}(Ey_{ij}^3) = \sigma(Ey_{ij}^2)$[13] and $\mathcal{O}(\pi_{ij}^2) = \sigma(Ey_{ij}^2)$, using $Ey_{ij} = 0$, and neglecting terms of smaller order than $\tau_i^2(D_{ij})$, we have

$$\pi_{ij} = \tfrac{1}{2}\,\tau_i^2(D_{ij}) \times r_i(z_{ij}), \tag{15}$$

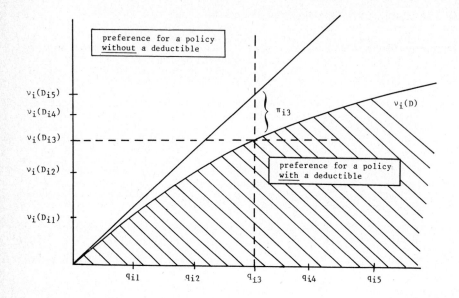

Figure 2. Expected expenditures $v_i(D)$ as a function of the premium reduction q for family i.

where

$$r_i(z_{ij}) = -\frac{U_i{}''(z_{ij})}{U_i{}'(z_{ij})} = -\left[\frac{\delta}{\delta z}\log U_i{}'(z)\right]_{z\,=\,z_{ij}}.\tag{16}$$

Estimation of Risk Aversion

From equations (12) and (15) we see that family i is prepared to take a deductible D_{ij} ($j = 1,2,\ldots,5$) if the premium reduction q_{ij} equals at least the mean value of the risk plus $\frac{1}{2}r_i(z_{ij})$ times its variance. Using the estimated values for the coefficients α, β, σ, and ρ (as presented earlier in this chapter), we are able to calculate for each family i and for each deductible D an estimate of the expected value $v_i(D)$ and the variance $\tau_i^2(D)$ by means of the following formulae:[14]

$$v_i(D) = E_{y_i}\left[y_i(D)\right] , \tag{17}$$

$$\tau_i^2(D) = E_{y_i}\left[y_i^2(D)\right] - \left[v_i(D)\right]^2 , \tag{18}$$

where

$$E_{y_i}\left[y_i^j(D)\right] = \exp\left[j\mu_i + \frac{1}{2}j^2\sigma^2\right] \cdot \Phi_2\left[\frac{\ln D - \mu_i - j\sigma^2}{\sigma}, A_i + j\rho\sigma; -\rho\right]$$
$$+ D^j \cdot \Phi_2\left[\frac{\mu_i - \ln D}{\sigma}, A_i; \rho\right] , \qquad j=1,2 \tag{19}$$

where μ_i and A_i are as previously defined in (1) and (3), and $\Phi_2(x,y;\rho)$ is the bivariate normal distribution function with correlation coefficient ρ.

In the questionnaire we asked the policyholder "If you would get a premium reduction q, what maximum amount D would you be prepared to take as a deductible?" Using for family i the answer D_{ij} corresponding to the premium reduction q_{ij}, $j = 1,2,\ldots,5$, and using the estimated values for $v_i(D_{ij})$ and $\tau_i^2(D_{ij})$, we can make an estimate of the risk premium π_{ij} [eq. 12] and of the measure of risk aversion $r_i(z_{ij})$ [eq. 15].[15]

In estimating the family health care expenditures we have not included the expenditures for medical assistance by the general practitioner, so we will only present the estimates of π_{ij} and $r_i(z_{ij})$ for those families who are not insured against general practitioner expenses.

The average[16] estimated risk aversion equals 0.0067, and the median value is 0.0048 (in 1976 guilders). These results imply a high degree of risk aversion.[17] For instance, a family with a risk aver-

W.P.M.M. van de Ven and B.M.S. van Praag

Table 5. Risk Premium as a Proportion of Premium Reduction (in guilders)

Premium Reduction Interval	Number of Observations (1)	Average Premium Reduction (2)	Average Estimated Out-of-Pocket Expenditures (3)	Average Risk Premium (2) - (3) (4)	(4) : (2) (5)
0-100	70	74.40	40.64	33.76	0.45
101-200	353	158.32	97.13	61.19	0.39
201-300	344	255.22	139.59	115.63	0.45
301-400	294	352.63	208.54	144.09	0.41
401-500	283	448.06	263.64	184.42	0.41
501-600	342	550.91	310.66	240.25	0.44
601-700	250	653.99	376.14	277.85	0.42
701-800	174	749.16	399.11	350.46	0.47
801-900	216	847.16	462.40	384.76	0.45
901-1000	102	949.94	495.65	454.29	0.48
1001-1100	89	1039.13	539.38	499.75	0.48
1101-1200	41	1149.17	613.23	535.94	0.47
1201-1300	38	1244.45	683.24	561.21	0.45
1301-1400	15	1346.42	604.74	741.68	0.55
1401-1500	20	1436.67	737.38	699.29	0.49
> 1500	27	1781.41	994.10	787.31	0.44
Total or Average	2658	536.22	297.60	238.62	0.44

sion r = 0.005, and with a .2 probability of at least one hospitalization (in a year) and a .5 probability of 400 guilders for
outpatient care, is only prepared to exchange the insurance policy
without a deductible for one with a deductible of 1000 guilders if
there is offered a premium reduction of at least 700 guilders, i.e.,
a risk premium of 300 guilders (for details, see note 15).

There are, however, reasons to assume that our estimates exceed the
true value of risk aversion. First, our data stem from a survey
carried out in cooperation with the insurance company, so the policyholder might not have told the whole truth in giving the maximum
deductible amount he was prepared to accept for a given premium
reduction, even though the respondent was explicitly told that his
(individual) response would not be made known to the insurance company. Second, we made an estimate of the risk aversion only for a
selected subsample, viz., those who were willing to take a deductible, i.e., those who were relatively healthy (see van de Ven and
van Praag, 1980). At the time we sent the questionnaire, all families had the same insurance without a deductible, so the "more
healthy" families subsidized the "less healthy" families.
Therefore, the relatively healthy families might consider a part of
the premium reduction as an allowance for the "over-premium" they
pay. Third, the policyholder might consider a part of the premium
reduction to be a compensation for the reduction of administrative
costs for the insurance company. The last two arguments imply that
the policyholders "accept" a part of the premium reduction without
weighing it against some expected health expenditures, which results
in an overestimation of the risk premium and the risk aversion.

Before looking in more detail at the risk aversion estimates, we
must note the limited information we used in assessing the expected
out-of-pocket family expenditures, whereas the policyholder might
have more relevant information at his disposal--e.g., a good
knowledge of the family's morbidity, or knowledge about the heatlh
care expenditures in the near future, because, for instance, of an
already planned hospital admission or an expected birth.[18]

Table 5 shows that the risk premium is an increasing fraction of the
premium reduction. Table 6 shows the estimated measure of risk
aversion by income group and family size.[19] In a previous study
(van de Ven and van Praag, 1979) we concluded that high income
groups and large families have a relatively high demand for deductibles. From Table 6 we may now conclude that these groups, given
their willingness to take a deductible, also want a lower risk premium for taking a risk than do low income groups and small families.
Friedman (1974) also found some evidence that higher-salaried
employees display a lesser degree of risk aversion.

CONCLUSIONS

In this chapter we have estimated from a data base of 6068 privately
insured families the distribution function of family health care
expenditures, the parameters of which are a function of relevant
explanatory variables. The model we have used is an adjusted tobit

Table 6. Estimated Risk Aversion by Income Group and by Family Size

Family Income (thousands of guilders)	Number of Families	Average Estimated Risk Aversion	Family Size	Number of Families	Average Estimated Risk Aversion
<20	121	0.0079	1	82	0.0148
20-25	126	0.0076	2	181	0.0082
25-30	233	0.0067	3	141	0.0070
30-35	155	0.0069	4	331	0.0055
35-40	157	0.0065	5	164	0.0046
40-50	117	0.0056	6	67	0.0039
$\geq$50	92	0.0049	$\geq$7	35	0.0044
Total	1001			1001	
Average		0.0067			0.0067

model, which deals with some of the shortcomings of the classical tobit model. A theoretical model is developed in order to assess the expected utility gain in case of a health insurance with deductibles as compared to one with complete coverage. Using the estimated parameters of the distribution function of family expenditures and the revealed preferences of policyholders with respect to a policy with a deductible, we have constructed an estimate of their risk aversion.

NOTES

[1]We measure y_i as all claims the insurance company paid in 1976 as reported in the files of the insurance company.

[2]Friedman (1974) found that the gamma distribution gave a relatively good fit to the distribution of health care expenditures. Newhouse, Rolph, et al. (1980) used a three-parameter distribution function which covers the log-normal ($\theta = 0$) and gamma distribution ($\theta = 1/3$) as special cases. They found an estimated value $\hat{\theta} = 0.11$ and stated that their finding was consistent with that of researchers using both the log-normal and the gamma distribution to fit medical expenses distributions. Although both null hypotheses ($\theta = 0$ and $\theta = 1/3$) were rejected,

we cannot directly relate the conclusion of Newhouse, Rolph, et al. to our assumption of log-normally distributed nonzero health care expenditures. Newhouse, Rolph, et al. estimated the <u>unconditional</u> distribution function of nonzero expenditures over 11,737 claimants, while we are concerned with the <u>conditional</u> distribution function of nonzero family expenditures, conditional upon the value of the variables that are used as explanatory variables for the parameter(s) of the lognormal distribution function.

[3]In Table 1 some variables (including DIST) are defined after a logarithmic transformation. This is given in equations (5) and (6).

[4]For details of the hypotheses about the influence of PINS on health care expenditures and for the interpretation of the estimated coefficients of PINS, see van de Ven and van Praag (1980).

[5]Formally, in the case that $\rho \neq 0$ this argument is only valid with respect to those X_2 variables that are not included in the X_1 vector (see Note a, Table 3).

[6]Details about the difference between the adjusted tobit model as we defined it and the classical tobit model, and about the simple estimation method as devised by Heckman for models with limited dependent variables or with sample selection, are given in van de Ven and van Praag (1980).

[7]Griliches et al. (1978, p. 147) found that the MLE estimates turned out to be between the OLS and "OLS with Heckman's λ" estimates, indicating that the latter may overshoot somewhat in correction-adjustment, but the changes (between MLE and "OLS with Heckman's λ") were not very large.

[8]This example roughly corresponds to a simultaneous "normal" change, or vice versa, of BED, SPEC, GP, and DIST (Table 3).

[9]In calculating this effect we used the results in Rutten (1978, pp. 84, 92, 100, 103, 143). For details, see van de Ven and van Praag (1980).

[10]In a previous study (van de Ven and van Praag, 1979), we have analyzed the answers to this question in detail. Our main findings are that income, education, and family size have a positive influence on the demand for deductibles; for the ratio of benefits to premium we found a negative influence.

[11]At the time we sent the questionnaire, the insurance company did not yet sell health insurance policies <u>with</u> a deductible, so all families had an insurance <u>without</u> a deductible. All policies are family policies (no group insurance). There exists no relationship beween the (potential) employer's contribution to the premium and the premium paid.

[12]We implicitly use the fact that $\nu_i(D)$ is an increasing function of D.

[13] $\mathcal{O}$ means "terms of order at most" and $\mathcal{o}$ means "terms of smaller order than."

[14]For details about the derivation of these formulae, using equations (1) through (4), (7), and (11), see van de Ven and van Praag (1980).

[15]The approximation we make in calculating the risk aversion r by using equation (15) instead of solving equation (13a) seems quite good for the range of the risk aversion and deductibles under investigation. E.g., a family with a

deductible D (D = 1000 guilders) has the following probability distribution of out-of-pocket health care expenditures $y_i(D)$:

$p[y_i(D) = 1000] = .2$ (hospitalization);
$p[y_i(D) = 400] = .5$ (outpatient care); and
$p[y_i(D) = 0]   = .3$

For the utility function with constant risk aversion $U(z) = 1 - e^{-rz}$ and r = .005, we find from equation (15) a risk premium

$$\pi = \tfrac{1}{2} \times (0.005) \times 120000 = 300 \text{ guilders, while solving}$$
equation (13a)

$$.2 \times e^{1000r} + .5 \times e^{400r} + .3 \times e^0 = e^{(400 + \pi)r}$$

(which is given in algebraically simplified form) yields a value π = 303.36 guilders.

For most reasonable values of D and the probability distribution of $y_i(D)$, the difference is less than 10%.

[16]The average risk aversion over 1001 families. If in the questionnaire more than one deductible was filled in, we took only one of them, viz., the highest value. The reason is that the policyholder might anticipate the reduction of administrative costs for the insurance company in case of a deductible, and might consider a part of the premium reduction as a result of those lowered costs. The relative importance of this component of the premium reduction decreases with increasing values of the deductible. The average deductible amount under investigation is 1035 guilders.

[17]Friedman (1974) estimated from health insurance data a risk aversion r = 0.0026 (1968 dollars) and considered this as a seemingly high degree of risk aversion. Other authors (e.g., M.S. Feldstein and Friedman, 1977; Keeler, Morrow, and Newhouse, 1977; Keeler, Newhouse, and Phelps, 1977) used as theoretically acceptable values a risk aversion r ranging from .0001 to .0025.

[18]After receiving from the health insurance company the annual family health care expenditures after 1976, we will be able to make a more accurate estimate of the expected out-of-pocket expenditures in case of a deductible.

[19]The results of Table 6 should be interpreted with caution because of some tax-related arguments which may reduce the real out-of-pocket costs for high-income groups and large families; therefore the estimated risk aversion for these groups may somewhat underestimate the true risk aversion. For details of the tax-related arguments, see van de Ven and van Praag (1979).

HEALTH, ECONOMICS, AND HEALTH ECONOMICS
J. van der Gaag and M. Perlman (editors)
© *North-Holland Publishing Company, 1981*

ANALYSES OF DEMAND AND UTILIZATION THROUGH
EPISODES OF MEDICAL SERVICE

Greg L. Stoddart
Morris L. Barer

INTRODUCTION

The role of the provider in the market for medical services has been
the subject of frequent debate among students of health care delivery systems, and with good reason.* The extent of supplier-induced
utilization, or alternatively the degree of imperfection in the
agency relationship governing physician-patient interaction, has
significant implications for the design of policies to achieve
rational utilization of scarce resources, whether the policies are
directed at cost control or access improvement.

Economists have given the subject substantial direct attention
recently (Evans, 1974; Pauly, 1975; Evans and Wolfson, 1978; Green,
1978; Fuchs, 1978; and Reinhardt, 1978b, for example); however, for
the most part it has been a debate staged largely in the implicit
assumptions underlying most segments of health economics literature.
While "broad" economists[1] have always maintained that supplier inducement is an "indisputable and inseparable characteristic of medical services provision," "narrow" economists have clung steadfastly
to their principles textbooks. The two groups have managed to bring
this debate smartly along to the point where there now seems to be a
grudging consensus that this market is not simply the aggregation of
numerous perfect agency relationships (Fuchs and Newhouse, 1978).
The health economics literature seems to be slowly converging with
observed facts.

In view of the growing body of empirical (instead of earlier
anecdotal) evidence suggesting that medical services utilization may
bear only a second or third generation resemblance to the
economist's notion of demand,[2] it is surprising to find the distinction between demand and utilization so seldom made explicit in the
demand analysis literature. Of particular concern is the observation that the empirical "demand" literature has grown, like an
inverted pyramid, almost entirely on the controversial assumption of

*This research was supported in part by National Health Research Scholar Award No.
6606-1373-48, Health and Welfare Canada. We also wish to acknowledge Robert
Evans, A. J. Culyer, and Kjeld Pedersen, each of whom provided helpful comments on
the original paper. Remaining deficiencies are, alas, entirely our responsibility.

no supplier inducement. The common _modus operandi_ involves first
specifying a demand equation from a conventional microeconomic model
of a sovereign consumer, and then estimating the equation with some
measure(s) of volume of services utilized as the dependent
variable(s). This amounts to an empirical misspecification to
whatever extent supplier inducement actually occurs in the given
delivery setting or data set.

If the utilization process is viewed as consisting of a patient-
initiated stage and a physician-generated stage,[3] then ideally one
would wish to employ measures of patient-initiated utilization (if
they existed) to estimate conventional "demand" equations and relevant elasticities. Measures of overall volume of services consumed
as a result of both stages of the utilization process would still be
appropriate dependent variables for "utilization" equations, though
the independent variables in these equations would presumably no
longer be restricted to prices and consumer characteristics.
Although it may be tempting to dismiss the demand/utilization
distinction as a matter of semantics, growing discomfort with the
no-inducement hypothesis supports the search for demand, not utilization, data with which to test predictions.

More than the internal consistency of health economics literature is
at stake. Empirical "demand" analyses are commonly undertaken with
one or more policy objectives in mind, such as cost control and
removal of impediments to access. If these analyses are to be used
as a means of assessing the impact of various economic policies on
total costs, then indeed, total utilization (or expenditure) may be
the appropriate dependent variable. One may be genuinely interested
in estimating utilization elasticities which include the responses
of both consumers and suppliers alike. If, however, one is primarily interested in issues of access, or wishes to disaggregate the
utilization response to phenomena such as the introduction or extension of health insurance, then an empirical analysis of overall utilization is considerably less useful and perhaps even misleading.
For these interests one must identify and explain patient demand.

It is the purpose of this paper to illustrate one potentially fruitful approach to demand measurement. In the first section, we
discuss the demand/utilization distinction in the context of two
bodies of literature. First, with respect to existing empirical
studies of factors influencing the "demand" for medical services we
illustrate the need for a measure of demand in the presence of inducement. Second, with respect to the theoretical discussion of
welfare burdens associated with health insurance we comment on the
implications of the distinction for estimates of those burdens.
While these bodies of literature are not usually combined in
discussions of demand analysis, they share the common effect of
channelling policy formulation toward levers aimed at the consumer
side of the market for medical services, often on the basis of analyses of utilization instead of demand.

In the second section, we outline an approach to demand measurement
through episodes of medical service, proceeding from a definition
of episodes to an application of the concept in a primary care
setting which resulted in the disaggregation into episodes of one
year's utilization experience for approximately 1300 urban fami-

lies. The episodes thus delineated were employed to estimate demand
equations and to investigate the potential bias involved in substituting utilization for demand measures in such equations. The
results of these empirical analyses are reported in the third section.

The empirical work reported in these two sections represents a first
attempt to employ an episodic approach to demand analysis of primary
care. Accordingly, it is subject to several limitations, yet also
offers the opportunity for several refinements and extensions.
These and the policy significance of a fully operationalized
episodic approach to demand analysis are discussed in the final section.

DEFINITION OF DEMAND IN DEMAND ANALYSIS LITERATURE

The literature on correlates and/or determinants of medical service
utilization is extensive.[4] Studies of the same general phenomena
differ along several dimensions. The independent variables of major
interest may be economic (Rosett and Huang, 1973; van der Gaag and
van de Ven, 1978; Guzick, 1978), organizational (Densen, 1960, 1962;
O.W. Anderson, 1972), or social-psychological (Rosenstock, 1966;
Becker, Drachman, and Kirscht, 1974). The approach may rely on
general systems (Kaitaranta and Purola, 1973), aggregate survey or
insurance claims data (Berki and Kobashigawa, 1978; Beck, 1974) or
microdata (Lairson and Swint, 1978). The analyses may purport to
explain overall utilization patterns (Fuchs and Kramer, 1972; Berki
and Ashcraft, 1979) or just variation in consumer demand (Wirick and
Barlow, 1964; Guzick, 1978). Variable selections may be based on
different underlying models, two of the most frequent being
Andersen's (1968) behavioral model and Grossman's (1972) human capital model.

Furthermore, the specific formulation of dependent variables may
reflect volume of utilization, including or excluding non-utilizers,
(Hershey, Luft, and Gianaris, 1975) or likelihood of any utilization
(Lairson and Swint, 1978). Econometric technique may also differ
(van der Gaag, 1978). The unit of analysis may be the family or the
individual (Andersen and Benham, 1970; Newhouse and Phelps, 1976),
and recently the utilization of services by children and adults has
been examined separately (Lairson and Swint, 1979). Finally, the
type of service examined, especially illness/injury versus preventive visits (Hershey, Luft, and Gianaris, 1975; Berki and Ashcraft,
1979), also varies across studies.

For purposes of this brief review we wish to focus primarily on the
model specifications in economic studies which attempt to explain
variation in consumer demand. The review illustrates that, while
the specifications in most "demand" studies may be appropriate in a
world of perfect agents, they are likely to be inappropriate
wherever physicians exercise discretionary power over any utilization which deviates from that of a fully-informed consumer/patient.
They are inappropriate because, with few exceptions, they employ
utilization data (physician visits or dollar expenditures per year)

generated by both provider and consumer decisions in attempts to
explain the relative significance of prices, income and socio-
demographic factors on demand.

Since even restricting consideration to economic "demand" studies
still produces more candidates for review than space warrants,[5] and
since these studies all share common roots in the conventional
microeconomic model, we shall attempt to illustrate the
demand/utilization distinction with respect to three frequently
cited analyses.

The conventional microeconomic model views the consumer's role in
the medical care market as one of rational choice under a budget
constraint. That is, medical care is but one, not particularly
unique, product available to the utility-maximizing consumer. While
many studies take as their starting point the specification of a
demand equation, such an equation arises from solving the first
order conditions which characterize this utility maximizing framework. The model predicts, _ceteris paribus_, a negative own price
effect and a positive impact of income on medical services
consumption.

The work of Andersen and Benham (1970) represents one of the
earliest comprehensive applications of the conventional microeconomic model. They concentrated on the role of family income in
explaining medical care consumption and employed two dependent
variables: (a) dollar expenditures on physician services, and, to
adjust for systematic bias introduced by differential fees for
similar services, (b) quantity of services consumed. The latter
measure was an aggregation of services weighted by relative values
established from the California Relative Value Fee Scale.
Considerable effort was expended to sort out the implications of
using each dependent variable, the effects of permanent versus
reported income, and the impact of price (types of health insurance
and premium cost), quality, demographic characteristics, illness
levels and attitudes toward preventive care.

Andersen and Benham reported income elasticities ranging from 0.17
to 0.41 (depending upon the particular specification of independent
variables) with an estimate of 0.30 based on permanent income
adjusted for illness level. These estimates are best viewed as utilization elasticities, however (even though neither their theoretic
nor empirical framework allows any direct role for the provider of
care), since their dependent variables refer to overall volume of
services consumed by families during the survey period. In the
absence of more sensitive measures of demand, the relationship between demand and utilization elasticities remains unknown.

One particularly elegant and influential approach to explaining the
demand for medical care is the human capital model developed by
Grossman (1972a). Since the details of this model will undoubtedly
be familiar to most readers, they will not be discussed here.
Suffice it to note that the demand for medical care is derived from
the demand for health. Although health does enter consumers' utility functions directly, it is viewed primarily as an investment
commodity with the return to investment in health capital being the
increased amount of healthy time available to the consumer for work
or leisure activities. Individuals combine medical care and own
time to produce gross investment, and when the model is formally

developed, the demand for medical care can be seen to depend upon
the price of care, and the consumer's age, wage rate and education.

The model is obviously one of autonomous consumer decision-making,
yet the empirical investigation is a subtle blend of a demand-
theoretic framework with a dependent variable (aggregate expenditures on medical care) measuring utilization.

When demand equations consist of a measure of utilization regressed
upon a set of independent variables reflecting prices and consumer
characteristics, either the assumption of no supplier inducement[6] is
being made (usually implicitly), or the empirical formulation would
appear to be misspecified. If demand is the true phenomenon of
interest, then the dependent variable must be refined. If utilization is the primary interest, however, then the specification can
usually be improved significantly by adding supplier-related independent variables.

Recent contributions to the demand literature by Newhouse and Phelps
(1974, 1976), which extend the work of Grossman while retaining its
spirit and conceptual base, perhaps best exemplify this approach.
In their 1974 study they estimate separate equations for hospital
days (weighted by an average room-type specific price) for those
with one or more admissions, and physician office visits (adjusted
for average price by type of provider), in what is essentially an
attempt to assess the impact of coinsurance rates on utilization.
They find negative or zero price and positive wage income elasticities in both utilization equations. In the 1976 study they add an
analysis of the hospital admissions phenomenon,[7] increase their
sample size and incorporate a number of analytic adjustments.
Negative own-price and positive income elasticities are derived.

Of more importance to this paper is their inclusion of supply-side
variables in both studies. By employing bed/population and
physician/population ratios as explanatory variables, they have
taken an important step toward specifying utilization equations
which realistically represent the market for medical and hospital
services. They have correspondingly moved a step away from producing accurate demand results, even though the theoretic underpin-
nings of their econometric analyses are very much concerned with
explaining demand. Supply-side variables are critical components of
a utilization analysis; but on the other hand, one has some difficulty explaining their presence in an analysis of constrained
choice by sovereign utility-maximizing consumers.

From a policy perspective, as noted earlier, there is nothing wrong
with estimating utilization equations. Indeed, further research is
required on both utilization and demand phenomena. The danger arises
when the conceptual "demand" framework is bootlegged past the
econometric specification and estimation to reappear at the policy
formulation stage. If the results are then viewed as those deriving
from a demand model, little attention is likely to be given to
potential supply-side policies aimed at impacts on utilization.

The policy focus on demand levers such as coinsurance has resulted
in part from a second body of literature, namely the theoretic
discussion of the welfare cost of health insurance. Attention here
has centered on moral hazard associated with consumer behavior; the
role of providers in determining aggregate utilization has been
largely ignored. While the assumptions that underlie welfare cost

analysis in general are well known (Harberger, 1954), difficulties
may arise in the market for health services when one addresses ways
of shrinking the welfare burden under the assumption that observed
utilization is in fact identical to demand. If supplier inducement
exists, the actual impact of policies such as coinsurance or
deterrent fees on aggregate expenditures, for example, may be quite
different from expectations based on demand analysis.[8]

The welfare burden literature has its historical roots in Arrow's
1963 article on the roles of risk and uncertainty in the medical
care market. There it was argued that the absence of insurance
markets to cover all risks leads to a sub-optimal allocation of real
resources. In addition, the peculiar and distinguishing characteristics of the market for medical services could be explained in
terms of these missing risk-bearing markets "and the imperfect
marketability of information" (1963, p. 947).

It would appear that the blurring of the demand/utilization distinction is also rooted in that same paper. In discussing the moral
hazard problem of insurance, Arrow explicitly recognizes the role of
the supplier in one sentence, only to dismiss it in the next:

> [T]he cost of medical care is not completely determined by the
> illness suffered by the individual but depends on the choice of
> a doctor and his willingness to use medical services. It is
> frequently observed that widespread medical insurance increases
> the demand for medical care (p. 961; emphasis added).

While Arrow noted the potential role of moral hazard in explaining
the absence of some insurance markets, it was left to Pauly (1968)
to show that this phenomenon (i.e., non-random "demand") may be a
sufficient reason for the absence of a complete set of risk-bearing
instruments. He argued that if the demand curve is sufficiently
elastic, and the consumer may purchase actuarially fair insurance,
the existence of moral hazard could leave the consumer better off
bearing the risks himself.

The weakness of this analysis stems from its traditional use of the
term "moral hazard" to refer to consumer response to declining
marginal cost without due regard to two factors. First, it is
assumed that pre-insurance utilization patterns are constrained
demand responses to relative prices. Thus, "even if the incidence
of illness is a random event, whether the presence of insurance will
alter the randomness of medical expenses depends on the elasticity
of demand for medical care" (p. 532, emphasis added). Moreover,
they are responses based on perfect information about the marginal
utility of additional consumption. Naturally the last unit of care
consumed is assumed to be of least benefit, and supplier inducement
is assumed away. Second, there may also be a moral hazard response
by suppliers who know their patients are no longer at risk (or are
bearing less of the risk). This may affect post-insurance inducement patterns.

Empirical attempts to estimate the welfare burden associated with
consumer moral hazard seem to be natural extensions of Pauly's 1968
analysis. Pauly himself (1969) took the first step by estimating,
"on certain standard assumptions, ... the welfare cost of excess
usage under a given kind of insurance." From a policy perspective,
however, this analysis also contains some unfortunate weaknesses.

While we resist the temptation to challenge further the assumptions underlying his model,[9] we do wish to point out an apparent analytic error.

Figure 1 portrays the basics of Pauly's model, with the welfare cost of health insurance being the area ABC, while d_h denotes demand for hospital care, P_h = MC, the price in a no-insurance market, and h represents homogeneous units of care being purchased in that market. With a coinsurance rate of OD/P_h, an additional $\Delta h(h' - h)$ units of care are purchased, and the insuring agency covers a share $i_h = I_h/P_h$ of per-unit price.

Pauly claims that "the total insurance benefit payment is equal to $hP_h i_h$," which, ironically, seems to underestimate total benefits by exactly the amount of moral hazard-induced excess benefit payments $\Delta h P_h i_h$. It can easily be shown that the greater the moral hazard effect on "demand", the greater will be Pauly's overestimate of welfare cost as a share of total insurance benefits.[10] Also, the lower the share of risk borne by the consumer, the greater will be that overestimate.

Assuming that the demand curve d_h represents consumer response to price variation, the area ABC as an estimate of total welfare cost ignores potential supply-side inducement both before and after introduction of the coinsurance. That area may, then, be an under- or over-estimate of total welfare cost resulting from traditional moral hazard plus supplier inducement adjusted for any provider moral hazard response. There is nothing conceptually incorrect about that model, if one is interested in separating the consumer and producer segments of "excess" utilization. If, however, one goes on as Pauly does to apply total insurance benefits and utilization elasticities[11] in the empirical/policy application of the model, internal inconsistency results. Either one must couch the underlying analysis in terms of utilization relationships, or one of the empirical tasks must be to identify benefits paid in response to stochastic demand.

What are the potential policy implications of this analytic/empirical discrepancy? Pauly's work provides an estimate of the magnitude of the aggregate welfare burden resulting from the moral hazard associated with the introduction of a particular type of health insurance. Because of the explicit model from which that estimate is derived, the welfare cost can only be the result of consumer price response. The only policy prescriptions for reducing welfare burden which logically emerge from that type of analysis relate to raising prices (increasing coinsurance) faced by consumers. In view of the problems with copayment policies which are identified in other analyses (Barer, Evans, and Stoddart, 1979; Badgley and Smith, 1979), the results of this research seem potentially hazardous to the health of policymakers.

A graphic illustration of the distinction between Pauly's framework and a similar analysis in an inducement context is provided in Figures 2 and 3. The former illustrates the welfare cost associated with supplier inducement in the no-insurance situation (indicated by the shaded triangle). U denotes the relationship between the price for services and total utilization. Thus at price P_h, consumers demand h units of care, and are provided with μ units of care. The difference, μ - h, is a measure of inducement-related utilization.

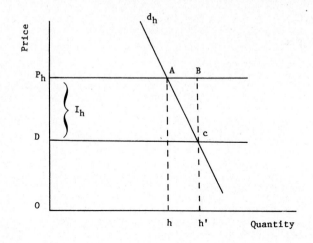

Figure 1. From Pauly (1969, p. 284) with minor modifications.

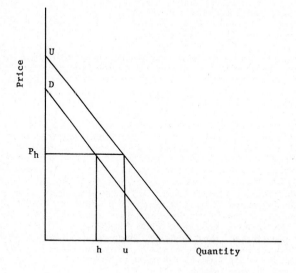

Figure 2.

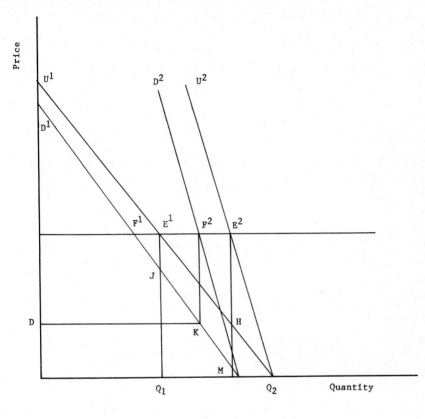

Figure 3.

Figure 3 illustrates the introduction of a coinsurance feature in an
inducement "market". It is assumed that suppliers do not markedly
alter their inducement activities even in the face of increased
quantities demanded at any given price paid to them. Clearly, other
assumptions may be equally (un)realistic. D^2 represents the relationship between the price received by suppliers, and quantities
demanded by consumers. Thus the introduction of coinsurance
(consumer price per unit = OD/OP) causes the demand curve to pivot
from D^1 to D^2 in the supplier-price framework. The area F^1E^1J
represents welfare cost as a result of inducement in the no-
insurance setting (i.e., Figure 2). An area equal to F^1F^2K represents the extent of consumer moral hazard-induced welfare cost.
Total welfare cost resulting from insurance in this type of induce-

ment setting is F^1E^2M. The share attributable to inducement is F^2E^2MK. When Pauly estimates the welfare burden, he applies a utilization elasticity estimate, consequently his empirical estimate of welfare cost will correspond to the area E^1E^2H. But the total increase in the welfare burden resulting from introduction of the coinsurance is given by E^1JME^2. Therefore, not only is it unlikely that Pauly's estimate will coincide with the total welfare cost resulting from health insurance, but it is also the case that his estimate will be equivalent to the consumer moral hazard-derived welfare cost (F^1F^2K) only if the extent of inducement is invariant with respect to price (i.e., if the D and U curves are pairwise parallel).

In a similar attempt to estimate the net welfare gain from reducing insurance coverage (after adjusting for welfare loss from the direct disutility of increased individual risk-bearing), M.S. Feldstein (1973) initially acknowledges the potential of supplier reactions to lowered prices. Building on his earlier work, in which he found that physicians tend to raise their fees as insurance coverage becomes more comprehensive, Feldstein describes the vicious cycle which may develop:

> [E]ven the uninsured individual will find that his expenditure
> on health services is affected by the insurance of others.
> Moreover, the higher price of physician and hospital services
> encourages more extensive use of insurance. People spend more
> on health because they are insured and buy more insurance
> because of the high cost of health care (1973, p. 252).

But the price response is quite separate from the supplier inducement response. Additional costs resulting purely from price increases are merely transfers of wealth from consumers to suppliers, and will not affect the above analysis except insofar as price increases are related to extent of inducement.

Feldstein focuses primarily on the determinants of the demand for health insurance, arguing that it acts in a complementary but inverse fashion to expenditures for health services. As the price of health services faced by consumers increases, the demand for those services falls and/or the demand for health insurance increases (assuming that price increases lead to expenditures increases). But again the entire analysis is laid out in terms of consumer demand responses to increased insurance, and welfare loss is computed in an analogous manner to that of Pauly (1969). Feldstein does incorporate a shift in the "demand" curve. It is not a shift from demand to utilization, but rather a response to quality increases resulting from higher prices! The empirical results relate to the magnitude of changes in welfare loss resulting from consumer responses to coinsurance rate changes.

It should by now be clear that the failure to distinguish demand from utilization in the welfare burden literature may seriously undermine the usefulness of that literature for policy purposes. The blurring of the concepts there parallels the fuzziness in the empirical literature reviewed above, which results in inconsistency between the theoretic base for demand equations and their empirical specifications. These are problems which would not arise if we were able to identify and measure the economist's definition of demand in the market for medical services.

MEASUREMENT OF DEMAND THROUGH EPISODES OF MEDICAL SERVICE

For consistency with models of autonomous consumer decision-making, an operational measure of demand must meet at least two criteria. First, it should discriminate between the patient-initiated phase and the physician-generated phase of the utilization process. Second, it should be a richer measure than the likelihood of using any medical care during a given period. In addition, it is desirable that a measure of demand reflect as accurately as possible the nature of the product being demanded. In this respect, P.J. Feldstein (1966) pointed out some time ago that consumers in the market for medical services do not in general demand specific services such as office visits or hospital bed days. Rather, they demand "treatment", combinations of services deemed by their physicians (or themselves) to be likely to resolve their medical problems.[12]

Consequently, we define an "episode of medical service" to be a set of medical services received continuously by a patient in response to a particular request. The utilization of medical services by an individual during any given period may then be regarded as one or more episodes for a variety of medical problems or requests. It seems reasonable to suggest that the number of episodes (i.e., the number of requests for treatment) represents a measure of demand. Since a request is normally presented in the initial contact of an episode, the episodic approach is consistent with a two-stage view of the utilization process and preserves the flexibility to generate overall utilization measures such as dollar expenditures or total visits in cases where they would be more relevant for policy purposes. Yet it simultaneously affords a useful measure of demand.[13]

It should be stressed that, with respect to the concept of demand, it is the set of services that is important, rather than specific components of the set. In fact, there is good reason to believe that in the absence of knowledge regarding the relative effectiveness and discomfort of alternative procedures, the consumer is either indifferent to the combination of services used to treat the presenting problem/request, or prefers less to more procedures. The provision of services in a continuous flow is another important characteristic of an episode, for this continuity distinguishes an episode of service from an episode of illness.[14] Note also that episodes of service may be provided for acute conditions, chronic conditions or reasons of prevention, depending upon the initial problem or request.

In order to operationalize the concept of a medical service episode, one requires several pieces of information. For each physician contact[15] it is necessary to know the date, the nature of the presenting problem or request, and the specific procedures or services provided to the patient. In addition, a set of rules (algorithms) must be specified which will allow episodes to be delineated from this aggregate utilization data base.

Although some arbitrary judgments will be unavoidable in algorithm design and data interpretation, information on service provision generally allows clear delineation of episodes. The purpose (or type) of episode is normally identifiable from either the patient's presenting problem, the practitioner's diagnosis, the specific service or procedure provided, or a combination of these.

Identification of the beginning of a new episode often, though not always,[16] amounts to confirmation that an earlier episode has terminated. Signals include new presenting problems or diagnoses, or new patient-initiated objectives.

A specific set of algorithms was developed and applied to the utilization records of approximately 1,300 families residing in the city of Vancouver, British Columbia. A one-year study period during 1973-74 was employed, during which time all families received ambulatory primary care from a university-affiliated family practice unit located in a residential area of the city and staffed by a multidisciplinary team consisting of salaried family practice physicians and several other health professionals. The application of the algorithms to the utilization data allowed the derivation of individual and family demand variables, while socioeconomic and demographic information for demand analyses on individuals and households was gathered through a combination of registration information and household survey.

Very briefly, the rules governing episode delineation were as follows:

(a) A new presenting problem implies a new episode unless closely related to a current or recent presenting problem of another episode. If ambiguous, consult diagnostic information, wherein an unchanged diagnosis indicates the continuation of a previous episode and a changed diagnosis initiates a new episode.

(b) Contacts for the same problem but 15 days or more apart constitute separate episodes. Exceptions to this rule include contacts separated by holiday periods, and situations in which extended periods are required to assess treatment effectiveness (e.g., fractures, birth control advice, antibiotic regimen).

(c) All regular contacts for desensitization or obesity counselling constitute one episode.

(d) All contact for regular monitoring and/or maintenance of chronic conditions, or emotional problems, constitutes one episode. Contacts for 'flare-ups' may generate separate episodes subject to the above algorithms.

(e) All contacts leading to the diagnosis of pregnancy constitute a single episode. Pregnancy-related contacts during the period from diagnosis through normal delivery to immediate postnatal care for the mother constitute another episode. During pregnancy, contacts for unrelated conditions and problems may generate separate episodes subject to the above algorithms.

In the few situations where the detailed algorithms summarized above provided an insufficient basis for episode delineation, consultation from family practice unit personnel was obtained. As a result of the delineation exercise, all visits, contacts and procedures during the study period were grouped into episodes of medical service by individual and family.[17]

ESTIMATION OF DEMAND AND UTILIZATION EQUATIONS

In view of the issues emphasized in the selective review of demand-analysis literature in the first section, the existence of an empirical demand measure (number of episodes of service) for individuals in the family practice unit sample suggests numerous investigations. In this section we shall briefly consider three specific questions which arise from the substitution of an episodic demand measure for more customary utilization or expenditure measures as the dependent variable in "demand" equations, based on a conventional microeconomic model of consumer behavior: (1) Does the substitution of an episodic-demand measure for utilization/expenditure measures increase the ratio of explained to total variance, as one would expect if episodes represent a more sensitive and accurate measure of consumer behavior? (2) What effect does the substitution have on income and price elasticities? and (3) How do demand elasticities computed with an episode approach compare with existing estimates?

Table 1 describes the variables employed in the analyses. The dependent variables employed in both individual and family equations are number of episodes of medical service (IES,FES), number of contacts (ICONTCS,FCONTCS) and dollar expenditures (IEXPINS,FEXPINS). The last two variables may require further explanation. Since this study was undertaken on a data base generated by a medical unit staffed by salaried practitioners, surrogate prices (fees) were assigned to all services provided. The two variables IEXPINS and FEXPINS are, therefore, "mocked up" estimates of the amounts which would have been billed to the provincial medical services plan under fee-for-service. We have postulated that the episodes equation will show a higher $\overline{R}^2$ than equations which proxy demand with contacts or expenditure as dependent variables, even within this salaried setting. Belief in the inducement hypothesis would lead one to expect even greater $\overline{R}^2$ differentials from comparable analyses undertaken in fee-for-service settings.

Price and income were the independent variables of primary interest. Since dollar prices at point of service are effectively zero in the Canadian setting of universal, first-dollar-coverage health insurance (and premiums are not utilization-related) an attempt was made to specify an indirect price variable. TRAVTIM was defined as the average time taken to travel from an individual's residence to the family practice unit.[18] With respect to income, an attempt was made to allow for transitory influences by specifying variables for the presence of a household head who was either a full-time student or unemployed during the study period.

Additional independent variables were included for socio-demographic factors, the effects of which might otherwise be confounded with price and income effects. These included age, sex, education and occupation (based on the Blishen scale). It should be noted that no variables pertaining to supplier characteristics were included in the specifications, since the objective was to estimate demand equations and to assess the changes which occurred when utilization measures were regressed on the same set of independent variables. Consequently, the contact and expenditure equations in Tables 2 and 3 should not be interpreted as attempts to explain utilization itself, since for this purpose their specifications would be incomplete.

Table 1   Variable Acronyms and Descriptions

Symbol		Mean	Standard Deviation
Dependent Variables			
IES	number of episodes of medical service for an individual	3.23	2.39
FES	number of episodes of medical service for a family	6.07	5.07
ICONTCS	number of contacts for an individual	6.79	7.61
FCONTCS	number of contacts for a family	12.66	12.09
IEXPINS	dollar expenditures for an individual	71.09	67.86
FEXPINS	dollar expenditures for a family	131.31	130.14
Independent Variables			
TRAVTIM	average travel time between residence and clinic	23.98	16.03
FY2	family income (hundreds of dollars)	160.23	108.65
STUHEAD	household head a student	.06	.23
UNEMPLOY	household head unemployed	.23	.42
SEX	females	.58	.49
SAG	females 18-40 years	.28	.45
AG1	under 1 yr./base: 41-60 yrs.	.02	.11
AG2	1-5 yrs.	.09	.29
AG3	6-15 yrs.	.12	.33
AG4	16-22 yrs.	.12	.32
AG5	23-40 yrs.	.38	.49
AG6	over 60 yrs.	.09	.29
BL1	unskilled and blue collar/base: white collar	.17	.37
BL2	professional	.20	.40
BL3	missing	.19	.39
EDSA[a]	less than high school/base: high school	.23	.42
EDSB[a]	tech. or voc. school, commun. college	.15	.36
EDSC[a]	at least some university	.41	.49
HAG1	age of head of household, 18-22 yrs./ base 41-60 yrs.	.04	.20
HAG2	age of head of household, 23-40 yrs.	.50	.50
HAG3	age of head of household, over 60 yrs.	.14	.35
FAMSIZE	family size (number of members)	2.45	1.48

[a]For individuals under 18 years, all EDS variables were assigned values denoting the mother's education. If this was unavailable, the household head's value was used. The household head's value was used for education variables in the family equations.

Equations 1 through 6 in Tables 2 and 3 report OLS results for individuals and families respectively.[19] While the $\overline{R}^2$ values are low
for all equations, they are within the customary range for this
genre of study. More importantly, the $\overline{R}^2$ values are higher for the
episodes than for the contacts or expenditure equations in both the
individual and family samples. The common set of independent
variables, theorized to be determinants of demand, appear better
able to explain variance in demand measured by episodes than by contacts or expenditures. This is consistent with our expectations if
utilization is supplier-influenced, since the equations contain no
supply-side variables. It should also be noted that the $\overline{R}^2$ values
in the contacts equations are markedly higher than those in the
expenditure equations. Thus contacts would appear to be an improvement over expenditures as a measure of demand. This may be partly
accounted for by the observation that episodes may often consist of
only one contact.

Throughout Tables 2 and 3, the replacement of demand by utilization
measures generally results in a loss of significance for most explanatory variables in these specifications. This is particularly true
for the income variable, as indicated in Table 2. In the absence of
significant income coefficients in Equations 2 and 3, it is not clear
that a comparison of demand and "utilization" elasticities computed
from Equations 1-3 would have any meaning.

With respect to price and income effects on demand, Equation 1 indicates that the indirect price effects of travel time are relatively
insignificant, though the coefficient exhibits the expected sign.
This contrasts with Acton's (1973) estimates of travel time price
elasticities. He found elasticities of between -0.25 and -1.0 for
care provided privately and through public clinics to insured, low-
income New York families.[20]

The family income variable, on the other hand, enters Equation 1
significantly, with an elasticity of -0.15 (computed at the means of
FY2 and IES). The inverse relationship between income and demand
certainly does not support the enabling effect of income postulated
by conventional economic theory, nor is it consistent with the
"demand" estimates of Grossman (1972a), or Newhouse and Phelps (1974,
1976) which range from 0.1 to 0.7; however, this is not an altogether unexpected finding given that all families possessed first-
dollar insurance coverage. The negative sign may be consistent with
the hypothesis that the opportunity cost of seeking care is higher
for higher income individuals, though this requires further investigation. It is also consistent with the suggestion that higher
income families tend to be healthier, due perhaps to greater use of
preventive services or to life-style.[21]

Although our focus in this paper is upon price and income effects,
the remainder of Equation 1 reflects the increased demand for services associated with maternal and infant care. It also indicates
some non-linearity in the effect of education on demand; individuals
with both more than high school and less than high school education
have lower demand than the baseline high school group.

Table 2 Demand and Utilization Equations: Individuals (N = 418)

Variable	Equation 1 IES (episodes)		Equation 2 ICONTCS (contacts)		Equation 3 IEXPINS (expenditures)	
	coeff.	t-value	coeff.	t-value	coeff.	t-value
TRAVTIM	-0.008	(1.08)	-0.035	(1.48)	0.055	(0.10)
FY2	-0.003	(2.61)	-0.006	(1.52)	-0.036	(0.40)
STUHEAD	-0.605	(1.20)	-1.552	(0.94)	-45.969	(1.25)
UNEMPLOY	0.717	(2.28)	1.207	(1.18)	20.458	(0.89)
SEX	0.451	(1.54)	1.313	(1.38)	26.881	(1.26)
SAG	1.272	(3.12)	3.427	(2.58)	63.585	(2.13)
AG1	2.123	(2.03)	-1.785	(0.52)	5.059	(0.06)
AG2	0.001	(0.03)	-2.660	(1.78)	-10.643	(0.32)
AG3	-0.568	(1.38)	-1.282	(0.96)	-12.132	(0.40)
AG4	-0.495	(1.08)	-2.467	(1.66)	-13.870	(0.42)
AG5	-0.497	(1.25)	-2.086	(1.61)	14.346	(0.49)
AG6	-0.362	(0.74)	-1.135	(0.72)	-6.223	(0.18)
BL1	0.642	(1.93)	4.039	(3.72)	57.938	(2.38)
BL2	0.571	(1.79)	1.090	(1.05)	15.764	(0.68)
BL3	0.044	(0.13)	-0.011	(0.00)	-7.272	(0.30)
EDSA	-0.532	(1.51)	-1.164	(1.01)	-29.179	(1.13)
EDSB	-1.112	(2.93)	-2.259	(1.82)	-19.056	(0.69)
EDSC	-0.279	(0.91)	0.262	(0.26)	-11.455	(0.51)
CONSTANT	3.690		7.949		42.150	
$\overline{R}^2$	.113		.074		.044	
F	3.96		2.85		2.07	

Table 3 Demand and Utilization Equations: Families (N = 224)

Variable	Equation 4 FES (episodes)		Equation 5 FCONTCS (contacts)		Equation 6 FEXPINS (expenditures)	
	Coeff.	t-value	Coeff.	t-value	Coeff.	t-value
FY2	-0.006	(1.56)	-0.012	(1.21)	-0.081	(0.39)
STUHEAD	-1.344	(1.12)	-2.956	(0.91)	-72.541	(1.12)
UNEMPLOY	1.489	(1.87)	2.720	(1.27)	39.710	(0.92)
EDSA	-1.227	(1.36)	-2.625	(1.08)	-43.625	(0.90)
EDSB	-2.044	(2.23)	-5.387	(2.18)	-47.046	(0.95)
EDSC	0.096	(0.13)	0.526	(0.25)	-18.329	(0.44)
HAG1	-1.510	(0.96)	-4.802	(1.13)	-17.260	(0.20)
HAG2	1.491	(2.10)	3.493	(1.82)	94.010	(2.45)
HAG3	-0.482	(0.44)	-0.804	(0.27)	-5.275	(0.09)
FAMSIZE	1.957	(8.48)	4.355	(6.99)	40.440	(3.25)
CONSTANT	1.865		3.359		20.380	
$\bar{R}^2$	.294		.223		.052	
F	10.28		7.39		2.23	

LIMITATIONS, EXTENSIONS AND SIGNIFICANCE OF THE EPISODIC APPROACH

Although the results discussed above represent a rather crude first
attempt to operationalize an episodic approach to demand analysis,
they are encouraging in that they are consistent with the expected
empirical impact of the theoretic distinction between demand and
utilization. Nevertheless several notes of caution are in order.

The empirical estimation was undertaken on a data set deriving from
a salaried primary care unit. This necessitated the estimation of
expenditures for the IEXPINS and FEXPINS equations. While the
actual application of provincial-fee-for-service schedules to family
practice unit service data is operationally simple, it is quite con-
ceivable that actual service patterns might have been different in a
fee-for-service environment.

The analysis was somewhat restrictive in other respects. Episode
delineation applied only to primary care services, to the exclusion
of telephone contacts, referrals, and hospital care. While this
particular application was determined by available data, in principle episodes entail the _entire_ set of services used to treat a
problem or request. Inclusion of hospitalization in a comparison of
episode and contact/expenditure measures, however, would require a
significantly larger sample size. In fact, if the validity and utility of the episodic approach are to be fully investigated, it will
probably need to be applied on a much larger, perhaps provincial,
data set. Before attempting this, we should give attention to
refining the delineation algorithms outlined in the second section,
especially algorithm (ii) concerning the critical time period for
separation of contacts continuing an episode. Although the 15-day
period adopted for this initial study was arrived at in consultation with clinicians, the sensitivity of episode delineation
to the period selected needs to be established. Ideally, a specific
critical time period should be detailed for each diagnosis or presenting problem.

While these caveats are important, none of the empirical refinements
appear insurmountable. With such refinements in place, the differential impact of various policies on number of episodes and episode content might be addressed. For example, one might expect
changes in a fee schedule, in a fee-for-service environment, to
impact differently on the number of episodes than on their
service/procedure composition. Those differences will be of very
real policy importance to parties involved in fee schedule nego-
tiations. In a non-universal insurance setting, changes in the
structure of benefit coverage will again be likely to induce different impacts on number of episodes and content of episodes.

An operational episodic approach might also assist in resolving the
current debate in the United States over whether certain forms of
national health insurance would foster patient "abuse" (more
episodes) or changes in service mix within episodes (supplier
inducement).[22] At the very least, the use of episodes might give
some empirical content to what have traditionally been very loosely
defined terms.

Indeed, the value of an episodic analysis further disaggregated by disease category and stage of contact is that it might enable us to identify (in the absence of a formal theory of supplier inducement) the circumstances in which supplier inducement appears most significant. Disaggregation by disease category would remove one source of variation in the service intensity of episodes which might otherwise be attributed to patient decisions or physician discretion. Disaggregation by stage of contact might also enable us to assess whether the measurement of demand by number of episodes is overly restrictive--i.e., to what extent are "first" visits in an episode supplier induced, and subsequent visits patient determined.

The other areas of policy and research interest in which both empirical results and the conceptual framework of an episodic approach to demand and utilization would be useful include manpower planning and cost-effectiveness analyses. The ability to measure and apply demand rather than utilization information as a basis for manpower planning would provide a significant refinement to this area of policy analysis. It seems intuitively more reasonable to undertake manpower planning not on the basis of provider-determined "appropriate" utilization levels, but rather on the epidemiologic likelihood of the number of episodes of specific types requiring treatment capacity. The linkage between roles for episodes in manpower planning and in cost-effectiveness analysis is provided by their potential utility in investigating alternative delivery mixes for a given set of epidemiologic needs.

The episode of service is perhaps the most appropriate unit of analysis for cost-effectiveness studies of alternative treatment patterns. The extent to which an episode of service satisfies a patient's request, removes symptoms, or restores a normal level of functioning can be viewed as a measure of effectiveness. Furthermore, for a given diagnosis, if the costs of achieving a specified level of effectiveness via alternative episodes of service can be calculated, then well-defined episodes of service with documented effectiveness at acceptable cost might be viewed as desirable treatment technologies.

Moreover, since episodes of service appear to be an appropriate definition of physician output, delineation of episodes would allow much more detailed analysis of the characteristics of medical care production processes than at present. Episode data would be useful in analyzing changes in technology or service mix, by type of provider and/or organizational setting, over time. Finally, costs of standardized episodes of service might provide an alternative index of the price of medical care, resolving some of the difficulties in price index construction noted by Scitovsky (1964, 1967).

The methodology and preliminary results underlying this discussion of potential policy and research applications represent, in our opinion, an important building block in the construction of a realistic framework for analysis of the medical marketplace. Effective future policies will depend on such a framework.

NOTES

[1]The designations "broad" and "narrow" have been employed by Evans (1976b) to refer to groups of economists whose works proceed from fundamentally different views of the market for medical services. The primary difference between the two is that "narrow" economists accept the view that resource allocation in the market for medical services responds to and reflects expressed consumer preferences, while so-called "broad" economists reject consumer sovereignty as an appropriate theoretic base for analysis of this market.

[2]For further examples of evidence of the significance of supplier influence on utilization, see Monsma (1970), Fuchs and Kramer (1972), Vayda (1973), Gertman (1974), Boutin and Bisson (1977) and Kronenfeld (1980).

[3]Unless otherwise indicated, the term "demand" is hereafter used to refer to the patient-initiated stage of this process, while utilization refers to the entire process, i.e., the sum of both stages. If the agency relationship is in fact perfect, then demand and utilization are identical. Note that no assumptions regarding the motivation for inducement are necessary (nor are any made) for the purposes of this paper.

[4]In fact, even surveys of the topic are numerous. In addition to Lloyd's selective review of economic literature (1971) and a bibliography by Aday and Eichhorn (1972), taxonomies of various approaches to the topic have been suggested by Andersen (1968), Greenlick et al. (1968), McKinlay (1972), J.G. Anderson (1973) and Stoddart (1975).

[5]Specifications of the demand for medical services date back at least to Wirick and Barlow (1964) and Klarman (1965). They are characterized in general by a failure to distinguish demand from utilization which continues up to the present as illustrated in Guzick (1978).

[6]This, in turn, implies either (a) that consumers are able to make fully informed decisions and can control the utilization process (both of which may on occasion be true--witness the amount of primary care subject to repeat purchase, and the concern among physicians about non-compliance with regimens) or (b) that although these conditions do not in general prevail, where they fail to exist the agency relationship is in fact perfect. In view of studies such as those mentioned in Note 2 above, it is difficult to accept either of these assumptions as the rule rather than the exception.

[7]See Barer et al. (1980) for a slightly different treatment of the same problem in the Canadian context.

[8]A more detailed analysis of this case is provided in Barer, Evans and Stoddart (1979), including discussion of the experience of the province of Saskatchewan with deterrent fees--an experience in which the utilization of middle-aged, middle-income groups appears to have increased after the introduction of direct charges into what had previously been first-dollar coverage.

[9]He assumes the equality of price and marginal cost, non-interdependence of utilities, and that market demand fairly reflects economic welfare.

[10]In fact, the relationship between what we believe to be the correct ratio of

welfare cost to insurance benefit payment (W/B_{BS}) and Pauly's ratio (W/B_p) is given by

$$\frac{W}{B_{BS}} = \frac{W}{B_p} \cdot \frac{h}{h'}$$

[11]Pauly adopts the "demand elasticity" of 0.25 estimated by P. J. Feldstein (1964), using aggregate medical care expenditures as a dependent variable.

[12]Klarman (1965) suggested that consumers might simply be assumed to be demanding to be seen by a doctor, believing that the doctor would then handle the entire situation. This would appear to be a crude version of the episodic approach. Solon et al. (1960, 1969) and Fink (1973) have illustrated the clinical significance of an episodic approach to utilization. Certain of the delineation algorithms mentioned below stem from considerations first discussed, though not operationalized, by Solon. More recently, health service researchers have employed an episodic approach in quality of care appraisal. See, for example, Kane et al. (1977), Moscovice (1977) and Lohr et al. (1980).

[13]Implicit in the use of the number of episodes to represent demand is the assumption that suppliers do not generate entire episodes of service as well as additional services in an episode already initiated. While the assumption is certainly violated in iatrogenic cases, and perhaps challenged by the "programming" of patients to respond to certain symptoms, overall these are not felt to be of major significance.

[14]It has long been recognized that illness is episodic in nature, and, as Richardson (1970) noted, the use of episodes of illness as a health measure allows meaningful comparison of instances of "getting sick." Indeed, one of the strongest endorsements for the use of episodes of service as a demand measure is that they correspond to the natural history of medical care. Although illness and service episodes are related, they differ in two important respects. First, they may differ in duration, i.e., the onset of illness normally precedes service, while an illness episode may terminate either before or after service. Furthermore, some illness episodes (especially those for chronic conditions) may contain more than one service episode. Second, illness episodes may occur in the absence of service episodes, and vice versa. A more detailed discussion is given in Stoddart (1975), Chapter 6.

[15]"Contact" is employed instead of "visit" since, in a group practice or clinic, a patient may receive services from more than one medical care provider during a given visit.

[16]Episodes may overlap or be interleaved. In these cases patients receive treatment for two separate problems during the same, or alternate, contacts. In general, delineation algorithms accommodate these situations by operating either to define new episodes or to allocate specific services to existing episodes. Episodes terminate, in retrospect, when services cease to be added to them.

[17]There were approximately 3200 individuals registered with the family practice unit during the period July 1, 1973 - June 30, 1974. They accounted for 7,092 visits, 8,330 contacts, and 10,859 specific services/procedures. The delineation exercise indicates that these were provided during 3,862 episodes of service.

[18]In other estimated equations TRAVTIM was replaced by a variable measuring distance from residence to the family practice unit; however, results were even less significant. Ideally one wishes to measure the indirect cost (including lost earning, transportation expenses, etc.) of seeking care. An attempt to create such a variable from supplementary household survey data was unsuccessful due to a prohibitive number of non-responses to the relevant questionnaire items.

[19]These samples represent individuals (N = 418) and families (N = 224) who were registered with the unit for the entire study period, who had at least one episode, and for whom income information was available.

[20]It may, however, be more consistent with the findings of Bashshur et al. (1971), and Salber et al. (1971) which imply that distance exerts a more significant effect upon the choice of a medical care source than it does upon the volume of services consumed.

[21]The complex interrelationship of income, life-style, health status, and medical care utilization (one could also add education)--and the specific question of whether poverty causes sickness or vice versa--are unfortunately beyond the scope of the present paper. We note, however, that the negative income elasticity of demand does not support Grossman's acknowledgment that if income acts as a proxy for life-style, it is not inconsistent to find higher-income consumers demanding more medical care though less health. (Newhouse and Phelps also suggest that their positive elasticities provide support for the Grossman life-style hypothesis.)

[22]Similarly, had episodic data existed on a larger scale in Canada, Evans (1976a) might have been able to disaggregate post-Medicare utilization increases into changes in patient demand and changes in provider practice patterns.

PHYSICIAN BEHAVIOR

HEALTH, ECONOMICS, AND HEALTH ECONOMICS
J. van der Gaag and M. Perlman (editors)
© *North-Holland Publishing Company, 1981*

THE BEHAVIOR OF HEALTH CARE AGENTS: PROVIDER BEHAVIOR

Alain C. Enthoven

INTRODUCTION

Spending on health care services in the United States increased from
$43 billion or 6.2% of GNP in 1965 to $192 billion or 9.1% of GNP in
1978 (Gibson, 1979). This was a doubling in real per-capita
spending. Over the same years, public sector spending on health
care increased from $11 to $78 billion. A recent survey of health
care expenditures in nine industrialized countries reveals a similar
pattern in all of them (Simanis and Coleman, 1980). The average
increase for the group was 2.4 percentage points of GNP between 1965
and 1975. So it seems appropriate to focus this review on factors
contributing to the growth in health care spending in the U.S.

The measures of cost of health care services that should be of most
interest to those who must pay for them, directly or indirectly, are
total spending and per-capita spending. Total spending is the product of unit prices and quantities of services or utilization.
Economists and public policy-makers have tended to focus on unit
prices or unit costs of health care services because those are the
variables their tools can measure and control. Their interest in
utilization has been largely confined to price elasticity of demand,
sometimes supplemented by investigation of the influence on the
patient of time-cost to obtain services. Such a focus on unit
prices and costs produces an incomplete view. Provider-determined
variations in utilization may be of much greater interest from the
point of view of cost-reduction. Inducing providers to curtail the
rendering of those services which yield very low or no marginal
health value may be a far more effective and acceptable way to limit
spending than attempts to reduce the price or unit cost of services,
or to make consumers pay a larger fraction of the price.

Indeed, a focus on unit costs such as a hospital's cost per patient-
day or cost per stay may produce perverse results from the point of
view of total costs. For example, a hospital may exhibit a comparatively high cost per day because its medical staff keeps
patients in the hospital for a relatively short time. Or it may
exhibit a comparatively high cost per stay because its medical staff
hospitalizes only very sick people, while another hospital may have
a low cost per stay because its physicians hospitalize people who
could have been treated equally well on an outpatient basis. The
behavior of the physicians associated with the hospital exhibiting
higher cost per day or stay may be associated with lower total cost
of health care. Similar remarks apply to the cost per doctor's

office visit. Behavior that produces low cost per day, stay or
visit may or may not be consistent with behavior that produces low
cost per capita. It all depends on the associated effects on use of
services.

In the United States, the largest and (with the exception of nursing
home care) the fastest growing component of health care spending is
hospital services, which increased from $14 billion or 32% of the
total in 1965 to $76 billion or 40% of the total in 1978 (Gibson,
1979). Spending on physician services increased from about $8.5
billion or 20% of the total to $35 billion or 18% of the total.
While physicians' services account for less than one fifth of the
grand total, physicians control or exert a very strong influence
over most of the rest of health care spending, especially hospital
spending. Physicians recommend hospitalization and admit patients.
They recommend and perform surgery. They order and may perform
other diagnostic and therapeutic procedures. They prescribe drugs,
and they decide when to discharge patients. Blumberg (1979) has
estimated that physicians control 70% of total health spending.
Thus, physician propensities to prescribe costly services are of
particular interest from the point of view of total health care
spending.

FACTORS SUGGESTING THAT PROVIDER BEHAVIOR IS CRUCIAL

Variations in Per-Capita Utilization

In the United States, there are wide variations in the per-capita
use of various health care services that have, so far, not been
explained by differences in income, insurance coverage, medical need
or health produced. For example, Lembcke (1952) compared per-capita
rates of appendectomy and death rates from appendicitis (including
dying from surgery) in 23 different hospital service areas in New
York State. The age-sex adjusted rate of appendectomy per 1000
population varied from 2.9 in the lowest to 7.1 in the highest. He
found no evidence of differences in the incidence of appendicitis in
these rather homogeneous areas.

Gittelsohn and Wennberg (1977) found variations in the per-capita use
of various health services in thirteen different service areas of
Vermont, despite the similarity of the populations in terms of rates
of illness, income, racial and social background, insurance
coverage, and number of physician visits per capita. The overall
age-adjusted rate of surgery per capita in the highest area is twice
that in the lowest. The variation was much higher for some
operations. For example, tonsillectomy rates varied from 4 to 41
operations per 1000 children per year.

A recent report by the Health Care Financing Administration shows
variations in the per capita rates of hospital admission, average
length of stay, and days of care per 1000 Medicare enrollees (aged 65
and over) in different areas (Deacon et al., 1979). For example,
the 10 areas with the longest average lengths of stay ranged from

14.9 to 17.1 days, while the 10 with the shortest ranged from 7.1 to
7.9. The 10 areas with the highest days of care per 1000 enrollees
ranged from 4,644 to 5,123 (omitting one extreme case), while the 10
with the lowest ranged from 2,022 to 2,448. These differences cannot be explained by differences in hospital insurance coverage.

These variations illustrate that the professional standards whose
existence is implicitly assumed by economists and policy-makers do
not, in fact, govern health care utilization. The study of other
possible explanatory variables such as physician characteristics and
organization should be an especially important area for future
research.

Evidence of Low Marginal Health Benefits

Do the higher rates of utilization yield a positive "marginal
product" in terms of health status? There is a substantial body of
evidence that suggests that, at least in many cases, higher utilization rates yield zero, or possibly negative health benefits. In
other cases, higher utilization rates yield marginal benefits that
are too small or too elusive to be measured. In still other cases,
it appears that utilization of costly services has been expanded in
the absence of evidence of efficacy (Enthoven, 1980a).

For example, Lembcke, in the study just mentioned, found a higher
death rate from appendicitis in the eight service areas with the
highest appendectomy rates than in the rest of the state. Since the
purpose of appendectomy is to prevent death from appendicitis, it
would appear, at least in this case, that the marginal productivity
of a higher rate of operations in terms of health status was
negative.

Newhouse and Friedlander (1977) and Miller and Stokes (1978) examined the relationship between the health of people living in different areas and the quantity of available medical resources,
controlling for demographic and socioeconomic characteristics of the
populations. Both found little or no significant positive relationship between health and health resources.

Hutter and his colleagues at the Massachusetts General Hospital
(1973) reported a study of early hospital discharge after myocardial
infarction. Uncomplicated patients were randomly assigned to either
a two- or a three-week total hospital stay. During the six-month
follow-up period, there was no difference between the two-week and
three-week patients in frequency of return to work, anxiety or
depression, heart condition, or survival. A more recent study tried
sending half the uncomplicated patients home on the seventh day, with
similar results (McNeer et al., 1978). British randomized studies have
compared home and hospital care for acute myocardial infarction
patients and found no discernible benefit from hospital as compared
to home care for most patients (Mather et al., 1976; Hill, Hampton
and Mitchell, 1978).

There were more than 380,000 hospital admissions for acute myocardial infarction in the United States in 1974. (Not all of these are

"uncomplicated" and thus suitable candidates for short stays or home care.) The average length of stay was 14.4 days. Patients with this diagnosis accounted for about 5.5 million hospital days. So the amount of resources devoted to care apparently yielding no marginal benefit in these cases may be quite large.

Electronic fetal monitoring has become a widely used technology in the United States. Associated with its use has been an increase in deliveries by Cesarian section. The percentage of deliveries by Cesarian section increased from 5.5 in 1965 to 12.5 in 1976. In the mid-1970s, monitoring added about $35 to $75 to the cost of a delivery, while Cesarian section raised the hospital cost of delivery by from $700 to $3000.

Neutra et al. (1978) did an analysis of 15,846 live-born infants, 47% of whom were monitored, to assess the effect of monitoring on newborn death rates. They developed a numerical risk score based on eighteen factors believed to influence the likelihood of death of newborns, and classified all the births into five risk categories. They then compared the death rates for those monitored and those not monitored in each category. They found that for the three-quarters of one percent of the births in the highest risk category, monitoring was associated with a reduction in death rate from about 304 to 195 per 1000 live births. In the 76% of the births in the lowest risk category, the death rate was 0.5 per 1000 for those not monitored and 1.1 for those who were. These differences were not statistically significant, which illustrates the difficulty of obtaining adequate sample sizes when one is looking for small differences in small risks. And the research design was not prospective and randomized so the possibility of bias remains. Nevertheless, the results suggest that monitoring the low-risk deliveries yields no health benefit.

A costly medical technology put into widespread use before its efficacy was established is Coronary Artery Bypass Graft surgery (CABG). This operation was first introduced in the late 1960s. By 1977, its annual volume exceeded 70,000 at a cost of roughly $1 billion.

The Veterans' Administration started a randomized clinical trial in the early 1970s with more than 1000 patients, roughly half of whom were treated medically, the other half with CABG. The results were published in 1977 (Murphy et al., 1977). Surgical treatment was found to prolong life for the 11% of patients having diseased left main coronary arteries. In the rest, there was no statistically significant difference in survival between the two treatment groups at follow-ups 21 and 36 months after entry into the trial.

There has been considerable debate over the significance of these results. Some have argued that surgical technique has improved considerably since the trial was conducted, and that there are important quality-of-life benefits not measured by survival rates. Be that as it may, the point remains that a great deal of spending took place in the absence of any scientific evidence that this use of resources produced better health.

These examples are suggestive, not conclusive. Each of them remains subject to debate or uncertainty. The lack of evidence of marginal health benefits may be explained in part by our inability to measure

health benefits that patients value. More research is needed to
clarify the extent of marginal health benefits and to establish the
overall magnitude of expenditures yielding essentially no marginal
health benefit.

Nevertheless, we may proceed with the hypothesis that it is possible
to reduce the utilization of some services without harm to the
health of the population served, and examine what is known about the
influence of different types of physician organization and payment
on the use of services.

Relationship of Physician Organization to the Use of Services

Monsma (1970) called attention to the relative importance of physician organization and method of payment, compared to price paid by
the consumer, in determining per-capita use of surgery. He
contrasted per-capita rates of surgery under insured fee-for-service
and prepaid group practice. Under insured fee-for-service, beneficiaries are usually subject to some coinsurance or copayment. So
the marginal cost to the patient of an operation is likely to be
positive. Marginal revenue to the physician is positive. Under
prepaid group practice, marginal cost to the patient is practically
zero, as is marginal revenue to the physician. The ordinary model
of consumer demand would predict less per-capita use of surgery
under insured fee-for-service. Yet the opposite is the case.
Marginal revenue to the physician appears to be the decisive
variable.

INSURED FEE FOR SERVICE

The fee-for-service or piecework system of payment is the major
payment system presently operating in the U.S. It rewards physicians with more revenue for rendering more services, and/or more
costly services, whether or not these improve the health or well-
being of the patient. Insurance typically reduces the marginal
financial cost to the patient for more services, after an annual
deductible is satisfied, to an amount ranging from 25% of the fee or
charge to zero, depending on the insurance scheme. (Time costs and
psychic costs of receiving medical care remain.)

Supplier-Induced Demand

Perhaps the most interesting and significant empirical finding about
provider behavior in the insured fee-for-service context is the
supplier-induced demand hypothesis. Fuchs and Kramer (1972)
reported: "supply factors, technology, and number of physicians
appear to be of decisive importance in determining the utilization
of and expenditures for physicians' services. The number of physicians has a significant influence on utilization, quite apart from
the effect of numbers on demand via lower fees. Indeed, we find

that the elasticities of demand with respect to income, price, and
insurance are all small relative to the direct effect of the number
of physicians on demand."

Specifically, using 1966 cross-section data among states, and aggregate indices of average prices received by physicians and average
physician visits per capita, they found that visits per capita are
positively associated with number of physicians per capita when
income, price, insurance benefits and hospital beds per capita are
held constant. The estimated elasticities under different specifications range from .34 to .51, and are significant at the .01 level.
They also found that visits per physician are negatively related to
average price and number of physicians per capita, though the
elasticities were not significant in all specifications of the
model. (There was a small insignificant positive elasticity of
supply with respect to price in one specification of their model.)
Elasticities of supply of services with respect to physician-population ratios ranged from -.49 to -.67, suggesting that an increase in
physicians per capita leads to a less than proportional decrease in
visits per physician.

Evans (1974) reported similar findings, though with substantially
smaller (in absolute value) elasticities of physician workload with
respect to physician-population ratio.

Such findings undermine the normative significance of neoclassical
demand theory. Proponents of regulation of health care services on
the public-utility model use this finding to argue that the private
market cannot allocate health care resources efficiently, and hence
regulation is necessary. While I find the Fuchs-Kramer view
persuasive, I do not accept the implication that a private market
cannot allocate resources efficiently in the health care sector. I
will argue later in this paper that, while there is good reason to
expect market failure in the purchase of individual medical care
services by insured consumers, an effective and reasonably efficient
private market can be organized around the annual purchase of membership in a competing comprehensive health care financing and delivery program, as exists in a few places in the United States.

Numerous criticisms of the physician-induced demand hypothesis have
been made both on logical and empirical grounds. For example, Yett
(1978) asked: "After all, if physicians really do have the power to
raise fees and sell more of the same services to a small number of
patients in areas where the physician density is high, why don't
they do this sort of thing under all circumstances? If the answer
is that they aim for target incomes, what determines the height of
the target?" Of course, to argue that the hypothesis leaves important questions unanswered is not to argue that it is wrong. As for
the height of the target, Evans (1974) argues that the origin of
such targets is no more unclear than the origin of the utility function.

Sloan and Feldman (1978) criticize Fuchs and Kramer for their lack
of a completely specified model, and they point to other empirical
findings that fail to confirm Fuchs and Kramer. For example, they
cite a study by May (1975) which reports significant positive
elasticities of utilization with respect to physician-population

ratios, but which finds much lower elasticities for follow-up visits
than for total visits (including first visits). The physician-
induced demand hypothesis would predict higher elasticities for
follow-up visits. But their main criticism is that Fuchs and Kramer
and other proponents of the supplier-induced demand hypothesis
failed to rule out quality-amenity variables as an explanation for
the positive association of utilization and physician supply. That
is, higher physician-population ratios could lead to higher observed
utilization in the absence of reduced fees in a manner completely
consistent with the neoclassical model if they led to reduced travel
times, reduced waiting times, and longer, better-quality visits for
the same price. Put alternatively, the total price to the consumer
for a quality-adjusted visit might be reduced in a situation in
which the reported unadjusted price was unchanged or increased.

To add to the criticisms on empirical grounds, Yett (1978) deplored
the use of aggregate data on physician services and prices rather
than more specific data on utilization patterns for patients with
the same diagnosis in areas with high and low physician-population
ratios.

To respond to these criticisms, Fuchs (1978) re-examined the
supplier-induced demand hypothesis using in-hospital surgery rates
and the supply of surgeons. As he noted, "Time costs... are likely
to be less relevant for in-hospital operations because the psychic
costs of surgery and the time costs of hospitalization are likely to
be large relative to the time costs of search, travel and waiting."
Moreover, the quality-amenity hypothesis seems unlikely in the case
of surgery since what evidence we have suggests that busier surgeons
produce better results (Luft, Bunker and Enthoven, 1979). Moreover,
in this study, Fuchs controlled for demographic factors including
age, sex, race, and education. Fuchs found that "other things
equal, a 10% increase in the surgeon/population ratio results in
about a 3% increase in per-capita utilization. Moreover, differences in supply seem to have a perverse effect on fees, raising them
when the surgeon/population ratio increases." Surgeon supply is in
part determined by factors unrelated to demand, especially by the
attractiveness of the area as a place to live.

If physicians can induce demand for their services, what limits
their ability or willingness to do so? Reinhardt (1978a) offered the
important distinction between services requiring substantial inputs
of the physician's own time and ancillary services produced primarily by non-physician personnel and requiring little or no input
of the physician's time. In the former case, the physician's
unwillingness to expand his workload indefinitely limits
demand-inducement; in the latter case, it does not.

While Fuchs's evidence seems persuasive, the supplier-induced demand
hypothesis continues to lack foundations in a completely specified
model of rational consumer and provider behavior. Fuchs (1978) con-
ceded that Yett's question remains unanswered: "If surgeons can
raise prices where they are more numerous, why don't they raise them
even higher where the surgeon/population ratio is lower? One
possible answer is that their incomes are already satisfactory."
However, a recent paper by Sweeney (1980) makes the point that a
maximum demand curve representing quantity demanded at each price

when (a) doctors encourage demand to the maximum extent, (b) physicians adjust price and quantity to achieve a target income, and (c)
a stable equilibrium exists (i.e., there is excess supply above the
equilibrium price), implies that an increase in the number of physicians must lead to a decrease in price and an increase in expenditure on physicians' services.

In searching for an explanation, one might be tempted to drop the
assumed stability of equilibrium and revert to the permanent excess
demand hypothesis enunciated by M.S. Feldstein (1970). However, Fuchs
(1978) cites very persuasive evidence that "the average number of
operations per surgeon is far below the level that surgeons consider
a full workload, and below the quantity that surgeons would be
willing and able to perform at the going price." So the paradox
remains. Happily for our profession, more research is needed.

The supplier-induced demand hypothesis has profound implications for
public policy. First, it exposes as naive the idea of reducing the
cost of medical care by increasing the supply of physicians. (This
belief was a powerful motivating factor behind the decisions in the
1960s to double the capacity of American medical schools and to
change immigration laws to encourage the entry of foreign
physicians.) On the contrary, more doctors appear to mean more doc-
toring and higher fees. It also exposes as naive the notion that
the medical monopoly artificially restrained the supply of physicians in its own interest. (It is interesting to contrast the lack
of opposition by the medical profession to the expansion of medical
schools with its sustained and effective opposition to the growth of
alternatives to fee-for-service practice.)

Second, it suggests that price controls applied to physicians' fees
may be counterproductive from the point of view of restraining total
health care spending. They may merely increase utilization,
including the substitution of costly procedures for comparatively
simple ones, and they may produce substantial external diseconomies
such as increased hospital use. In a review of the American
experience with price controls between 1971 and 1974, Dyckman (1978)
observed that "the greatest two-year change in physicians' services
occurred during the two-year period when price controls were in
effect, FY1973 and FY1974. While fees, as measured by the CPI, rose
2.4 and 4.0%, respectively, during FY1973 and FY1974 [compared to
increases in the CPI for all items less medical care of 6.4% in
CY1973 and 11.1% in FY1974] physician utilization increased 6.3 and
5.5% respectively." Utilization increased by 3.9 and 4.3% in the
two previous years and by 2.5 and 2.8% in the two subsequent years.
"The substantial increase in measured utilization during only
those years when price controls were in effect and the subsequent
resumption of more normal patterns of utilization increases suggest
that physicians may have increased billings to compensate for their
inability to raise fees." Evans (1975) described a similar
phenomenon, including "procedural multiplication," in Canada.

Third, as Evans (1974) noted, supplier-induced demand calls into
question the efficacy of deterrent charges as a means of reducing
utilization and moderating cost-increases under a national health
insurance plan. Deterrent charges might appear effective if applied

to a small subset of the population, for in that case the effect on physicians' incomes would be small, and an offsetting increase in supplier-induced demand might not be apparent. But if a substantial deterrent charge were applied to the whole population, physician incomes would be reduced, and an offsetting physician-induced demand shift might render the deterrent fee ineffective.

Recognition of physician-induced demand should lead economists and policy-makers interested in the utilization of health care services to give at least as much attention to provider incentives as they do to consumer incentives.

Fourth, as noted earlier, physician-induced demand undermines the normative significance of the demand curve for individual units of medical service. This is compounded by the substantial element of moral hazard inevitably present in a system of universal health insurance. All this suggests that the purchase of individual units of service by the insured consumer is not a good subject for economic calculation. Those who would prefer a private market to a government regulatory system of resource allocation need to look to other ways of organizing a market.

Physician Pricing

We do not have a satisfactory theory of physician pricing under insured fee-for-service. Measuring, or even defining, "price" of physicians' services can be very difficult. The "usual and customary fee" may not measure actual price because of price discrimination and/or variable collection ratios. Prices are ratios with dollars in the numerators and units of service in the denominators. The notion of a stable price for a service rests on the assumption that there is a stable meaningful denominator. But the "doctor visit" is not a precise or standard unit of service. Its duration and content may vary widely. A doctor may raise fees simply by "unbundling," i.e., by charging separate fees for separate services performed on the same visit. One would expect such problems to be less the more precisely defined and uniform the service is. For example, an all-inclusive fee for an uncomplicated delivery is a much more precise concept than "a follow-up office visit."

Despite these difficulties, various studies have provided evidence in favor of certain generalizations. First, several studies have found that fees are higher where physicians are more numerous. Newhouse (1970) found a positive partial correlation between physicians per capita and fees of .55. Fuchs (1978), in the study discussed above, found a positive effect of supply of surgeons on price. He explained surgeon location by various exogenous variables measuring attractiveness of the area as a place to live. Predicted price was found to have no effect on surgeon supply. Thus, Fuchs was able to "reject the view that the high correlation between price and surgeon supply reflects a causal relation running from price to supply." Reinhardt (1975b) and Blumberg (1979) also found higher fees where physicians were more numerous. Burney et al. (1979) observed that Medicare, whose payment system is based on a combination of "usual and customary charges" by the individual physician and "prevailing charges" in each area, paid an average of 33% more for services in counties with more than 1.75 doctors per 1000 population than in counties with less than 0.75 physicians per 1000. However, this finding is not universally accepted. Using a variety of specifications, Sloan (1976) quite consistently found a negative and usually significant relationship between fees and physician supply across states. The negative relationship between appendectomy fees and supply of surgeons was quite strong. This discrepancy in results remains to be explained.

Second, under insured fee-for-service, physicians earn considerably more per hour doing surgery and other complex procedures than they do in ordinary office-based patient care (Blumberg, 1979; Hsiao and Stason, 1979). For example, Hsiao and Stason found wide differences in hourly rates of remuneration for different services implied by prevailing Medicare charges. They reported, "For office visits in 1978, the general practitioner and specialist grossed $40 and $60-68 per hour, respectively. Corresponding rates for time spent in surgery depend on which assumption is accepted with regard to the value of pre- and post-operative care. When no adjustment is made for pre- and post-operative care, the hourly rate of remuneration ranges from $310 per hour for an inguinal hernia repair to $788 per hour for a lens extraction. Even under the most conservative assumption the time in surgery is remunerated at between three and seven times that in office practice, with wide variations between specialties."

This finding overlaps substantially with the finding that physicians' net earnings per hour are substantially greater in hospital care than in office care (Blumberg, 1979).

The public policy significance is clear: the fees now in widespread application reward physicians considerably more for providing costly, resource-consuming kinds of care. Of course, as Blumberg, Hsiao and Stason suggest, it would not have to be that way. A system of fees could be devised that would provide physicians equal profit margins for all types of services in order to eliminate the cost-increasing incentives.

ALTERNATIVES TO INSURED FEE-FOR-SERVICE

In the system of insured fee-for-service, there is little or no financial incentive for well-insured patients to seek out a physician who is economical in the use of resources. Hence, there is little or no reward--more likely a penalty--for the physician for being economical. If every insurance plan offers "free choice of doctor," there can be no economic competition among physicians, for each insured person's premium will be virtually the same whether he goes to the most expensive or most economical doctor. But there are alternatives to insured fee-for-service with "free choice of doctor." In the United States, many people choose voluntarily to limit their choice of doctor, usually for a year at a time, in exchange for what they perceive to be better care and/or lower cost.

Prepaid Group Practice

The largest alternative to insured fee-for-service in the United
States is prepaid group practice (PGP). In 1978, there were 130
PGPs serving about 6.4 million members. In a PGP, an organized
group of physicians, working together full time, agrees to provide
comprehensive health care services for a per-capita payment, fixed
in advance, to a defined population of voluntarily enrolled members.
There are many variations on this theme. The physicians may be
salaried or may receive a per-capita payment plus a share of the
program's net income. Some PGPs own their own hospitals. Others
do not. Some of the physician groups include a broad range of
specialties; others emphasize primary care and refer patients to
outside physicians (and pay for the services) when specialty care is
needed (Enthoven, 1980a).

Luft (1978) reviewed and re-analyzed 38 studies comparing costs and
utilization of people enrolled in PGPs with costs and utilization of
similar people cared for under insured fee-for-service. Generally
speaking, these studies compare people in the same employee group
and adjust for age and sex composition of the groups being compared.
Some of the studies examine Medicare and Medicaid beneficiaries. In
general, Luft found that total costs of health care services
(premium and out-of-pocket) for persons enrolled in PGPs are some 10
to 40% below those for similar people cared for under insured
fee-for-service. PGP enrollees have as many or more ambulatory
visits. But they typically experience some 25 to 45% fewer hospital
days per capita. Since the cost per visit and per hospital day in
PGPs and in fee-for-service settings appears to be similar, the
reduction in total cost is mainly explained by reduced hospital use.
There is no evidence that PGP enrollees are any worse off for
undergoing fewer days of hospitalization.

Luft (1979) has offered four hypotheses to explain the lower hospital use in PGPs and other Health Maintenance Organizations (HMOs):
(1) HMO physicians more effectively screen patients and decide which
ones really need to be hospitalized; (2) HMOs may undertreat, or
fee-for-service providers overtreat, nondiscretionary cases; (3)
HMOs may provide preventive care that reduces the need for hospitalization; or (4) persons who self-select HMO membership may be in
better health or have greater aversion to hospital admissions than
others. Luft noted "sufficient evidence is not yet available to
allow for a comprehensive evaluation of these hypotheses." There
are other possible explanations (see below).

Summarizing what evidence there is, Luft found (1) "the average HMO
offers care comparable or somewhat superior to the 'average' fee-
for-service practitioner;" "outcomes in HMOs are much the same as or
slightly better than those in conventional practice;" (2) the preventive care explanation seems unlikely: many new HMOs have exhi-
bited low hospitalization rates from the outset; and (3) "in general
these studies have shown few differences between people enrolling in
HMOs and in conventional plans."

The self-selection by healthier people hypothesis may remain a
source of controversy for a while. Eggers (1980) recently reported

a small sample case study in which Medicare beneficiaries who joined
a PGP in an open enrollment had a hospital use rate before joining
over 50% below the comparison group. However, the study design contained large potential sources of bias (Enthoven, 1980b). The groups
being compared were not equal in survivorship. Moreover, "new
joiners" may be unrepresentative of the whole group. Other broadly-
based studies have found no significant differences between PGP
enrollees and members of comparison groups in health status perceived or number of chronic conditions (Gaus, Cooper and Hirschman,
1976; Blumberg, 1980).

Multi-Specialty Fee-For-Service Group Practice

Economists naturally think in terms of the financial incentives
inherent in the per-capita method of financing as the explanation
for lower hospital use by PGP enrollees (Monsma, 1970). However,
some recent studies have compared per-capita hospital use in multi-
specialty group practices that are paid largely on a fee-for-service
basis with per-capita hospital use in PGPs. These studies have
found that the hospital use of the former closely resembles that of
the latter (Scitovsky and McCall, 1980; Christianson and McClure,
1979).

By way of explanation, Scitovsky and McCall suggest (1) "in a
group practice, the number of physicians and their distribution by
field of specialty are likely to be planned largely on the basis of
demand for the group's services...[it] is unlikely to add a surgeon
to its staff unless its surgeon members have more work than they can
or are willing to perform... Thus... they are much less likely to
be faced with the temptation to generate demand for their services
than their solo practice colleagues;" and (2) "peer presence is
quite likely...to make for relatively conservative use of hospitals
and especially of hospital surgery." That is, the professional
checks and balances inherent in the multi-specialty group practice
style appear to limit hospital use. A third explanation may be that
the large multi-specialty groups in question are equipped and organized to provide on an ambulatory basis services for which solo
practitioners must hospitalize their patients.

Individual Practice Associations

The next largest alternative to insured fee-for-service is the individual practice association (IPA). In 1978 there were about seventy
IPAs in operation with about one million members. In an IPA, each
physician continues to practice in a private office on a fee-for-
service basis. However, as members of the IPA, the physicians agree
to provide comprehensive health services to the enrolled membership
for a fixed monthly payment. To be sure the services are provided
at a cost that does not exceed the IPA's revenue, the physicians
agree to accept (1) a maximum fee schedule, (2) "peer review" and
controls on hospital use such as "pre-admission certification," and
(3) varying degrees of financial risk such as a pro-rata reduction
in fees if the money runs low (Enthoven, 1980a).

Luft (1978) found "no documented evidence that costs for enrollees
in individual practice associations are lower than those for people
with conventional insurance." Hospital use appears to be reduced by
IPAs by between zero and 25%. The key to IPA cost control may be
the presence or absence of sufficient competition to make cost
control an economic necessity for IPA physicians. For example,
Christianson and McClure (1979) report that in Minneapolis-St. Paul,
where seven HMOs compete, the larger of the two IPAs has hospital
use rates about 26% below the average of six comparison groups on
insured fee-for-service, though 30% above the average of the seven
HMOs.

Primary Care Networks

A third type of alternative to insured fee-for-service is the
Primary Care Network (PCN). In this model, which is comparatively
new and small, the enrolled beneficiary agrees to get all of his
care from or on referral by the participating primary care physician
of his choice. There is no deductible or coinsurance. The participating primary care physician agrees to provide all primary care
services directly, to arrange referrals for specialty care, and to
supervise all specialty and hospital care. For his or her own
services, the physician is paid a negotiated monthly capitation
payment based on the age and sex of the patient. For the referral
services, the physician manages a budgeted amount for all his or her
patients in the PCN. At the end of each year, the physician shares
in the difference between the budgeted amount and the actual
expenses. (There are "stop loss" provisions to protect the physician in the case of "catastrophic expenses.")

Moore (1979) reported that the SAFECO Life Insurance Company's PCN
in Seattle experienced 293 hospital days per 1000 enrollees per
year, compared to 350 days in Group Health Cooperative of Puget
Sound, a large PGP, and 479 days for Blue Cross insured fee-for-
service in the State of Washington. (These figures are not age-sex
adjusted. But when SAFECO's age-specific rates are applied to the
Blue Cross age distribution, its hospital use increases only to 310
days.)

There are several possible explanations for this reduced hospital
use. One is simply a response to the financial incentives. Self-
selection by patients presenting a favorable risk cannot be ruled
out, though the absence of coinsurance should make this option
attractive to high-risk patients. More likely, physicians who elect
to join such a plan are those who are more comfortable with a conservative practice style and therefore recognize that they can profit by joining a PCN. And there is "peer review" or "checks and
balances" in the interaction between the primary care physician, who
is acting as the patient's purchasing agent, and the specialist.
However, the experience with PCNs is too new and on too small a
scale to permit the drawing of any firm conclusions.

It should be emphasized that there are many variations on each of
these themes. And there are other "limited provider plans."
Ellwood and McClure (1976) have proposed the Health Care Alliance.

Newhouse and Taylor (1971) described Variable Cost Insurance. In
each case, the beneficiary agrees to limit his sources of care to
one or another set of providers; the premium he pays depends on the
ability of those providers to control cost. Physicians may be paid
on a salary or fee-for-service basis, but the "limited provider"
aspect subjects them to market forces.

COMPETITION OF ALTERNATIVE DELIVERY SYSTEMS

If in fact some physicians and medical care organizations can provide comprehensive health care services of a quality that is equal
to or better than that of others for a substantially lower cost, how
can they be identified and their growth encouraged?

One possibility now attracting support in the United States is to
organize a fair economic competition among alternative comprehensive
health care financing and delivery organizations. Such a competition can be defined by the following principles. First, there
would be <u>multiple choice</u>. Once a year, each consumer would be
offered the opportunity to enroll in any of the health care organizations operating in his area. Second, <u>subsidies</u> to assist consumers in the payment of premiums would be in <u>fixed-dollar amounts</u>.
Such subsidies would replace the almost open-ended entitlements
characteristic of most government- and employer-provided health
care financing plans today. Such subsidies would be usable only as
premium contributions to qualified health care plans. They could be
related to financial and predicted medical need. Third, <u>a uniform
set of rules</u> would apply to all health care plans. Rules would
govern premium setting practices (nondiscriminatory pricing), minimum benefit packages, catastrophic expense protection, etc. For
example, all plans eligible to receive subsidies would have to agree
to participate in an annual open enrollment. The point of such
rules would be to curtail such practices as preferred-risk selection
or the selling of deceptive or inadequate coverage. (If health
plans are free to select only good risks, the poor risks become
uninsurable. However, higher-risk people, if separately identified,
might be charged higher premiums and receive correspondingly higher
subsidies.) Fourth, <u>physicians</u> would be organized <u>in competing
economic units</u>, the "limited provider plans" discussed above, so
that the premium each health care plan charged would reflect the
ability of its physicians to control costs. Consumers would voluntarily limit their choice of doctors, for a year at a time, to those
participating in one or another health care plan, or to specialists
to whom they are referred by participating doctors (Enthoven,
1980a).

In such a system, physicians would have incentives to control costs
and to act in the best economic interests of their enrolled members.
Utilization of services would be limited to the level at which
marginal units were valued by the enrolled members at their marginal
cost. Moral hazard would be controlled by various combinations of
copayments, waiting times, and providers instructing patients in the
appropriate use of the health care system. Consumers choosing more
costly health plans would pay the difference between the premium and

the subsidy level; thus they would pay the full incremental cost of the more costly health plans. Consumers would make a purchase decision once a year, usually when they were well, rather than attempting to make economic decisions under stress at the time of medical need. Such a market would be organized around the annual choice of comprehensive health care financing and delivery organizations, whose reputations and practices consumers could reasonably be expected to be able to evaluate, and not around the purchase of individual units of medical care service.

Such markets are emerging in several places in the United States. For example, in Minneapolis-St. Paul the leading employers adopted the market strategy in the early 1970s. In 1970, there was one HMO in the area serving 36,000 people. Today, there are seven HMOs serving 370,000 enrollees, five of which are group practices, and two of which are IPAs. From 1972 through 1979, they sustained an annual compound growth rate in membership of 29%, an increase in market share from 3 to 16% (Christianson and McClure, 1979). Several leading employers have 60% or more of their employees enrolled in HMOs (though all have the choice of insured fee-for-service).

Competition among HMOs is also emerging in the main metropolitan areas of the West Coast. However, its growth has been attenuated by the fact that most employers either do not offer their employees choices or, if they do, pay 100% of the premium whichever choice the employee makes. This practice is encouraged by the income tax laws which make such employer contributions tax free to the employee. Competition is also attenuated by Medicare and Medicaid which do not allow the beneficiaries to keep for themselves the savings that would be generated if they were to join an HMO.

Several bills have been introduced in Congress to eliminate these barriers to fair economic competition among alternative health care plans. If any should pass, the accelerated development of such competition should provide many attractive research opportunities for health care economists.

CONCLUSION

When you consult a physician for care of a serious illness, what financial incentives do you want him or her to have? Let us assume that you must bear your share of the expected per-capita cost generated by his incentives and clinical policies. In that case, it is far from obvious that the fee-for-service system is best. What is clear is that you want him to be seeking to maximize your utility, not his. But exactly how does one translate that into a system of payment? Would you prefer that your doctor be paid fee-for-service, capitation, or salary, and be in a PGP, IPA, or PCN? If one of the latter, in which of their many variations? Nobody has worked out a priori what is an optimal payment system from the patient's point of view. Because of the great variety of ailments and treatments and the pervasiveness of uncertainty, I doubt that it can be done. In fact, I believe there will be dif-

ferent "bests" for different consumers, depending on tastes and
beliefs about medical care. Thus, overall consumers' surplus is
likely to be greater if there are choices. It seems likely that the
only way we will find good payment systems is empirically, through
trial and error, in an economically fair private market. The United
States now has the opportunity to try that approach.

HEALTH, ECONOMICS, AND HEALTH ECONOMICS
J. van der Gaag and M. Perlman (editors)
© *North-Holland Publishing Company, 1981*

THE INDUCEMENT HYPOTHESIS:
THAT DOCTORS GENERATE DEMAND FOR THEIR OWN SERVICES

J. Richardson

INTRODUCTION

The conventional economic model is based upon the assumption that
price and output may be explained by the interaction of independent
supply and demand.* For a number of years there has been doubt
about whether the assumption is correct in the market for medical
services. The alternative "demand-shift" or inducement hypothesis
is that medical practitioners have the ability to generate demand
for their services directly--that they have the ability to shift the
position of the consumers' demand curve.

The implications of this hypothesis are profound. Most of the
welfare conclusions of the conventional model are derived from the
fact that the self-interested behavior of both supplier and consumer
is held in check by the self-interested behavior of the other.
Under idealized conditions the interaction of the two groups results
in Pareto efficiency, and with even moderately imperfect conditions
an acceptable level of efficiency may be expected to result from it.
By contrast, the interdependence of supply and demand postulated by
the demand-shift hypothesis implies that little normative significance can be attached to the outcome of the freely operating medical
market. The "revealed preference" of consumers may have more to do
with producer than consumer welfare.

Despite its importance, there has been comparatively little testing
of the theory.[1] Much of the early support was obtained from casual
observations of an association between the supply and demand for
surgical procedures and doctors' services generally, and from the
weak association between doctor density and doctor incomes. These
observations, however, are also compatible with the competitive

---

*The author is indebted to a large number of persons for their assistance with
this project; in particular to Professors V. Fuchs and D. Throsby, Drs. J. Deeble,
J. Newhouse and G. Withers, Messrs. B. Ferguson, R. Harvey and G. Madden for comments and to E. Golder and S. Manefield for assistance with computing. The
research was financed by a Health Program Grant from the Australian Commonwealth
Department of Health.

model. The limited number of econometric studies to date produced
results consistent with inducement, but all have encountered
problems with either the quality of data used or the specification
of the models tested. Econometric results are also unconvincing
unless there is a "micro theory" of consumer and producer behavior
compatible with the hypothesis. This aspect of inducement has
received surprisingly little attention (see Evans, 1973, 1974,
1976c).

The present paper is in two parts. The first tests two models of
demand-shift, using 1976 pooled cross-section data from the final
six-month period of the Australian compulsory health insurance
scheme (Medibank). Its objective is to establish whether the data
are consistent with the inducement theory. The second part
discusses the "microeconomics" of demand shift.

TESTING DEMAND-SHIFT WITH AUSTRALIAN DATA

The empirical study reported in this section is based upon the
framework used by Fuchs and Kramer (1972). The price and utilization data were obtained from a one in ten sample of the persons
receiving benefits during the final six months of the Australian
compulsory health insurance scheme, Medibank. This provided medical
insurance to the entire population from July 1975 to September 1976.
Fixed rebates were determined so that when doctors charged the
"schedule fee," there would be a patient copayment of 15% or $5.00
per item billed, whichever was least. However, the actual copayment
was dependent upon the unconstrained fees charged by doctors.[2] For
about one third of services it was zero, as doctors accepted the
benefit as full payment. The average copayment varied between statistical divisions from $0.42 to $1.80 for general practitioner consultations and from $2.30 to $5.51 for consultations with
specialists. The national average copayment was 11% for both types
of service.

In June 1976 a population census was conducted which also collected
information on household income, ethnicity and education. The combination of these two sources provides a data set of exceptional
reliability.[3] Relevant information was aggregated to provide 58
observations corresponding to the statistical divisions (S.D.)
across Australia. Definitions and data sources of other variables
used in the study are given in Appendix 2 and summary statistics in
Appendix 1.

Two Models of the Medical Market

Two models, 1 and 2, are tested. In both, there is a demand
equation containing the usual independent variables and, in addition, the estimated doctor supply is included to detect any shifting
of the demand curve which might be attributed to doctors after standardizing for the effect of other variables.

The chief difference between the two models is that the first
assumes that doctors are price-takers: prices are determined by the

interaction of supply and demand. By contrast, in Model 2, doctors
are assumed to have the ability to set prices as they wish.
However, it is postulated that price will rise with both the doctor
density and with the patient's capacity to pay (INC), and that they
will be raised to reduce excess <u>exogenous</u> demand, Q_E. A major difference in the models is that in the first, the doctor supply is
assumed to be a function of the gross price: the traditional market
information mechanism is assumed to apply. An increase in the exogenous demand for doctor services will increase price and this in
turn will increase the supply of doctors. (It should be noted,
however, that the comparative statics of the model do not imply that
an exogenous increase in the supply of doctors will necessarily
depress the price level. If demand-shift is sufficient, prices
might rise with supply.) By contrast with this, in Model 2 the doctor supply is a direct function of the demand for services: an exogenous increase in demand is postulated to result in some form of
non-price information mechanism attracting doctors into the area.

The Equations and Variables

The demand equation is identical in both models. In addition to net
price and income, the independent variables include a measure of the
expected use of services, Q, which is based upon the age/sex composition of the statistical division and the average use of services
by each demographic sub-group across Australia. The education
variable, EDUC, measures the percentage of the population in a statistical division with higher degrees or diplomas. The theoretical
rationale for the inclusion of this variable is discussed by
Grossman (1972a). Some allowance is made for time costs by the
inclusion of the variables DIST, WAGE and QUE. The first of these
is the proportion of services received by residents of a statistical
division (S.D.)--that is, it indicates the average distance travelled to obtain a service.[4] WAGE is an estimate of the hourly rate
of remuneration for employed persons. Since those outside the work
force are normally assumed to be there voluntarily, it measures the
opportunity cost of the time required to receive medical services.
Without the inclusion of this variable, the coefficient on income
(INC) would confound the pure income and time cost effects.[5] QUE is
defined as the percentage of a specialist's income derived from GP
items. Since specialist work is more rewarding, it is assumed that
the higher this percentage, the more easily patients may obtain a
specialist consultation and so the lower the queuing time. The
variable is the least reliable one employed in the study. It is
only included in the demand equations for specialist visits.

The supply of doctors is predicted by Equation 2. It is assumed
that the supply is influenced by either demand or gross price (see
above) and that doctors also locate themselves in congenial environments. This latter aspect is proxied by the level of economic and,
hence, social status of populations, INC, and a set of exogenous
variables, X_i. These include urban and state dummies[6] and variables
for educational attainment, an index of climatic comfort and--
following Fuchs (1978)--hotel receipts per capita. The equation
also includes the number of services per doctor. Fuchs and Kramer
(1972) suggested that physicians may have an aversion to locating
themselves in an area where a high exogenous demand for services may
force them to work excessively long hours. Hospital beds per capita
are included in the equation since, in the case of specialist doc-

J. Richardson

MODELS 1 AND 2

Model 1: Demand Shift with Market Determined Fees

$$Q_D = f^1(\hat{P}_n, \text{INC}, \text{EDUC}, \hat{DOC}, \text{DOCRAT}, \text{HB}, \bar{Q}, \text{DIST}, \text{QUE}, \text{WAGE}) \qquad (1)$$

$$DOC = f^2(\hat{P}_G, \text{INC}, \frac{\hat{Q}}{DOC}, \text{HB}, X_i) \qquad (2)$$

$$Q_s \equiv (DOC\,(\frac{Q}{DOC}) + Q^{ji} - Q^{ij})\, \text{POP}^{-1} \qquad (3)$$

$$P_N = \hat{P}_G - R \qquad (4)$$

$$\frac{Q}{DOC} = f^3(\hat{DOC}, \text{DOCRAT}, \text{AGE}, \text{SEX}, \bar{Q}) \qquad (5)$$

$$Q^s = Q^D \qquad (6)$$

Model 2: Demand Shift with Doctor Determined Fees

$$Q_D = f^1(\hat{P}_N, \text{INC}, \text{EDUC}, \hat{DOC}, \text{DOCRAT}, \text{HB}, \bar{Q}, \text{DIST}, \text{QUE}, \text{WAGE}) \qquad (1)$$

$$DOC = f^2(\hat{Q}_D, \text{INC}, \frac{\hat{Q}}{DOC}, \text{HB}, X_i) \qquad (2)$$

$$P_G = f^3(\hat{DOC}, Q_E, \text{INC}) \qquad (3)$$

$$P_N = \hat{P}_G - R \qquad (4)$$

---

tors, these are a complementary product. In equations where the dependent variable is GP services per capita, the number of out-patient departments per capita is included, since these are competitive with the services of general practitioners.

Results

The two models were tested in linear form and also using a log transformation of all variables. Both OLS and 2SLS regressions were

KEY TO MODELS 1 AND 2

$\hat{}$ = Denotes a variable whose value is predicted in State I when 2SLS estimates are used

$\frac{Q}{DOC}$ = Doctor productivity

INC = Average family income

Q_D = Demand for medical services per capita

EDUC = Education attainment of the population

Q_s = Supply of medical services per capita

HB = Total hospital beds

Q^{ij} = Services given in the S.D. (i) to residents elsewhere (j)

DIST = Distance travelled to obtain a consultation

WAGE = Estimated wage rate in an S.D.

Q^{ji} = Services given elsewhere (j) to residents of the S.D. (i)

QUE = A proxy variable for queuing time

$\bar{Q}$ = Demand for medical services predicted from the age sex composition of an S.D.

X_i = Variables indicating the desirability of the S.D. as a residence

AGE = Average age of doctors

Q_E = Exogenous demand variables

SEX = Proportion of male doctors

DOC = Doctor supply in an S.D. per 1000 population

$P_N;P_G$ = Net and Gross Price of a doctor's visit

DOCRAT = The ratio of specialists to GPs

R = The insurance rebate

run. Variables were retained despite large standard errors either when they were essential to the model, or when the signs obtained were consistent and as expected on theoretical grounds in each of the four formulations of the model. Other variables were eliminated from the analyses.[7]

In Tables 1 and 2, the results of the two models are presented for all doctors (GPs plus specialists). In the key demand equation (Equation 1) only one of the exogenous demand variables--distance-- is significant. The sign on DIST is negative as expected; that is, as the time taken to obtain a consultation rose, the demand for doctor services fell. Neither family income nor the net price of doctor visits proved to be significant. The former result is not

J. Richardson

Table 1. Results from Model 1: All Doctors

	2SLS				OLS			
	LINEAR		LOG		LINEAR		LOG	
Equation 1: Quantity Demanded								
DOC	1.72	(2.57)	1.10	(5.59)	1.74	(6.14)	.82	(8.49)
HB1	.02	(1.41)	−.01	(−.10)	.02	(1.85)	.02	(0.26)
HB2	−10.90	(−2.04)	−.02	(−.90)	−10.87	(−2.57)	−.02	(−1.37)
DIST	−.78	(−0.73)	−.44	(−2.23)	−.75	(−1.38)	−.43	(−2.69)
EDUC	−.07	(−1.88)	0.08	(0.52)	−.07	(−2.50)	−.11	(−1.16)
					(R^2 = .74)		(R^2 = .77)	
Equation 2: Doctor Supply								
P_G	.04	(1.21)	.66	(0.74)	−.02	(−.95)	−1.00	(−1.48)
Q/DOC	.01	(2.43)	1.73	(2.35)	−.002	(−1.46)	−.37	(−1.32)
QLD	−.38	(−3.44)	−.63	(−3.50)	−.21	(−3.30)	−.27	(−1.82)
WA	−.15	(−2.09)	−.27	(−1.54)	−.25	(−3.63)	−.54	(−3.37)
NT	−.08	(−.36)	−.62	(−1.37)	−.58	(−4.15)	−1.62	(−4.83)
URBAN	.04	(0.78)	.08	(0.68)	.04	(0.75)	.06	(0.51)
MS	.40	(4.84)	.42	(2.24)	.34	(4.08)	.42	(2.11)
EDUC	.03	(1.99)	.58	(2.11)	.03	(1.74)	.56	(1.97)
					(R^2 = .58)		(R^2 = .51)	
Equation 3: Net Fee								
P_G	.99	(.14)						
R	−.99	(−.16)						
Equation 4: Doctor Productivity								
AGE					3.00	(2.70)	1.37	(3.55)
SEX					−227.9	(−1.81)	−2.60	(−1.35)
					(R^2 = .14)		(R^2 = .19)	

surprising in a market in which there is widespread and comprehensive insurance, since the resource constraint upon individual utilization is largely removed. The latter result does not imply that price was an unimportant determinant of individual demand. In the aggregation of individual utilization some other factor--presumably the doctor supply--may have offset any price effects. That is, price variation within a statistical division may simply have redistributed a volume of services which was doctor-determined.

By contrast with these results, doctor supply (DOC) is highly significant in all regressions and the coefficients obtained are comparatively stable. The linear models indicate that an increase of one doctor per 1000 population resulted in an increase in the number of visits per capita in the six month period of between 1.02 (Model 2, 2SLS) and 1.70 (all other runs). The log equations show that a 10% increase in the doctor supply was associated with an increased utilization of between 7.2% (Model 2, 2SLS) and 11.0% (Model 1, 2SLS). Since elasticities greater than unity are implausible, it appears that the OLS coefficient is more reliable than the comparatively unstable 2SLS estimate.

The variable reflecting the educational attainment of the population (EDUC) is significant and with one exception (Model 1, 2SLS) has the expected negative sign. _Ceteris paribus_, more educated populations were less likely to use medical services than less educated ones. HB1, the hospital beds per 1000 population, displays a positive sign in these results, suggesting that hospital beds may be a complementary good. By contrast, the sign of HB2 (the number of hospitals per capita with beds greater than 200) is negative. This suggests that as the number of out-patient departments rises, the demand for private services falls. However, since these last two results are

---

NOTE TO TABLE 1, FACING

For definitions, see Key to Models 1 and 2, and Appendix 2.

      t-values in parentheses.

    MS: a dummy variable for the location of a medical school in an S.D.

    NT, QLD, SA, WA: dummy variables for the Northern Territory and the States of Queensland, South Australia and Western Australia respectively

    URBAN: a dummy variable for a predominantly urban S.D.

    HB1: hospital beds per capita times 10

    HB2: outpatient departments/1,000 population

J. Richardson

Table 2. Results from Model 2: All Doctors

	2SLS				OLS			
	LINEAR		LOG		LINEAR		LOG	
Equation 1: Quantity Demanded								
DOC	1.02	(1.92)	.72	(3.76)	1.74	(6.14)	.82	(8.49)
HB1	.03	(1.59)	.04	(0.28)	.02	0.02	.02	(0.26)
HB2	-12.04	(-2.21)	-.02	(-1.05)	-10.87	(-2.57)	-.02	(-1.37)
DIST	-1.80	(-2.01)	-.42	-1.89	-.75	(-1.38)	-.43	(-2.69)
EDUC	-.05	(-1.48)	-.17	(-1.09)	-.07	(-2.50)	-.11	(-1.16)
					(R^2 = .74)		(R^2 = .77)	
Equation 2: Doctor Supply								
Q_D	.37	(6.51)	1.15	(6.66)	.30	(11.06)	.98	(15.77)
Q/DOC	-.004	(-4.75)	-1.02	(-4.90)	-.003	(-5.67)	-.92	(-8.31)
WA	-.02	(-.30)	.08	(0.60)	-.06	(-1.42)	.01	(0.10)
NT	-.13	(-1.05)	-.01	(-0.5)	-.21	(-2.58)	-.24	(-1.54)
URBAN	.04	(1.08)	.02	(0.26)	.04	1.40	.03	(0.65)
MS	.12	(1.73)	.03	(0.20)	.16	(3.31)	.08	(0.95)
EDUC	.02	(1.72)	.16	(0.79)	.02	(2.42)	.20	(1.74)
					(R^2 = .87)		(R^2 = .91)	
Equation 3: Gross Fee								
DOC	6.48	(4.82)	.10	(1.88)	2.94	(2.98)	.04	(1.14)
INC	.0002	(1.62)	.32	(2.56)	.0003	(2.06)	.26	(2.19)
$\bar{Q}$	-1.80	(-1.12)	.18	(0.56)	.73	(0.43)	.21	(0.65)
DIST	8.61	(3.86)	.04	(0.94)	3.59	(1.92)	.001	(0.02)
					(R^2 = .24)		(R^2 = .13)	

not repeated in the models for general practitioners and specialists separately, they cannot be accepted with confidence.

In the second equation in Tables 1 and 2, the two most notable results are the failure of gross price to be associated with the doctor supply (Model 1) but the highly significant relationship between demand for medical services (Q_D) and the supply of doctors. These results, which are repeated in the equations for general practitioners and specialists separately (Tables 3 and 4) strongly support the view that the supply of doctors does not respond to gross price, as postulated in the simple text-book market model, but responds to non-price signals.

While Fuchs and Kramer (1972) failed to find support for their hypothesis that doctors avoid areas where the workload forced upon them is too great, the results here are consistent with the suggestion. With two exceptions (Model 1, TSLS), the coefficient on Q/DOC is negative, and in Model 2 it is highly significant. Subsequent regressions (Tables 3 and 4) clearly indicate that it is general practitioners who displayed this behavior. The significant positive coefficient in the specialist equations (Table 4) is probably due to the fact that in Australia specialists locate their practices close to hospitals where they have access to publicly provided technology which increases their productivity.

The other results reported in Equation 2 are as expected. Doctors revealed a preference for living in urban centers (URBAN) and locating their practice near a medical school (MEDSCHOOL). Despite lower demand, more doctors were located in the better educated centers where the social environment was presumably more congenial to them. There was a disinclination to be located in the Northern Territory or Western Australia. Results from Model 1 also suggest an aversion to Queensland.

The other noteworthy result in Tables 1 and 2 is the outcome of the equations for gross fee in Model 2. These show that there is a consistent, positive relationship between fees charged and the doctor supply, which is highly significant in the linear formulations of the model. However, since these results do not allow for the composition of the doctor supply--the percentage of doctors who are general practitioners and specialists--they could reflect the positive association between total doctor supply and the percentage of specialist doctors in the supply. Subsequent results in Tables 3 and 4 support this view. Only GP fees are shown to rise with the doctor supply and the standard errors of the estimated coefficients are larger than in Tables 1 and 2. Despite this, the results contradict the hypothesis that, ceteris paribus, an increase in the doctor supply will be associated with decreasing fees.

The results in Equation 3 also reveal a consistent positive relation between income and fees. Subsequent results in Tables 3 and 4 show that this positive association also exists for general practitioners and for specialists separately--that the results are both consistent and stable for both groups, but significant in the statistical sense only for general practitioners. Linear equations show an average increase of 11 cents in GP fees for each $1000 increment to family income, and a 26 cent rise in specialist fees. Log results imply an

J. Richardson

Table 3. Results for GPs

	2SLS				OLS			
	LINEAR		LOG		LINEAR		LOG	

MODEL 1

Equation 1: Quantity Demanded

P_N	.44	1.23	.67	(2.22)	.09	0.47	.30	1.85
DOC	1.45	(2.26)	.46	(2.53)	1.61	(4.18)	.51	(4.79)
$\bar{Q}$	.13	(0.23)	.42	(0.51)	.01	(0.02)	.39	(0.55)
DIST	-1.46	(-1.78)	-.35	(-2.41)	-1.25	(-2.14)	-.30	(-2.81)
WAGE	-.23	(-2.90)	-1.57	(-3.32)	-.19	(-3.01)	-1.30	(-3.44)
EDUC	-.02	(-.49)	-.26	(-1.06)	-.02	(-.56)	-.19	(-.98)
					(R^2 = .69)		(R^2 = .76)	

Equation 2: Doctor Supply

P_G	.06	(0.94)	-.60	(-.41)	.05	(1.18)	-.23	(-.19)
Q/DOC	-.002	(-4.00)	-.82	(-3.12)	-.001	(-4.20)	-.72	(-3.75)
SA	.07	(1.27)	.14	(0.69)	.07	(1.34)	.16	(0.84)
WA	-.09	(-1.67)	-.38	(-1.93)	-.09	(-1.88)	-.35	(-1.95)
NT	-.40	(-4.47)	-1.62	(-4.93)	-.39	(-4.79)	-1.58	(-5.09)
MS	.17	(3.09)	.29	(1.38)	.18	(3.43)	.29	(1.47)
EDUC	.01	(0.76)	.37	(1.26)	.01	(0.90)	.37	(1.33)
					(R^2 = .63)		(R^2 = .52)	

MODEL 2

Equation 1: Quantity Demanded

P_N	.42	(0.95)	.98	(2.85)	.09	(0.47)	.30	(1.85)
DOC	1.06	(1.73)	.28	(1.71)	1.61	(4.18)	.51	(4.79)
$\bar{Q}$	.30	(0.53)	.67	(0.81)	.01	(0.02)	.39	(0.55)

Table 3 (continued)

	2SLS				OLS			
	LINEAR		LOG		LINEAR		LOG	
DIST	-1.87	(-2.35)	-.48	(-3.52)	-1.25	(-2.14)	-.30	(-2.87)
WAGE	-.23	(-2.72)	-1.95	(-4.20)	-.19	(-3.00)	-1.30	(-3.44)
EDUC	-.01	(-.21)	-.24	(-.96)	-.02	(-.56)	-.19	(-.98)
					(R^2 = .69)		(R^2 = .76)	

Equation 3: Gross Fee

DOC	1.31	(1.77)	-.001	(-.04)	1.04	(1.90)	.004	(0.20)
$\bar{Q}$	1.10	(1.22)	.41	(2.09)	1.25	(1.46)	.40	(2.07)
INC	.0001	(2.02)	.18	(2.39)	.0001	(2.15)	.18	(2.44)
DIST	1.02	(0.97)	-.01	(-.56)	.70	(0.80)	-.01	(-.47)
					(R^2 = .19)		(R^2 = .14)	

income elasticity of GP fees of 0.18 and for specialists of between
0.10 and 0.12. The results are rather more compatible with the view
that doctors charge according to an 'ability-to-pay criterion'
rather than, as often claimed, in accordance with the 'Robin Hood'
principle of increasing charges to the wealthy and correspondingly
decreasing charges to the poor. If only this latter principle were
applied, average fees would remain unchanged between geographic
areas, since the difference in fees would by subsumed in the
aggregation of the data.

There was little support for the hypothesis that fees rise with exogenous demand. Q, the age-sex predicted use of services per capita,
is significant in the logarithmic equations for GP fees but not in
the linear model or in the equations for specialist fees. Gross
fee is also positively related to DIST--the distance travelled to
obtain a consultation. This result, which is only consistent and
significant for specialist fees, was unexpected, since as distance
rises demand would be expected to fall. A possible explanation is
that as time costs rise, monetary costs become relatively less
important and higher fees may be charged without deterring patients.
However, since in Equation 1 fees do not appear to be a significant
determinant of the aggregate use of services, a more probable explanation is that as distance increases and the quantity of services
declines, the complexity, length, and hence cost of consultations
all rise.

J. Richardson

Table 4.   Results for Specialists

	2SLS		OLS	
	LINEAR	LOG	LINEAR	LOG

MODEL 1

Equation 1:   Quantity Demanded

P_N	-.02 (- .81)	.07 (0.26)	-.01 (- .74)	-.27 (-1.26)
DOC	1.55 (7.51)	1.19 (9.80)	.96 (6.69)	.76 (8.09)
DIST	-.02 (-.36)	-.003 (- .06)	-.14 (-2.92)	-.16 (-2.35)
EDUC	-.008 (-1.39)	-.44 (-2.64)	-.003 (-.61)	-.39 (-2.05)
QUE	-.20 (-1.31)	-.10 (-2.77)	-.30 (-1.82)	-.04 (-.95)
			$(R^2 = .73)$	$(R^2 = .75)$

Equation 2:   Doctor Supply

P_G	.004 (1.03)	.83 (1.22)	.001 (.032)	.54 (0.77)
Q/DOC	.001 (3.81)	.22 (3.87)	.001 (1.10)	.12 (2.59)
QLD	-.02 (-1.01)	-.09 (- .69)	-.03 (-1.01)	-.13 (-.88)
WA	-.05 (-1.90)	-.18 (-1.24)	-.06 (-2.27)	-.25 (-1.62)
NT	-.09 (-1.70)	-.99 (-3.20)	-.12 (-2.18)	-1.13 (-3.47)
URBAN	.04 (1.88)	.22 (1.98)	.03 (1.57)	.22 (1.85)
MS	.12 (3.83)	.41 (2.08)	.13 (3.75)	.46 (2.19)
EDUC	.01 (2.52)	.54 (2.08)	.01 (2.23)	.62 (2.25)
EMPLOY	.001 (3.50)	.30 (2.91)	.001 (3.21)	.31 (2.80)
			$(R^2 = .55)$	$(R^2 = .61)$

The supply and demand equations for general practitioners services
are reported in Table 3, and for specialist services in Table 4.   An
interesting result in the GP-demand equation is that the net price
variable has a consistent and sometimes significant positive sign--
possibly supporting the view that patients confuse price with
quality.   It certainly contradicts the hypothesis that the higher
demand observed in some Australian statistical divisions was a
result of lower consumer copayments.   By contrast, the coefficients
obtained for specialist services are negative and insignificant.

Table 4 (continued)

	2SLS		OLS	
	LINEAR	LOG	LINEAR	LOG

MODEL 2

Equation 1: Quantity Demanded

P_N	-.03	(-1.24)	-.14	(- .48)	-.01	(- .93)	-.32	(-1.53)
DOC	1.43	(6.68)	1.14	(9.07)	.95	(6.58)	.74	(8.00)
$\bar{Q}$	.34	(0.81)	.94	(1.22)	.40	(0.94)	1.41	(1.65)
DIST	-.03	(-.55)	.001	(0.01)	-.13	(-2.70)	-.13	(-1.98)
EDUC	-.006	(-.98)	-.37	(-2.12)	-.003	(-.42)	-.31	(-1.58)
QUE	-.19	(-1.18)	-.09	(-2.41)	-.27	(-1.64)	-.03	(-.86)
					$(R^2 = .73)$		$(R^2 = .76)$	

Equation 3: Gross Fee

DOC	4.28	(0.60)	-.02	(-.58)	2.93	(0.60)	-.005	(-.17)
INC	.0003	(0.98)	.10	(1.06)	.0003	(0.99)	.12	(1.26)
DIST	4.47	(2.41)	.02	(1.06)	4.21	(1.74)	.03	(1.68)
					$(R^2 = .20)$		$(R^2 = .14)$	

This discrepancy may reflect a greater consumer component in the selection of a general practitioner (and hence the confusion of price with quality). Specialists are generally chosen by a general practitioner on the consumer's behalf, not by the consumer himself.

The key result in these tables is that the demand for both general practitioner and specialist services is strongly influenced by the doctor supply. However, the influence is far greater in the case of specialist services. While a 10% increase in the supply of general practitioners was associated with between a 4.6 and 5.1% increase in GP services, a 10% increase in the supply of specialists is associated with between a 7.6 and an 11.9% increase in services.[8] This result was expected since, as noted, a larger percentage of GP services are initiated by patients. Also, since the technical complexity of specialist services is generally greater, consumer ignorance and consequently their dependence upon a doctor's advice is correspondingly greater.

The variable $\bar{Q}$ measures the use of services predicted from the age
and sex composition of a statistical division, that is, it is a
measure of "biological need." With the exception of the demand
equation for specialist visits in Model 1, $\bar{Q}$ is given the expected
positive coefficient in the demand equations. While the magnitudes
of the coefficients are reasonable, they are unstable between different formulations of the models, and the standard errors of the
estimates are large. This suggests a comparative insensitivity of
realised demand to "biological need."

Three variables--DIST, WAGE and QUE--were included to measure the
cost of time to consumers. For both GP and specialist visits, the
coefficient for distance is consistently negative and comparatively
stable. However, its quantitative importance is far greater for GP
visits, and the variable is only significant in the statistical
sense in the GP equations. The greater importance of time costs in
determining GP visits is also reflected by the results of including
WAGE--the dollar cost of a unit of time--in the demand equations.
In each of the eight equations for GP visits in Table 3, the coefficient is significantly negative: as unit time costs rise, demand
falls. The four log equations produced coefficients less than -1,
that is, a 10% increase in the cost of time reduced demand for GP
visits by more than 10%. By contrast, the coefficient in the specialist equations was neither consistent nor significant.
Consequently, it was eliminated from the analysis. The discrepancy
in these two results probably reflects, once again, the greater
discretionary component in GP visits. Individuals feel less competent to evaluate the costs and benefits of the more complex and
potentially more important specialist service than they do to evaluate the costs and benefits of a GP visit. Consequently, as the
costs rise, they are less likely to be deterred from persevering
from a specialist consultation.

This explanation is supported by the results obtained for the education variable, EDUC. Its coefficient is consistently negative, but
the magnitude is greater in the demand equation for specialists, and
the result is only statistically significant in the log version of
this model. This could be interpreted as reflecting the greater
confidence of more educated populations in evaluating the benefits
obtained from specialist services and so their greater readiness to
depart from the advice of the referring GP. Alternatively the
result could simply reflect superior health on the part of more educated persons.

The final variable reported in the demand equation for specialists--
QUE--did not prove to be a satisfactory proxy for time costs. It
was argued earlier that the variable, which measures the percentage
of a specialist's income derived from GP items, would also measure
the accessibility of patients to specialist care. The negative sign
on the coefficient indicates that this is not so. The result might
simply reflect the fact that as specialists spend more hours
carrying out GP procedures, the effective supply of specialists
is reduced. However, in other regressions the same result was
obtained after the supply of specialists was scaled down to allow
for the proportion of income derived from nonspecialist items. This
might have underestimated the true reduction in the effective supply
of specialists if, as is probable, the time taken to obtain a given

level of income was greater in the delivery of GP items than in the delivery of specialist items.

Summary and Discussion

A number of conclusions may be drawn from this study. Firstly, the 1976 supply of doctors across Australia could be explained fairly adequately in terms of both the demand for their services and the professional and social characteristics of the location. Secondly, supply did not respond to the gross price of services, and price did not appear to be the outcome of interacting supply and demand. Thirdly, the wide variation in the demand for services across Australia appeared to be unrelated to either net price or income, although time costs were important, especially for GP services where individual decision-making was relatively more important. The absence of a price effect implies that, within the range of obser- vations here, variation in the price of individual services may have simply redistributed a doctor-determined volume of services within each statistical division. Fourthly, more educated populations appeared to demand fewer medical services and, in particular, fewer specialist services. Finally and most importantly, the results give further credence to the inducement hypothesis--that suppliers generate demand for their own services. After allowing for other relevant variables, there was a strong and significant association between the supply of doctors and the demand for their services. The association was much stronger for specialists than for general practitioners.

There appear to be three possible grounds for rejecting these results as supporting inducement. Firstly, the doctor supply might only proxy time costs since all of these were not included in the study. These costs result from the queuing time between the first attempt to obtain a consultation and the actual consultation; from the distance travelled to obtain the service; from the queuing time within the doctor's office, and from the value of time to the indi- vidual. Only two of these variables have been included in the pre- sent study--distance and the value of time. It is probable that for general practitioner services the first of these costs is not impor- tant. Individuals usually receive services on the first day of the attempted consultation. However, queuing times in the doctor's office might still have a significant effect upon demand. Conversely, specialist services are normally by appointment and so the second cost is unlikely to be significant, but the queuing time between first contact and the day of the actual appointment might, potentially, be a deterrent to utilization.

These factors do not, however, explain the present results very satisfactorily. A study by Sloan and Lorant (1977) revealed little variation in office queuing time as the doctor supply rose.[9] Similar results have been found by the present author.[10] Consequently the "queuing-time elasticity of demand" required to explain the association between doctor supply and demand is absurdly high. In the case of specialist services, it is the (nearly) uni- versal practice in Australia to be referred rather than to seek a direct consultation. The length of the queue is known to influence

the GP's choice of specialist, and it can result in a referral to
another statistical division, but it is unlikely to affect his medical judgement about the desirability of a consultation. Patients
may, of course, fail to follow the GP's advice if queuing time is
too long, but the marginal effort required to remember a consultation over a six- rather than a two-week period appears to be
too small to represent a serious deterrent.

Secondly, there may be a systematic variation in the quality of services with the doctor supply and this may generate an increased
demand for services. A second U.S. study by Sloan and Lorant (1976)
suggested that a 14-fold increase in the doctor supply would
increase the length of services by 12%. Analysis of other Medibank
data also suggests such a small increase in the length of consultations with supply that this aspect of the quality of services
can scarcely explain the observed variation in demand. However the
suggestion that the intrinsic quality of a doctor's service (per
minute) may be evaluated sufficiently well by a sufficiently large
proportion of the public so that poorer quality doctors are relegated to inferior (low doctor density) regions stretches the assumption of consumer rationality too far.

Finally, it could be argued that the results must reflect misspecification, since there is no sensible micro-theory compatible with
demand-shift. It will be argued in the following section that this
is not true, therefore allowing the conclusion that the present
results strongly support the inducement hypothesis.

THE MICROECONOMICS OF DEMAND SHIFT

A thoroughly satisfactory explanation of demand-shift should explain
the behavior of both consumers and producers. More specifically,
the theory should explain why consumers should abdicate responsibility for decision-making in the area of health care and why they
should hand this over to the self-interested producers. The theory
should further explain how producers, uninhibited by the counter-
vailing influence of independent consumers, use their additional
power, and what constraints prevent their increasing their income
without limit. The first of these questions has received a fairly
adequate answer in terms of the asymmetry in the information
available to producers and consumers. The second, more difficult,
question has received surprisingly little attention, and to date the
answers given have not been entirely satisfactory.

Consumer Behavior, Information and Market Failure

In the conventional market model, information is required, not
simply so that an initial purchase may be undertaken with adequate
knowledge of the utility value of the commodity, but also to permit
subsequent purchases to be evaluated in the light of the initial
experience. Consumers must evaluate products by attempting to compare their welfare with and without the product. The first of these

states is directly experienced after the receipt of the product.
Normally, the second may be assessed from the person's welfare prior
to the purchase, thus providing sufficient information to prevent
the repetition of an initial error and information which may be
relevant to other consumers. In other words, the market usually
contains a self-corrective mechanism.

Except for trivial illness, this is not the case with health care.
The course of events without treatment is uncertain. Homeostasis or
progression may occur which prevents consumers from equating welfare
without treatment with welfare prior to treatment. An assessment of
the most probable course of events is normally part of the medical
service being judged. This uncertainty hinders evaluation and the
process of error elimination.

Neither uncertainty nor an inequality in technical knowledge between
producers and consumers is an inevitable cause of market failure.
What principally distinguishes health services from most other products is the consumer's inability to assess adequately the probabilities in the uncertain areas. Since each episode of illness is, in
a very real sense, unique to the consumer, reliance on his own
experience is limited and, in the case of serious illness,
impossible. Patients could, presumably, consult with each other in
order to check diagnosis and attempt to assess the benefits of particular treatments or particular doctors. But other patients'
experiences are also limited; moreover, they are unique individuals
with varying homeostatic properties (homeostasis may make even the
worst medical care appear successful). Independent advice could
also be sought from a number of physicians, and judgments made on
this basis. However, since medicine is not an exact science, there
is ample scope for legitimate differences of opinion with respect to
both diagnosis and treatment, and the consumer has little ability to
judge. Despite this, individuals could, in principle, obtain a sufficiently wide range of opinions to make an accurate assessment, but
they would need, apart from time and money, to be aware of the
potential advantages of such an investigation and to have confidence
in their own ability to conduct the study and assess its results.
The first obstacle could be dismissed on the somewhat tautological
grounds that if people do not expend resources on information, then
the information cannot be worth those resources. However, the
second obstacle cannot be dismissed. While it is reasonable to con-
ceptualize a more or less idealized system of price-market institutions in order to assess whether market failure is inevitable, it is
not reasonable to assume that the market is populated with more or
less idealized people. The former assumption is useful, since it
abstracts from the influence of particular markets and thus indicates whether institutional changes alone would restore efficiency
(see Bator, 1958). The latter assumption would simply make analysis
irrelevant to any real-world situation.

A probable consequence of this informational impediment is the
substitution of a special relationship with a doctor for independent
consumer evaluation. There is considerable casual evidence to
suggest that in the provision of health care, patients want to trust
the doctor, and that consequently they will voluntarily hand over
decision-making even when some consumer input might be possible. A
large part of medical care is concerned with the receipt of comfort,

reassurance and sympathy, and it is difficult to receive these from
someone who is being treated in the way a second-hand car dealer
might be treated by Ralph Nader.

Producer Behavior

In the conventional market model, producer behavior is constrained
by the existence of a demand curve over which producers have little
control.[11] An increase in either quantity or price can only be
achieved at the expense of the other. Consequently, it is possible
to construct a plausible predictive model of business behavior by
assuming a single, simple objective: profit maximization.[12] If the
demand curve for medical services can be shifted, it is necessary to
explain why doctors do not increase their income without limit and
why, with such discretionary powers, doctors in different geographic
locations do not equalize their income and workloads. That is, it
is necessary to explain the nature of the constraints which operate
in the absence of fixed demand. Five possible explanations are
discussed below. The first three involve external constraints upon
behavior. In the last two cases, demand generation is constrained
by the nature of the doctors' own objectives.

   1. The first possibility is that doctors always shift demand as
far as possible. This in turn requires an explanation of the limits
to which the demand curve may be shifted and, in particular, whether
potential shift is a function of population characteristics or of
the number of doctors per capita. If it is the first of these,
then potential demand (D_{pot}) could be represented by the following
equation:

$$D_{pot} = \sum_i [\text{demand by age/sex group}_i] \, [1 + shift_i],$$

where shift i is the maximum amount by which a particular group's
demand can be shifted. However, if this term is independent of the
supply of doctors then so is the potential demand. The effect of
the shift factor would appear to be due to demographic variables and
there would be no unexplained association between doctors and
demand.

The hypothesis that potential shift is a function of the doctor
supply is equally puzzling. Why should more doctors increase the
extent to which otherwise identical populations will permit their
demand to be shifted? What prevents doctors in less doctored areas
from shifting demand to the same extent and increasing prices to
regulate excess demand? One answer is that the ability to shift
demand may be proportional to the time patients are in contact with
doctors, and that where there are more doctors, exposure time and so
the potential for shifting may increase. However, this explanation
is also unsatisfactory. Following an increase in the doctor supply,
exposure time to doctors must first be increased before additional
demand can be generated. If this occurred in the conventional way
then the increase would have to be associated with a decrease in

price or time costs, and the shift phenomenon would be
indistinguishable from the price or time cost elasticity of demand.

2. A second possibility is that doctors shift demand to the limit
in the long run but are constrained by political considerations in
the short run. This answer fails to explain the geographical
variation in demand-shift. There is no reason to suppose that the
over-doctored areas are closer to the long run than under-doctored
areas unless shift is proportional to the doctor supply--an argument
which again encounters the difficulty discussed above. It is not
clear why the "long run" has not already been reached, or why the
smaller doctor supply in the past faced greater political obstacles
than the larger doctor supply at present.

3. A third possibility is that doctors are individual maximizers
and "collective shifters"--that the collective, via the doctors'
organizations, set norms and that individual doctors maximize income
in the time they choose to work. This explanation simply transfers
the problem back one stage. What constrains the collective? Is the
potential shift a function of aggregate doctor supply or population
characteristics? Has the collective already exploited demand-shift
to its fullest? If so, how can it be distinguished from demographic
variables or from a simple price elasticity of demand? If
unexploited potential remains, what has constrained the collective
in the past? The explanation also implies the existence of price
elasticity of demand for the services of individual doctors which
exceeds unity. While this is not contradicted by the observation of
an inelastic aggregate demand curve, the majority of observers of
the medical market appear to agree that individual doctors could
increase their income, at least in the short run, by increasing
fees. Further, if such income maximization dominates the behavior
of the majority of doctors, it would be expected to be reflected at
the collective level, and there is little doubt that doctors, acting
in unison, could increase income in the short run by increasing
fees.

4. The fourth explanation is that doctors are "satisficers," not
maximizers--that there is no fixed constraint upon their demand-
creating potential, but that they will exploit this potential only
until they have achieved particular income and leisure targets. As
a consequence, demand generation would be directly proportional to
the doctor supply. The chief difficulty with this explanation is
that it fails to explain why there should be any systematic
variation in the income and work characteristics of doctors with
their supply. However, results published to date all show a systematic decrease in the number of services and income per doctor as
the doctor density rises. In the extreme case in which demand-shift
was totally unconstrained and doctor utility was a function of
income, leisure and their social environment, doctors would be
located entirely in the single most congenial location while less
pleasant environments would be doctorless. Incomes would be maintained at a constant level at the expense of the local population.

5. The most plausible explanation of doctor behavior appears to
be in terms of additional arguments which may enter their utility
function. Two which have been discussed in the literature are the
use of the doctor's discretionary power to shift demand (Evans,

1974; Sloan and Feldman, 1978; Green, 1978), and the patient's
income (Evans, 1976).

The usual assumption, that doctors dislike the use of their discretionary power, appears to reflect the belief that there is--or that
doctors believe that there is--a technically "correct" or "optimal"
behavior and that any conscious deviation from this must be a source
of disutility to a principled doctor. The argument is not convincing. Firstly, it implies that a significant proportion of the
profession--those in regions with a larger doctor-to-patient ratio--
are consciously behaving unethically. However, there are no other
a priori grounds for believing doctors to be less well endowed with
scruples than the remainder of the population. Secondly, the
assumption that there is generally a "correct" form of treatment is
implausible. Discretion is required in determining the length of
both the social and medical component of a consultation, the detail
of the background history to collect, the thoroughness of diagnosis,
the number of ancillary tests to conduct, the time to spend upon
patient education or counselling, and the need for repeated treatments and periodic monitoring of a patient's progress. In other
words, part of the doctor's task is to determine the number and
length of services, and the provision of an increased quantity may
simply be regarded as the provision of better-quality service.[13]
Finally, even if an "optimal" set of procedures were specified, the
demand-shift hypothesis would be compatible with doctors consistently recommending the "correct" level of treatment. Prices
could be raised so that patients would voluntarily purchase less
than the optimal volume. The doctor's influence could then be used
to shift consumption back to the correct level (at a higher price).
Since there are no objective criteria for determining either the
correct price or doctor's income, demand shift per se should cause
no moral qualms unless other objectives are postulated.

Evans's 1976c suggestion that patients' economic well-being (income)
might enter the utility function provides a more plausible explanation of the doctor's reluctance to shift demand to the limit. His
postulate that doctors are concerned with consumer welfare suggests
that both the price, P, and the quantity of services, Q, should also
be included directly in the utility function. If doctors believe
their services to be of value even on the margin, and doctors like
to help people, then, ceteris paribus, the provision of an increased
quantity should increase, not decrease their utility. If doctors
believe there is a price-elastic demand for their services, i.e.,
that higher prices would reduce some patients' access to medical
care, then price would enter the function, the partial derivative
being negative.

A less altruistic reason for including the two variables can be
obtained by assuming doctors to be concerned with their social
standing and the esteem with which patients regard them. The maintenance of low, "reasonable" prices in combination with long working
hours is more likely to achieve such objectives than the opposite.
While patients may be unable to judge the need for additional services, and so equate them with the quality of care, they are able to
appreciate the self-interested motivation behind higher fees.
Doctors are likely to be influenced by any resulting social
opprobrium, albeit on the margin.[14] Additionally, doctors' self-

esteem is likely to be dependent upon the same factors that determine their social standing. It is not improbable that many will
feel the need to justify the public investment in their education,
as well as their large incomes, by contributing to the achievement
of social objectives.

The resulting utility function would be given by Equation 1.

$$U = U [Y(DOC), Y(PAT), (P-R), Q, W] \tag{1}$$

$$Y(DOC) = P \times Q.$$

$$Y(PAT) = \bar{Y} - Q \times (P-R)$$

$$W = w \times Q.$$

where

Y(DOC) = doctors' income;	R = insurance rebate;
Y(PAT) = patients' economic well-being (income);	Q = total services/doctor
P = gross fee;	W = hours of work

Price and quantity are not shown as being interdependent since it is
assumed that the demand curve is shifted to reconcile the chosen
values for the two.[15] The first-order conditions corresponding with
Equation 1 are:

$$U_P = U_{Y(DOC)} \times Q - U_{Y(PAT)} \times Q + U_P = 0 \tag{2}$$

$$U_Q = U_{Y(DOC)} \times P - U_{Y(PAT)} \times (P-R) + U_Q + U_W \times w = 0 \tag{3}$$

Equation 2 states that price will be adjusted until the marginal
utility of income earned from raising price is equal to the disutility to the doctor arising from the adverse effect upon patient
income and access. Equation 3 implies that quantity will be
increased until, on the margin, the utility of income generated plus
the utility from assisting patients (U_Q) is offset by the disutility
arising from reduced patient income and the loss of leisure time to
the doctor.

The addition of some relatively minor assumptions about the partial
derivatives in Equations 2 and 3 suggests that, contrary to Sloan
and Feldman's (1978) assertion, the response to an increase in the
doctor supply may differ from the response to an increase in the
insurance rebate or patient income. In the first case, a falling
workload per doctor would initially reduce doctor income. Either
price or quantity would be increased. However, a given increment to

doctor's income would be achieved at greater expense to patients if
the adjustment was by price, since this would leave the insurance
rebate unchanged, whereas an increased quantity would induce a
greater insurance payment.[16]   Further, raising price would be a
direct source of disutility, whereas raising quantity would increase
utility.   As against these reasons for preferring an increase in
quantity, the volume of work would rise if this option was adopted.
However, it appears likely that U_W, the marginal disutility of work,
would fall with the absolute volume of work.   Consequently, there
would be a comparative preference for increasing the quantity of
services, rather than price.   If the workload fell sufficiently and
U_W became positive (since work is a source of social and self-
esteem) then the quantity option would be unambiguously preferred.

By contrast, following an increase in either insurance coverage or
patient income, workload would not decline and consequently the
disutility of work would not fall.   However, in this case it is
likely that both $U_{Y(PAT)}$ and U_P would decline as doctors become less
concerned with the impact of their actions upon patient income and
access.   Consequently, it is more probable that prices would be
increased in this case.   That is, the inclusion of patient welfare
in the doctor's utility function suggests that doctors will apply a
"capacity-to-pay" principle in setting their fees.

An unsatisfactory feature of the type of speculation here is that it
is extraordinarily difficult to test empirically the importance of
such nebulous (but nevertheless real) motivations as a doctor's concern with patient welfare, social and self-esteem.   While this is
unfortunate, it is not a fatal defect when the purpose of the argument is considered.   Aggregate statistical evidence supporting the
demand-shift hypothesis could legitimately be rejected as spurious
if there was no plausible micro-behavior compatible with the
hypothesis.   The purpose of this section has been to argue that the
theory cannot be rejected on these grounds.   It is at least as
plausible to suppose that doctors respond to a complex mix of social
motivations as it is to suggest that they relentlessly and single-
mindedly maximize only selfish objectives.

APPENDIX 1

Summary Statistics

Variable	Mean	Standard Deviation	Range
DIST(TOTAL)	0.25	0.13	0.05-0.70
DOC(GP)	0.43	0.16	0.04-0.83
DOC(SPEC)	0.21	0.09	0.02-0.40
EDUC	5.02	1.72	4.00-16.00
HB1	9.19	3.38	2.08-18.59
HB2	0.01	0.01	0.00-0.46
INC ($)	8799	1452	7092-14343
P_N (GP) $	0.86	0.22	0.42-1.80
P_N (SPEC) $	3.51	0.68	2.30-5.51
P_G (GP) $	7.39	0.45	6.70-8.82
P_G (SPEC) $	31.00	2.78	24.24-35.83
Q_D (GP)	1.30	0.48	.21-2.15
Q_D (SPEC)	0.34	0.14	0.07-0.64
$\bar{Q}$ (TOT)	2.08	0.12	1.79-2.62
Q/DOC (TOT)	110.05	23.30	38.5-179.8
WAGE	6.09	0.75	4.88-8.50

APPENDIX 2

Definitions and Data Sources

Sources
S1:   A one in ten sample of the full insurance record of persons sub-
        mitting a medical claim in Australia for the period June 1 to
        Sept. 30, 1976.
S2:   A 100% sample of doctor's records in the one-week period June 30
        to July 6, 1976.
Cens: The Australian census, June 1976
O.P.:   Official Government Publication

Variable (Source)	Definition

AGE (S2):   The average age of medical practitioners in a statistical division (S.D.), (GP, specialist or total).

DIST (S1):   The percentage of items delivered to patients resident in an S.D. from doctors practicing in another S.D., i.e., the percentage of items for which patients travelled to another S.D. (GP, specialist or total).

DOC (S2):   The effective full-time doctor supply per 1,000 population (GP, specialist or total).

There are no reliable statistics collected in Australia indicating the regional supply of doctors. Consequently, supply was calculated in the following way: (1) Doctors were classified as general practitioners or specialists. (2) They were divided into part-time or full-time doctors, the criterion being the receipt of $200 and $300 gross income respectively. Full-time doctors were attributed to statistical division in direct proportion to the percentage of their week's income earned in each statistical division. (For example, if a doctor delivered items valuing $400 in SD_i and $600 in SD_j then the doctor supply in statistical divisions i and j was increased by 0.4 and 0.6 respectively.) The income of all part-time doctors received in each statistical division was summed and divided by the average income of full-time doctors to yield an estimate of equivalent full-time doctors.

EDUC (Cen):   Percentage of population with higher degrees or diplomas.

EMPLOY (Cen):   Self-employed and employers as a percentage of the work force.

HB 1 (OP):   Hospital beds per 1,000 population.

HB 2 (OP):   Hospitals with more than 200 beds per 1,000 population.

INC (Cen):   Average family income per annum. This was preferred to income per capita as a measure of available resources.

MS: A dummy variable, 1 if S.D. has a medical school, otherwise 0.

NT: A dummy variable for the Northern Territory.

P_N, P_G(S1):   The net price, P_N, is equal to the (doctor-determined) gross price P_G less the (exogenously-determined) rebate, R. It is measured in dollars.

Q(S1):   The average number of medical services received per capita in a statistical division in the last six months of Medibank (GP, specialist and total). Since information was only available concerning the number of items billed, as distinct from visits, a sub-routine was used to collapse items into visits. In this, a second item received by the same patient from the same doctor specialty located in the same S.D. on the same day was assumed to have been delivered concurrently, and the fee and rebate were

combined with the basic fee and rebate. In cases in which
patients did not provide information on their health insurance
number, the items were attributed to the doctor's statistical
division and the total services scaled up by the ratio of total
to identifiable items. The magnitude of the error introduced
by the procedure is believed to be small.

$\overline{Q}$ (S1,Cen): The predicted quantity of services per capita was obtained by
dividing the population of each statistical division into 34
age/sex categories (17 age groups of five years each) and
summing the product of the resulting numbers in each group by the
Australian average use of medical services for the same group.

Q/DOC (S2): The number of services provided per full-time equivalent doctor
(GP, specialist and total).

QNS: A dummy variable for the state of Queensland.

QUE (S2): The percentage of a specialist's gross income derived from the
delivery of GP services.

R (S1): The insurance rebate, determined exogenously by the health
insurance commission.

SA: A dummy variable for the state of South Australia.

SEX (S2): The proportion of medical practitioners who were female.

URBAN: A dummy variable, 1 if S.D. is primarily urban, otherwise 0.

WA: A dummy variable for the state of Western Australia.

WAGE (Cen): The wage rate was estimated as the product of INC and the ratio of
total population to the number of employed persons times the
average number of hours worked per week times 46.

NOTES

[1]Sloan and Feldman review the literature up to 1977. Studies have sub-
sequently been published by Fuchs (1978) and Green (1978).

[2]It was legally possible for private insurance funds to offer additional "gap"
insurance for the (15% or smaller) difference between the "schedule" fee and the
Medibank rebate, but not for the amount by which fees exceeded the schedule fee.
Their officially reported annual payment was only $4 million, or 0.5% of the
annual medical bill. While this figure probably underestimates the actual
payment, the amount was so small that it is disregarded here.

[3]An estimate of doctors' incomes based upon Medibank payments was within 1%
of the figure derived from the Department of Taxation.

[4]Two other variables indicating travel within a statistical division were
insignificant and eliminated from the analysis.

[5]For a further discussion of this theory, see Owen (1969).

[6]There are no good a priori reasons for entering the state dummies into the demand equation. In Australia, there are no (known) significant state-specific disease patterns and the conditions attached to the federal funding of public health facilities ensure that these (potentially competitive) services are provided fairly equally by different state governments. Similarly, the regulations governing para-medical (and medical) services are similar throughout Australia so there are no grounds for believing that the level of other competitive services differ between the states. By contrast, there are strong grounds for believing that, on average, the statistical districts in the southeast of Australia would be preferred by doctors as residential locations.

[7]These included the specialist-to-GP ratio and average family income from all demand equations; and family income, the hospital variables, hotel receipts per capita, an index of climatic comfort and the dummy variables for the states of Victoria and Tasmania from all of the doctor supply equations.

[8]The higher TSLS coefficient again appears to be less reliable than the OLS result.

[9]The implied elasticity was in the order of 0.01.

[10]Unpublished results from a 1978-1979 survey of Sydney medical practitioners.

[11]Producers may attempt to shift demand by advertising. The inducement theory could be reformulated as a hypothesis that doctors can advertise effectively at very low or zero cost. However, conceptualizing demand-shift in this way is not helpful. The process and even the motivation behind inducement may be quite different from advertising elsewhere.

[12]Of course, other objectives can be assumed. The point here is that no problem arises in describing the limits to self-interested business behavior.

[13]The fact that in less doctored areas the same "quality" is not provided does not imply unethical behavior there, but simply the need for rationing of existing resources. Since doctors make these decisions, it is not the case that there is "excess demand" from patients.

[14]It is also probable that the collective is constrained in an analogous way. Several attempts have been made by governments in Australia to limit "excessive" fee arises by doctors, whereas the quantity of services has not been overtly identified in terms of the self-interested behavior of doctors.

[15]Since the empirical results show less than 100% demand generation, a full model of doctors' behavior should include a demand constraint over which doctors have some, but not unlimited, control. However, the purpose of the analysis here is solely to demonstrate the plausibility of constraints other than demand, and the omission is justified by the significant simplification in the argument which results.

[16]The argument is not true in aggregate in an unsubsidized insurance scheme, since premiums would rise as quantity rose. However, since the behavior of other doctors is given, the argument is valid in relation to each doctor's perception of his actions.

HEALTH, ECONOMICS, AND HEALTH ECONOMICS
J. van der Gaag and M. Perlman (editors)
© *North-Holland Publishing Company, 1981*

THE MAGNITUDE AND DETERMINANTS OF
PHYSICIAN-INITIATED VISITS IN THE UNITED STATES

Gail Roggin Wilensky
Louis F. Rossiter

Conventional wisdom regarding the demand for medical care holds that
it is the physician rather than the patient who determines the kind
and quantity of medical care which the patient receives.* Some have
argued that the degree of physician domination in the decision-
making will vary according to the type of service, the amount paid
by third-party payers, and the intensity of competition among physicians in the market area. In particular, it is believed that in a
fee-for-service system physicians are more likely to encourage
patients to return for visits or to order laboratory services and x-
rays when a third party pays for the services and when the number of
physicians in the population is high. To the extent that physicians
in fact determine demand, universal coverage under a national health
insurance plan, or manpower policies which increase the supply of
physicians, could result in substantial increases in the demand for
medical care. The role of the physician in determining the demand
for medical care has critical implications for the policymaker.

The purpose of this paper is to understand the following issues: Is
there empirical support for physician-initiated demand? If so, what
is the magnitude of this demand, however measured? Under what circumstances does it occur--that is, what medical conditions and what
market conditions are associated with physician-initiated visits?
Finally, when does induced demand become socially inappropriate?

The last issue is beyond the scope of this paper but it is an important one. In principle, providing advice on the level of medical
care required to satisfy individual demands for health is exactly
what the physician is expected to do as adviser and agent for the
patient. Of course, this arrangement has the risk of going against
the public good. According to the definition by Fuchs and Newhouse
(1978), demand inducement becomes questionable when services go
above and beyond what the patient would be willing to pay for if he
knew as much as the physician. While this provides a reasonable
rule for discussing the social welfare implications and the normative implications of physician-induced demand, it is a difficult
definition to apply or make operational. As a result, the present
research cannot measure the social implications of such demand,

---

*We gratefully acknowledge the comments received on earlier drafts of this paper
from Amy K. Taylor, Pam Farley, Roger Feldman, and Don House. The views expressed
in this paper are those of the authors, and no official endorsement by the
National Center for Health Services Research is intended or should be inferred.

and the findings presented here should not be used for such
interpretations. Nor can an evaluation be made of the medical
appropriateness of physician-initiated visits.

Instead, a model of physician behavior is presented which considers
two components of physician-initiated demand. Physician-initiated
demand has a "good" component, with the physician serving as a perfect agent, and a "bad" component, where demand induced by the physician is related to economic factors rather than to medical ones.
While the model and empirical evidence presented here cannot
entirely differentiate between these two components, it provides
direct evidence of the magnitude and determinants of physician-
initiated demand. The results are presented first in terms of
descriptive statistics and then in terms of the estimation of the
model. A final section discusses the findings.

A MODEL OF PHYSICIAN BEHAVIOR

In this section the theoretical determinants of physician-initiated
demand are developed on the basis of a variant of a model first presented by Evans (1974) and extended by Sloan and Feldman (1978).
The model is further extended, for present purposes, to include
several other factors which may influence physician-created demand
and which can be tested directly with the data available. The model
combines variables thought to influence supply and demand and places
them in the framework of a utility-maximizing physician.

In the model, the physician is thought to maximize utility, U, with
respect to income, Y, and to the disutility which arises from two
factors: first, the disutility from greater work effort (converted
to output, Q, through the production function) and second, the
disutility which arises from initiating demand--both medically
necessary and induced demand--expressed here as D. The utility
function is:

$$U = U(Y,Q,D) \qquad U_Y > 0, \; U_Q < 0, \; U_D < 0 \qquad\qquad (1)$$

where

$$D \equiv cPq^d. \qquad\qquad (2)$$

The term c is the coinsurance rate or the percentage of the full
money price paid by the representative patient in the practice, P is
the full money price of output, or the price the patient would pay
in the absence of insurance, and q^d is equal to the number of visits
in the practice initiated by the physician.[1]

Evans (1974) and Sloan and Feldman (1978) refer to D as "the extent
to which the physician exerts discretionary influence," and the
"physician's discretionary influence on patient demand." In our
model, D has a similar meaning but is measured as the financial bur-

den on the patient of physician-initiated visits, whereby the number of physician-initiated visits is weighted by the net money price, P^o. Thus, $P^o \equiv cP$.

D enters the utility function with a negative impact, which is clear from the first partials in Equation 1 where both $\partial U/\partial Q = U_Q < 0$ and $\partial U/\partial D = U_D < 0$. U_D is considered negative because increases in D imply the physician is giving poor medical advice or is prescribing unnecessary treatment. The physician receives disutility and is sensitive to these concerns because physician-initiated demand may not be associated with good medical practice and the physician may come under scrutiny by peer review procedures, insurers, or consumers. In addition, the physician risks having patients balk at increases in D. While patient demands do not influence inducement directly in this model, they nevertheless may enter in an indirect way; i.e., as a factor the physician considers as a part of the disutility derived from initiating demand. Patients are more likely to balk if out-of-pocket costs are high, and less likely to question the physician's advice when either c or P or both are low. The expression cP takes account of this influence and is used to weight physician-initiated visits accordingly. It is also consistent with the model and this formulation of D to consider cP as the patient's average welfare loss--a factor the physician considers with empathy while initiating demand.

This is the negative role of physician-initiated demand. The positive effects are seen in the full demand equation,

$$Q = q^d + q \ (P^o, \ R) \tag{3}$$

in which q^d is added to the consumer demand faced by the physician to yield the total demand, Q. As before, the net money price, P^o, is related to the full money price such that

$$P^o = cP \tag{4}$$

where c is the coinsurance rate for the representative patient in the practice and is predetermined. R is the number of physicians in the market for physician services relative to the number of demanders[2] and is constant in the short run.[3]

Finally, the physician's income is a function of output such that

$$Y = PQ - C(Q,W) + Y^o. \tag{5}$$

In Equation 5, income is the difference between total revenue and total costs plus outside income, Y^o. Total revenue is the full money price, P, times output, Q, and total costs, C, are a function of output, and factor prices, W, set in competitive markets:

$$C = C(Q,W).$$

Substituting Equations 2 through 5 into Equation 1 forms the objective function

$$U = U \{P[q^d + q(cP, R)] + Y^o - C(Q,W), q^d + q(cP, R), cPq^d\}. \quad (6)$$

Maximizing the objective function with respect to P and q^d yields the first-order conditions:

$$dU/dP = U_Y [q^d + q(cP, R) + Pq_p - C_Qq_p] + U_Qq_p + cq^dU_D = 0 \quad (7)$$

and

$$dU/dq^d = U_Y [P - C_Q] + U_Q + cPU_D = 0. \quad (8)$$

The first-order conditions suggest that the physician will set P such that the marginal disutility of work plus the marginal disutility of inducement equals the marginal utility of income from a change in price. Equation 8 indicates that the physician will induce demand until the marginal utility of the added income that comes from inducement equals the marginal disutility of work and the marginal disutility of engaging in inducement.

As Sloan and Feldman (1978) suggest, the sign of U_D gives stability to the model. This is clear from both Equations 7 and 8. If U_D were not negative, the last term in Equation 7 would be positive, suggesting that it would be possible to simultaneously raise q^d and the price of output without limit in such a way that output and the disutility of working would be held constant while maintaining or even raising income. This behavior would be counter-intuitive in that it would imply that the physician could induce, if the market would bear it, only one physician visit per year for which the price was equal to the physician's income, because there are no direct constraints or effects on the amount of inducement providers can exercise over consumers. The only check to inducement is through the disutility derived by the physician from the activity. Likewise, $U_D < 0$ in Equation 8 and the second-order conditions[4] ensure, in the extreme case, that the physician could not induce all visits from only one patient in order to maximize utility, since the marginal disutility of initiated visits is increasing for all patients as well as any one patient as it rises through more inducement. Thus, $U_D > 0$ plays an important role in this model.

Equations 7 and 8 can also be expressed differently. Dividing by U_Y yields:

$$Q + Pq_p - C_Qq_p - Mq_p - cq^dN = 0 \quad (9)$$

and

$$P - C_Q - M - cPN = 0 \quad (10)$$

where $M = -(U_Q/U_Y)$ and $N = -(U_D/U_Y)$. Here, M is the physician's shadow price of time and N is the shadow price of inducement. Rearranging Equation 10 gives:

$$P - C_Q - M = cPN \tag{11}$$

which guarantees that equilibrium occurs where price less marginal cost, less the price of the physician's time, equals the value of disutility caused by initiated visits.

The reduced form equation cannot be solved, but solving Equation 9 for q^d and Equation 10 for P, and substituting in Equation 9, gives the determinants of q^d. In general form:

$$q^d = f\ (c,\ P,\ R,\ q_p,\ C_Q,\ M,\ N)$$

or $\tag{12}$

$$q^d = f\ (c,\ P,\ R,\ q_p,\ C_Q,\ U_Y,\ U_Q,\ U_D).$$

In summary, the quantity of physician-initiated visits is a function of the coinsurance rate, the endogenous full money price of physician visits, the physician-to-population ratio, demand factors which influence the slope of the demand function, the marginal costs of physician visits, supply factors which influence the shape of the physician's utility function with respect to income and work, and the marginal disutility of physician-initiated visits.

THE EFFECT OF COINSURANCE RATE AND PHYSICIAN DENSITY ON PHYSICIAN-INITIATED VISITS

The two important exogenous parameters in this model of physician behavior are the coinsurance rate and the physician-to-population ratio (or physician density). To determine the effect of a change in these two parameters on P and q^d we totally differentiate the first-order conditions for utility maximization given by Equations 7 and 8. This yields

$$[F] \begin{bmatrix} dP \\ dq^d \end{bmatrix} = \begin{bmatrix} -U_{Pc}dc - U_{PR}dR \\ -U_{Dc}dc - U_{DR}dR \end{bmatrix}$$

where

$$[F] = \begin{bmatrix} U_{PP} & U_{Pq^d} \\ U_{q^dP} & U_{q^dq^d} \end{bmatrix}$$

and is positive by the second-order conditions.

The desired expressions for a change in physician density are given by:

$$dq^d/dR = [\overset{-}{-U_q}\overset{+}{d_RU_{PP}}] - [\overset{-}{-U_{PR}U_qd_P}]/|F|$$ (13)

and

$$dP/dR = [\overset{-}{-U_{PR}U_qd_qd}] - [\overset{+}{-U_qd_RU_{P}qd}]/|F|.$$ (14)

These are complex expressions which cannot be signed without some simplifying assumptions. By assuming a separable utility function, the marginal utility of income, the marginal disutility of work or the marginal disutility of inducement are not affected by a change in any of the other arguments of the utility function. Thus, by assumption,

$$U_{YQ} = U_{QD} = U_{YD} = 0.$$

Now, in Equations 13 and 14, $U_qd_R = U_{YY}P(Pq_R - Cq_R) + U_{QQ}q_R$, which is positive, and $U_{PP} < 0$ and $U_qd_qd < 0$ by the second-order conditions. Thus the first bracketed term in Equation 13 is positive. The expression for U_{PR} is also complicated, but by assuming a separable demand function (i.e., $q_{P_c} = q_{PR} = 0$) it reduces to $U_{YY}[\cdot]$ $[Pq_R - Cq_R] + U_{QQ}q_Pq_R + U_Yq_R$, which is negative.[5] Thus the first term in Equation 14 is negative. The expression for $U_{P}qd$ can likewise not be signed without assumptions.[6] The positive influence of P on the utility of initiating visits is seen by the terms suggesting that an increase in price raises income and reduces work effort, which both increase utility. The negative influence is seen in the terms which involve the disutility of initiating visits and suggests that a rise in price increases the disutility of initiating another visit, since the physician's disutility is related to the amount the patient pays. If the changes in the marginal utility of income (U_{YY}) and the marginal disutility of work (U_{QQ}) are small, and the physician is given the benefit of the doubt in terms of whether a change in P increases or decreases the disutility of initiating visits, then U_qd_P is negative. This reasoning makes the second term in Equation 13 negative and the second term in Equation 14 positive. Thus dq^d/dR is unambiguously positive and dP/dR is unambiguously negative, demonstrating that as physician density rises, the number of physician-initiated visits increases and the price of output falls. These are the "classic" predictions which are so often "contradicted" by empirical cross-section data, though it should be emphasized that what is true for this model of a single physician for a change in the physician density may not be true for data on a cross-section of physicians in markets with different physician densities.[7] However, as the comparative static results suggest, whether or not the magnitude of these changes is significant is related in part to the effect of R and P on the marginal disutility of initiating visits and the rate of increase in the marginal disutility of physician-initiated demand.

The effect of a change in c on q^d and P is seen from the following:

$$dq^d/dc = [\overbrace{-U_{q}d_cU_{PP}}] - [\overbrace{-U_{pc}U_qd_P}]/|F| \qquad (15)$$

and

$$dP/dc = [\overbrace{-U_{Pc}U_qd_qd}] - [\overbrace{-U_qd_cU_{Pqd}}]/|F|. \qquad (16)$$

More complicated than the above expressions for a change in physician density, both dq^d/dc and dP/dc are ambiguous because of opposing effects.

The first bracketed term in Equation 15, U_{qd_c}, is very similar to U_{qd_P} (in Equation 13),[8] with c having both positive and negative effects on the disutility of initiating visits since the disutility of physician-initiated demand is tied to c. By the same reasoning, $U_qd_P < 0$, U_qd_c is assumed to be negative. Assuming a separable demand function as before,

$$U_{Pc} = U_{YY} [\cdot] (Pq_c - C_{QQ}q_c) + U_{QQ}q_Pq_c + U_Yq_c + U_{DD}cP(q^d)^2$$
$$+ U_Dq^d$$

which is negative. Since $U_{PP} < 0$ and $U_qd_qd < 0$ by the second-order conditions and each term in brackets is multiplied by a minus sign, all terms in brackets are negative. The bracketed terms are subtracted from one another; thus dq^d/dc and dP/dc cannot be signed.

The comparative static result for dq^d/dc is important for present purposes and deserves some further comment. Previously, the sign for dq^d/dR suggested that if an increase in physician density occurred, the demand for a particular physician's output might decline and increase the quantity of physician-initiated visits as the physician moved toward a new maximum income. One should expect the same situation for an increase in the coinsurance rate, which would also lower demand. This would be true were it not for the negative terms in U_qd_c. These terms appear because the physician's disutility from initiating visits depends upon the financial burden on the patient. As a result, when the coinsurance rate goes up it lowers consumer demand, just as an increase in physician density lowers consumer demand and increases q^d. But an increase in c also increases D in the utility function. Thus, the positive consumer demand effect in dq^d/dc is offset by a negative effect on the marginal disutility of initiating visits ($U_qd_c < 0$). As a matter of speculation, the positive consumer demand effect is probably smaller than the negative disutility effect, with the result that if c falls, the reduction in physician-initiated visits that accompanies any increase in consumer demand will be more than offset by the greater willingness of the physician to initiate visits because the patient pays less. Thus dq^d/dc is expected to be positive.

THE INFLUENCE OF OUTSIDE PHYSICIAN INCOME AND FACTOR COSTS

The comparative static properties of the model enable us to explore two other factors which are included in this model of physician-initiated visits. The first is the possible influence of outside physician income on q^d; the second is the effect of an exogenous shift in factor costs. As the general expression for the determinants of q^d in Equation 12 demonstrates, both the marginal utility of physician income and marginal costs are determinants of q^d. The marginal utility of income is influenced by outside income and the level of factor costs influences marginal costs, so each is worthy of further exploration in their effect on physician behavior.

Recalling that

$$Y = PQ - C(Q) + Y^o, \tag{17}$$

totally differentiating the first-order conditions and using Cramer's Rule, the comparative static result is:

$$dq^d/dY^o = [-U_q dy^o U_{PP}] - [-U_{PY^o} U_q d_P]/|F|$$

$$= [-U_{YY} P U_{PP}] - [U_{YY} Y_P U_q d_P]/|F|. \tag{18}$$

Having signed U_{PP} and $U_q d_P$ previously, recognizing that U_{YY} is negative and Y_P is negative by the first-order conditions, we see that dq^d/dY^o is negative. Thus an increase in outside income reduces the number of physician-initiated visits.

Turning now to an exogenous shift in factor costs we recall that

$$C = C(Q,W) \quad C_W > 0 \tag{19}$$

and again by Cramer's Rule the effect on q^d is given by

$$dq^d/dW = [-U_q d_W U_{PP}] - [-U_{PW} U_q d_P]$$

$$= [-U_{YY} P(-C_W) U_{PP}] - [-U_{YY} Y_P(-C_W) U_q d_P]. \tag{20}$$

The first bracketed term is positive and the second is negative. Thus dq^d/dW is unambiguously positive, suggesting that higher factor prices, set in a competitive factor market, increase physician-initiated visits.

THE ROLE OF WAITING TIME

The model just presented can be extended further to include the waiting times associated with physician visits. As variables of choice available to the physician, waiting time to get an appointment and waiting time to see the physician can be utilized to influence demand for physician output. Accordingly, waiting time also has an effect on the costs of the practice. Thus waiting time, t, enters the physician-initiated demand model in two ways; first, as an argument in the consumer demand function,

$$q = q\ (P^o,\ t,\ R),\qquad\qquad\qquad\qquad (21)$$

where $q_t < 0$, and second, as an argument in the cost function,

$$C = C(Q,\ t),\qquad\qquad\qquad\qquad\qquad (22)$$

where $C_t < 0$. The role of t in Equation 21 is clear, since lengthening the time to get an appointment or increasing the waiting time in the physician's office raises the full (time plus money) price of receiving care. Waiting has a negative influence on costs, since longer waits to get an appointment and longer waits to see the physician mean that the physician can schedule appointments close to one another and reduce the risk of experiencing down time resulting from a patient missing, or being late for, an appointment. A busy appointment schedule with waiting patients will reduce the likelihood that support staff are idle or that the physician is available with no patients to treat (Savings et al., 1978). Thus, higher t can reduce consumer demand but also lower costs.

By including waiting time in the model and maximizing with respect to P, q^d (as before) and t, it can be shown that the physician maximizes utility when the marginal utility of income, which comes from changing waiting time and thus output and costs, equals the marginal disutility of work. The model becomes particularly complicated by including waiting time in terms of comparative static results, and these are not presented here. Because t is a physician choice variable, dq^d/dt, the effect of waiting time on the level of physician-initiated visits cannot be determined theoretically.

If the assumption is made, however, that waiting time is a parameter in the model and is exogenous to the physician, the expression for $d_q{}^d/dt$ can be determined.[9] Allowing t to enter the consumer demand equation and cost function, the first-order conditions are similar to Equations 9 and 10. Totally differentiating and using Cramer's Rule, we reach the desired expression:

$$dq^d/dt = [-U_q d_t U_{PP}] - [-U_{Pt} U_q d_P]/|F|.\qquad\qquad (23)$$

The sign for dq^d/dt is ambiguous because neither the sign of $U_q dt$ nor the sign of U_{pt} can be determined.[10] The expression $[P_{qt} - C_t - C_{Qq_t}]$ appears in both cross-partials and its sign depends on the relative magnitudes of the negative relationship t has on consumer demand (q_t) and the positive influence t has on practice costs (C_t).

DATA BASE

The data used to estimate this model are from the National Medical Care Expenditure Survey (NMCES), which is providing a comprehensive statistical picture to date of how health services are used and paid for in the United States. NMCES data were collected to supply the data for a series of analytical studies focusing on key national health policy issues such as the effects of alternative national health insurance proposals, access to care, and cost of illness. These studies are a major component of the National Center for Health Services Research (NCHSR) Intramural Research Program.

Data for NMCES were obtained in three separate, complementary stages which surveyed (1) approximately 14,000 randomly selected households in the civilian noninstitutionalized population; each household was interviewed six times over an 18-month period during 1977-78; (2) physicians and health care facilities providing care to household members during 1977; and (3) employers and insurance companies for their insurance coverage.

Funding for the National Medical Care Expenditure Survey was provided by NCHSR, which cosponsored the survey with the National Center for Health Statistics. (Both Centers are part of the Office of Health Research, Statistics, and Technology, Public Health Service, Department of Health and Human Services.) Data collection for the survey was done by Research Triangle Institute, Research Triangle Park, North Carolina, and its subcontractors, National Opinion Research Center of the University of Chicago, and Abt Associates, Incorporated, of Cambridge, Massachusetts.

The data in this paper on visits to physicians and on who initiated these visits were taken from household survey information reported for calendar year 1977 in personal interviews with household respondents during the period January 1, 1977 to June 31, 1978. During each interview, responses were received from the patient or another person in the patient's household concerning each visit to a physician. Detailed information about each visit included the total charge for the visit and the amount paid or to be paid by the family or by any other source; whether the person had an appointment; how long it took to get the appointment; who initiated the visit; and how long the person had to wait before seeing the provider among other items. (For further information about the data used in this paper, see Appendix I.)

A unique feature of these data is that they provide a direct measure, from the patient's perspective or the perspective of a member of the patient's household, of who initiated the demand for each visit. Specifically, those interviewed were asked whether an appointment had been scheduled for each visit they or members of their family had made to a physician, or if the visit was made without an appointment. If the visit was by appointment, they were asked whether the physician had arranged for it during a previous visit or whether the patient had made the appointment. Visits arranged by the physician are considered physician-initiated; those arranged by the patient, whether by calling for an appointment or walking in, are considered patient-initiated. By definition, a physician-initiated visit must be preceded by a contact in person or by a telephone call during which the physician instructed the patient to return at a later time. The series of questions which provides these data is replicated in Appendix II.

These questions provide an operational definition of physician-initiated demand from the patient's perspective; to our knowledge, it is the first time that such data have been available for a sample of physician visits representing all visits which occurred in the United States in 1977.

Data in this paper on physician characteristics were obtained in the NMCES Physicians' Practice Survey (PPS) of a 25% sample of the physicians named by household respondents as providing care to them during calendar year 1977. In this survey, physicians were asked about their place and mode of practice; their hours worked; the type of visits provided; age, specialty, and board certification; and practice income and outside income. Both Appendix I and Appendix III provide more information on the content of and sampling for the NMCES Physicians' Practice Survey.

EMPIRICAL RESULTS

Descriptive Statistics

Physicians initiated 38% of all visits to physicians during the first quarter of 1977 (Table 1). Patients initiated 54% of all visits--40% through appointments and 14% by walk-ins. The remaining 8% were initiated by unknown means.

The distribution for office visits is similar to that observed for all visits, since office visits constitute 84% of all visits (Table 2). Only 9% occurred in a hospital outpatient department, 6% in an emergency room and 2% in other settings. Slightly more than half of the visits to hospital outpatient departments were initiated by the physician (Table 1). Here, of visits initiated by the patient, approximately equal percentages were with appointment and walk-in visits, 16 and 17%, respectively. As one would expect, almost all visits to the emergency room were initiated by the patient and were walk-ins (Table 1).

The distribution of visits by selected patient characteristics and physician-to-population ratios according to who initiated the visit is shown in Table 3. The percentage of visits initiated by the physician increased with patient age; the reverse held for visits ini-

Table 1. Distribution of Physician Visits,
by Medical Setting and Type of Visit

Type of Visit	All	Physician's Office	Hospital Outpatient Clinic	Emergency Room
		Percentage Distribution		
All visits	100%	100%	100%	100%
Physician-initiated	38	38	57	9
	(0.6)a	(0.6)	(1.7)	(0.7)
Patient-initiated				
Appointment	40	43	16	4
	(0.6)	(0.7)	(1.1)	(0.5)
Walk-in	14	11	17	82
	(0.5)	(0.5)	(0.7)	(0.9)
Other or unknown	8	8	9	5
	(0.3)	(0.3)	(0.8)	(0.5)

Source: National Medical Care Expenditure Survey, United States, 1977.

Note: Physician-initiated visits were set by the physician in a previous visit; patient-initiated were those in which the patient independently called for an appointment or walked in.

aStandard errors, estimated as a function of the sample size of the domain, in parentheses.

Table 2. Ambulatory Visits to a Physician, by Medical Setting

Medical Setting	Percentage Distribution
Physician's office	84%
	(0.5)a
Hospital outpatient department	9
	(0.4)
Hospital emergency room	6
	(0.2)
Other medical settingb	2
	(0.2)

Source: National Medical Care Expenditure Survey, United States, 1977.

aStandard errors, estimated as a function of the sample size of the domain, in parentheses.

bIncludes military clinics, school clinics, and neighborhood health clinics or centers.

tiated by the patient, whether appointments or walk-in visits.
Approximately two-thirds of all physician visits for children under
13 were patient-initiated as compared to 45% of the visits for persons over 65 years of age. Visits by health status were similarly
distributed. The percentage of visits initiated by physicians
increased with poorer health status, and that for visits initiated
by the patient declined by this measure. However, the differences
by health status in rates of walk-in visits were very small.

Although physicians were as likely to initiate visits for whites as
for other groups in the U.S. population, there were substantial differences between the types of patient-initiated visit in this
respect. Whites were more likely to have an appointment and less
likely to have a walk-in visit than all other groups. There were no
differences between physician- and patient-initiated visits for
males and females, and no consistent pattern of differences for different levels of education.[11]

The percentage of physician-initiated visits increased with physician density.[12] Visits to a physician in a county with 175 or more
physicians per 100,000 population were approximately 15% more likely
to have been initiated by the physician than in an area with a density of 100 to 124 physicians per 100,000.

Estimation of the Model

The probability that an office or hospital outpatient visit in
the population was physician-initiated, holding other factors
constant, was estimated using (1) logit analysis, (2) a linear probability model, and (3) a least squares estimation procedure which
accounts for the complex sample design of the NMCES survey (Shah,
et al., 1977). The results of the logit analyses are presented in
Table 4, and the means and standard deviations of the variables used
in the model are shown in Table 5. In general, the results of the
other two estimating techniques were consistent with the logit estimations, except for three variables (physician density, patient age
and race). For a discussion of the relationship between the design
effects and the regression results, see Appendix III.

The independent variables can be arranged into several groups. The
first three--the proportion of the bill paid by the family, office
waiting time to see the provider, and physician density or the
physician-to-population ratio--are key variables in the model
explained above, and reflect the level of demand for medical care on
the part of the patient and market conditions. The full money
price, although a key variable in the model, is not included,
because it is endogenous and should be estimated using an instrumental variable technique. The next group of variables--age, color,
sex, health status and education[13]--represent characteristics of the
patient and are considered to reflect the parameters of the
patient's utility function. The characteristics of the physician
which reflect the physician's utility function are the physician's
age and outside income.

Table 3. Physician Visits by Selected Patient Characteristics and
Physician-to-Population Ratios, According to Type of Visit

Patient Characteristics and Physician-to-Population Ratios	Total	Physician- initiated	Patient-initiated Appointment	Walk-in	Other
		Percentage Distribution			
Age					
Less than 13 years	100[a]	23 (0.8)[b]	48 (1.1)	19 (0.8)	10 (0.7)
13-19 years	100	30 (1.5)	43 (1.1)	19 (0.9)	8 (0.7)
20-44 years	100	39 (0.8)	39 (0.7)	14 (0.5)	7 (0.4)
45-64 years	100	42 (0.9)	38 (0.7)	12 (0.5)	8 (0.4)
65 or more years	100	48 (1.2)	34 (1.0)	11 (0.7)	8 (0.5)
Color					
White	100	38 (0.6)	40 (0.6)	14 (0.5)	8 (0.3)
All other	100	40 (1.2)	33 (0.9)	20 (0.9)	7 (0.6)
Sex					
Male	100	37 (0.7)	39 (0.7)	16 (0.5)	9 (0.5)
Female	100	39 (0.6)	40 (0.6)	13 (0.5)	8 (0.3)
Health status					
Excellent	100	34 (0.7)	45 (0.7)	14 (0.5)	7 (0.5)
Good	100	38 (0.7)	40 (0.7)	14 (0.6)	8 (0.4)

Table 3 (continued)

Patient Characteristics and Physician-to-Populatio Ratios	Total	Type of Visit			
		Physician-initiated	Patient-initiated		Other
			Appointment	Walk-in	
Fair	100	42 (1.0)	34 (0.9)	14 (0.5)	10 (0.5)
Poor	100	51 (1.8)	27 (1.2)	12 (0.7)	10 (0.9)
Education					
Some high school (0-11 years)	100	44 (0.9)	33 (0.8)	15 (0.5)	8 (0.4)
High school graduate (12 years)	100	41 (1.1)	39 (0.9)	12 (0.6)	8 (0.5)
Some college (13-15 years)	100	41 (1.2)	42 (0.8)	11 (0.6)	6 (0.5)
College graduate (16 or more years)	100	43 (1.3)	42 (1.2)	9 (0.7)	6 (0.6)
Unknown	100	26 (0.7)	45 (0.9)	19 (0.7)	10 (0.6)
Physicians per 100,000 pop					
Less than 100	100	36 (1.1)	39 (1.3)	16 (0.9)	8 (0.5)
100 to 124	100	34 (1.4)	42 (1.4)	16 (1.2)	8 (0.6)
125 to 149	100	39 (1.5)	37 (1.0)	15 (0.7)	10 (0.8)
150 to 174	100	40 (1.7)	42 (2.4)	11 (1.0)	8 (1.3)
175 and over	100	40 (0.7)	41 (0.7)	12 (0.4)	7 (0.4)
Unknown	100	43 (2.8)	40 (3.0)	10 (0.7)	7 (0.8)

Source: National Medical Care Expenditure Survey, United States, 1977.

[a]Percentages may not add to 100% because of rounding.

[b]Standard errors, estimated as a function of the sample size of the domain, in parentheses.

Table 4. Logit Estimates for Persons 17 Years or Older of the Probability that the Physician Initiated the Visit, by Physician Specialty[a]

Independent Variables	Primary Care Specialties		Secondary Care Specialties		Other	
	B-value	t-value	B-value	t-value	B-value	t-value
Constant	-0.2210	0.87	1.1217**	2.95	-3.7419**	5.68
Proportion paid by family	-0.5572**	9.08	-0.5562***	6.30	0.2401	1.48
Time in physician's office[b]	-0.0044***	5.13	-0.0015	1.55	-0.0069**	3.04
Time to get an appointment	0.0137*	2.10	0.0268**	2.47	0.3108	1.55
Physicians per 100,000 population[c]	0.0015**	4.77	0.0009	2.06	0.0002	0.28
Personal Demand Characteristics						
Age	0.0140	1.57	0.0667	0.52	0.0548**	2.44
Age squared	-0.0000	0.16	-0.0000	0.12	-0.0004*	1.95
Sex (0 = M, 1 = F)	0.2346***	3.67	-0.2486***	2.99	0.3304*	2.15
"Good" health (0,1)	0.0514	0.73	0.1395	1.37	-0.1818	1.01
"Fair" health (0,1)	0.1074	1.21	0.1529	1.22	-0.0949	0.41
"Poor" health (0,1)[d]	0.3533***	3.25	0.7321*	5.07	1.1490**	3.26
High school graduate (0,1)	0.0102	0.15	-0.1112	1.13	-0.0460	0.25
Some college (0,1)	0.1321	1.40	-0.7709***	5.37	-0.1774	0.72
College graduate (0,1)[e]	0.0461	0.44	-0.3234**	2.20	0.5754***	2.48
Family income (000's)	-0.0058**	3.26	-0.0112***	3.74	0.0024	0.62
Color (0 = white, 1 = all other)	0.0928	1.04	-0.2342	1.54	1.3109**	4.28
Physician Characteristics						
Age	-0.0130**	4.81	-0.0111**	2.85	0.0194**	2.92
Outside income (000's)	-0.0005	1.59	0.0008	1.21	-0.0216***	3.82
No nurse inputs (0,1)	0.0569	0.75	-0.3227***	2.57	1.3347***	3.98
High nurse wages (0,1)[f]	-0.0060	0.08	-0.4953***	3.53	1.3411**	3.72

Source: National Medical Care Expenditure Survey, Physicians' Practice Survey Sample, United States, 1977.

aThe specialty categories include Primary care: general practice, general internal medicine, pediatrics, obstetrics/gynecology. Secondary care: general surgery, surgery subspecialties, medical subspecialties, neurology, opthamology, otolaryngology. Other: allergy, dermatology, physical medi- cine, psychiatry, osteopathy.

bEither waiting time or waiting time and treatment time.

cIn the patient's county of residence.

dThe omitted variable is "excellent health."

eThe omitted variable is "some high school."

fThe omitted variable is "low nurse wages." Wages less than $175 per week are low; those $175 or more per week are high.

* p < 0.05.

**p < 0.01.

G.R. Wilensky and L.F. Rossiter

Table 5. Means and Variances for Variables in the Logit Equation Estimates of Physician-initiated Visits, by Specialty[a]

Variables	Primary Care Specialties Mean	Variance	Secondary Care Specialties Mean	Variance	Other Mean	Variance
Proportion paid by family	0.56	0.217	0.47	0.220	0.60	0.208
Time in physician's office[b]	33.54	1211.87	37.17	1832.42	21.44	882.820
Time to get an appointment	1.40	22.825	1.59	49.195	2.19	86.8003
Physicians per 100,000 population[c]	147.83	8296.75	156.65	9726.27	145.39	8677.46
Personal Demand Characteristics						
Age	46.73	363.669	51.10	334.723	44.32	279.475
Age squared	2547.37	0.365E7	2945.81	0.34E7	2243.69	0.284E7
Sex (0 = M, 1 = F)	0.71	0.20	0.55	0.247	0.67	0.221
"Good" health (0,1)	0.40	0.241	0.39	0.237	0.39	0.239
"Fair" health (0,1)	0.19	0.155	0.18	0.150	0.16	0.134
"Poor" health (0,1)[d]	0.10	0.094	0.15	0.129	0.07	0.066
High school graduate (0,1)	0.35	0.228	0.35	0.228	0.42	0.244
Some college (0,1)	0.13	0.112	0.12	0.103	0.12	0.105
College graduate (0,1)[e]	0.10	0.09	0.10	0.092	0.16	0.134
Family income	18484.2	0.31E9	17964.7	0.250E9	18312.3	0.468E9
Color (0 = white, 1 = all other)	0.12	0.108	0.09	0.078	0.08	0.075
Physician Characteristics						
Age	50.36	120.81	49.48	113.361	53.35	146.816
Outside income	11288.1	0.128E11	7720.86	0.383E10	4254.81	0.165E9
No nurse inputs	0.46	0.25	0.62	0.237	0.73	0.196
High nurse wages (0,1)[f]	0.33	0.222	0.24	0.182	0.22	0.173

Source: National Medical Care Expenditure Survey, Physicians' Practice Survey Sample, United States, 1977.

aThe specialty categories include Primary care: general practice, general internal medicine, pediatrics, obstetrics/gynecology. Secondary care: general surgery, surgery subspecialties, medical subspecialties, neurology, opthamology, otolaryngology. Other: allergy, dermatology, physical medi- cine, psychiatry, osteopathy.

bEither waiting time or waiting time and treatment time.

cIn the patient's county of residence.

dThe omitted variable is "excellent health."

eThe omitted variable is "some high school."

fThe omitted variable is "low nurse wages." Wages less than $175 per week are low; those $175 or more per week are high.

The physician's practice income is not included in the equation
because it likewise is endogenous and needs to be estimated using an
instrumental variables technique.[14] The model also suggests that in
setting D, the cost of providing services is an important factor.
Characteristics of the physician's practice which proxy the
physician's cost function are the level of nurses' wages.
Physicians who do not employ nurses are treated as a separate
category.

Separate logit equations were estimated for primary care physicians
(general practice, internal medicine, pediatrics, obstetrics),
secondary care physicians (surgeons and medical and surgical
subspecialists), and "other" physicians. The latter group includes
psychiatrists, neurologists, dermatologists, and other specialties.
The equations were estimated separately for primary care and secondary care visits based on the belief that visits to these physicians
differ significantly in terms of medical conditions and practice
characteristics. It is also expected that the "other" equation will
be less easy to explain because of the heterogeneous mix of patients
and physicians.

Significant variables in the logit equations for primary and secondary care physicians are the proportion of the charge paid by family
(coinsurance rate), waiting time in the physician's office, waiting
time for an appointment, physician density, sex, poor health status,
family income, and the physician's age. In addition, two of the
education variables and the nurses' wage level are significant in
the secondary care equation. As predicted by the model, the larger
the proportion of the bill paid by the family, the less likely is
the physician to initiate the visit. Also, the higher the number of
physicians per 100,000 population in the county, the more likely is
the physician to initiate the visit. It should be noted that the
magnitude of this effect is very small.

There are two types of waiting time variables in these equations.
The model is indeterminate with respect to the expected signs for
these two variables, but if the costs to the patient are the dominant influence on each of these measures, the results are consistent
with the model. Waiting time in the office represents a distinct
time cost to the patient, while waiting time to get an appointment
does not. The latter is more likely to reflect the severity of the
patient's illness and also the general level of demand facing the
physician. Thus the dominant effect associated with longer waiting
times for appointments is a reduction in practice costs, by which
the physician's incentive to initiate visits is lessened. The dominant effect associated with longer office waiting times is the
increased time cost to the patient, which more than offsets the
reduction in practice costs to the physician. This reasoning
explains why the two waiting time variables have opposite signs.

Of the patient-related variables, the effects of sex on who initiates the visit has different signs in the two equations. Poor
health status (as reported by the respondent) is more likely to be
associated with a physician-initiated visit, and the magnitude of
the effect is large. In the secondary care equation, visits for
persons with some college education are less likely to be initiated
by physicians than visits for persons in the lowest education group.

Family income is consistently associated negatively with the probability that a visit was initiated by the physician. Family income
enters the model as a factor which influences the consumer's demand
function. Analogous to the physician-to-population ratio, higher
family income increases consumer demand and thus reduces the
physician's incentive to initiate visits in the same way that a
lower physician-to-population ratio increases demand and reduces the
physician's incentive to initiate visits.[15]

Of physician-related variables, physician age is negatively associated with the probability of a physician-initiated visit. This is
a factor which reflects the physician's marginal utility of income
and the disutility of work. Inasmuch as older physicians have
higher income and more established practices, they are less likely
to have an incentive to initiate visits because the marginal dollars
earned are of less value and the marginal value of leisure is worth
more. Outside income is not significant. Factor costs were
expected to be positively associated with the probability of a
physician-initiated visit. The variables used here are either statistically insignificant or have signs in an unexpected direction,
possibly because the absence of a nurse and the level of a nurse's
wages are not a good proxy for factor costs.

The significant variables in the equation for other specialties are
waiting time in the office, patient's age and age squared, sex, poor
health status, college education, and race; physician's age and outside income, and nurse's wage level. Contrary to expectation and to
the other equations, neither the proportion paid by the family nor
the physician-to-population ratio are significant. It is not obvious
why the coinsurance rate is insignificant here except that it may be
more difficult to explain behavior for this residual group. It may
also be that total physician density does not correlate well with
the density of other specialty physicians. The age effect is presumed to proxy poor health status. College education is more likely
to be associated with physician-initiated visits than lesser amounts
of education. It appears that for the other specialties, a great
financial commitment, higher education and higher income (although
not significant) are more likely to be associated with physician-
initiated visits. It is not obvious why this is so, but it may be
that psychiatrists are dominating the equation. The physician-
related variables are also somewhat perplexing for the other specialty physicians. Physician age is positively associated with the
probability of inducement, although outside physician income is
negatively associated with inducement. It seems likely that the
outside income variable is reflecting the same effect as the physician age variable in the other equations, i.e., a declining marginal utility of income. The factor cost variables are both significant and positive. While the level of wages was expected to be
positively related, the absence of a nurse was thought to be negatively associated with factor costs and thus inducement. Again, it is
likely that these variables are not good measures of factor cost.

Predicted Probabilities at the Mean

The logit coefficients can be converted into predictive probabilities. These are shown in Tables 6 and 7. Table 6 shows the changes

Table 6. Predicted Probabilities ($\hat{p}$) That a Primary Care Visit is Initiated by the Physician, Given Values for the Independent Variable

Proportion Paid by Family	$\hat{p}$	Physicians per 100,000 Population	$\hat{p}$	Physician Age in Years	$\hat{p}$
0	.509	60	.399	25	.514
.1	.495	80	.406	30	.497
.2	.481	100	.414	35	.481
.3	.467	120	.421	40	.465
.4	.453	140	.429	45	.449
.5	.439	160	.436	50	.433
.6	.426	180	.444	55	.417
.7	.412	200	.451	60	.401
.8	.399	220	.458	65	.386
.9	.385	240	.466	70	.370
1.0	.372				

Source: National Medical Care Expenditure Survey, Physicians' Practice Survey Sample, 1977.

in the predictive probabilities for changes in the proportion of the
bill paid by family, changes in the physician-to-population ratio,
and changes in the physician's age holding all other independent
variables constant. These probabilities are based on the primary
care equation which represents the majority of visits.

The predictive probabilities in Table 6 show that if a visit is paid
entirely by the family, the probability that it was initiated by the
physician is .37, other things held constant. If the visit is paid
entirely by a third party or parties, this probability increases to
.51. Thus a decline in the proportion paid by the family is predicted to increase substantially the likelihood that the visit was
initiated by the physician.

Table 6 also shows that a visit to a physician in a county with a
physician-to-population ratio of 60 is less likely to be initiated
by the physician than a visit to a physician in a county with a
ratio of 240. The increase in likelihood, however, is not great:
visits in the lowest density counties are physician-initiated with a
probability of .40; those in the highest density counties with a
probability of .47.

The last column in Table 6 indicates that changes in physician age
are associated with changes in the probability that a visit is
physician-initiated which are of a magnitude similar to changes in
the proportion of the bill paid by the family. The probability
declines from .51 for physicians aged 25 to .37 for physicians aged
70.

Table 7 shows changes in the predictive probabilities that a visit
is initiated by the physician for changes in outside physician
income. The first column is based on the primary care equation; the
second column on the other specialty equation. The differences between these two columns are striking. There is essentially no effect
from differences in outside earnings for primary care physicians.
The presumed decline in the marginal utility of income reflected in
the physician age variable is not captured in variations in outside
income. The probability that a physician initiates the visit
declines by a moderate amount with increases in outside income for
visits to other specialty physicians, from .76 with zero outside
income to .65 for outside income of $25,000. The implied level of
initiation is clearly higher for other specialty physicians than for
primary care physicians.

SUMMARY AND DISCUSSION

The focus of this paper is on physician-induced demand: does it
exist, and, if so, what is its magnitude and what factors determine
it? Data from the National Medical Care Expenditure Survey show
that the majority of visits to physicians (54%) during 1977 were
initiated by patients. More than one-third of the visits (38%),
however, were initiated by the physician. This suggests that while
there clearly is a place for traditional demand analyses in
explaining medical care utilization, the concept of induced demand

defined in terms of physician-initiated visits is relevant.
However, nothing about the medical appropriateness of these visits
can or should be inferred.

As our model suggests, economic factors and market conditions do
influence the probability that the visit is initiated by the physician. Decreases in the proportion of the bill paid by the family
are associated with increases in the probability that the physician
initiated the visit. Furthermore, this increase is not trivial.
For visits to primary care physicians, if the proportion paid by the
family goes from 75% (approximate percentage presently paid by family
for office visits) to 0 (what would be paid under a comprehensive
national health insurance plan), the probability of physician-
induced demand increases from .41 to .51, or 10 percentage points.

The impact of changes in the physician density model is also as predicted by the model, although the magnitude of the change is relatively small. The national physician-to-population ratio is
projected to increase from 179 to 220 per 100,000 from 1977 to 1985.
This would imply an increase in the probability of a physician-
initiated visit of less than 2 percentage points.

Waiting time is an additional measure of economic and market conditions. Waiting time in the office is negatively associated with
inducement, presumably reflecting the dominance of the increased
time cost to the patient; waiting time for an appointment is positively associated with inducement, presumably reflecting the dominance of a reduction in practice costs.

Some characteristics of the patient are important. As expected,
poorer health status is more likely to be associated with physician-
initiated visits; higher family income is less likely to be so associated.

Characteristics of the physician are also important. Increases in
physician age are associated with decreases in the probability that
the physician initiated the visit--like the share of the bill paid
by family, the magnitude of the change is not trivial. For visits
to primary care physicians, if the physician age increases from 25
to 65, the probability of a physician-initiated visit decreases from
.51 to .39. Although outside income does not appear to affect inducement, it is assumed that the negative relationship with age
reflects a declining marginal utility of total income and increasing
marginal disutility of work.

The rate of physician-initiated visits for visits to the other specialty physicians is more difficult to explain. Except for waiting
time in the office, economic and market conditions do not appear
important. Of patient-related characteristics, age, poor health,
and college education are all negatively associated with the likelihood of inducement. The most interesting finding is that outside
income is negatively associated with the likelihood of inducement.
As outside income increases from zero to $25,000, the likelihood of
a physician-initiated visit declines by 11 percentage points, from
.76 to .65. Although it is not possible to estimate precisely the
overall level of inducement by specialty with the weights used in
this analysis, it is clear that the level of inducement is much

Table 7. Predicted Probabilities That the Visit Is Initiated
by the Physician, Given Values for the Independent Variable

Primary care physicians	$\hat{p}$	Other specialty physicians	$\hat{p}$
		Outside Physician Income	
0	.433	0	.759
$1,000	.433	$1,000	.755
$3,000	.433	$3,000	.747
$7,000	.432	$7,000	.730
$10,000	.432	$10,000	.717
$15,000	.431	$15,000	.695
$25,000	.430	$25,000	.647

Source: National Medical Care Expenditure Survey, Physicians'
Practice Survey Sample, 1977.

higher for other specialty physicians than for primary or secondary
care physicians.

These findings are potentially important in terms of policy implications. They suggest that National Health Insurance proposals which
maintain a fee-for-service system and which decrease the proportion
of the bill paid by the family may, ceteris paribus, increase the
probability of physician-initiated visits, and that the magnitude of
the increase is not trivial. It should be noted that this increase
is in addition to any increase which might result from increased
consumer demand. Our findings also suggest that the increased
number of physicians projected for the 1980's should not result in
large increases in physician-induced demand as a result of increased
physician-to-population ratios. The change in the age structure of
physicians which results from the introduction of substantial
numbers of new physicians in the 1980's may have more impact in the
short run.

APPENDIX I

Data on Physician Visits in NMCES

The NMCES household survey. The NMCES questionnaire collected data on physician
visits in two steps. First, household respondents were asked a series of
questions which served to remind them of the number of times they had seen any
medical providers since January 1, 1977, or the last interview. Specific
questions were asked about 19 different types of medical providers. In the next
step, a series of 20 questions was asked about each encounter with a medical provider reported in the first step. Two important things should be noted regarding
the data used in this paper.

First, the data pertain not to all medical provider visits but to visits to physicians (M.D.'s) or doctors of osteopathy (D.O.'s) in the doctor's office, hospital outpatient clinic, or emergency room, based on information reported by respondents. This information is taken from the questions in the first step (above) and pertains to the type of provider, service or place connected with the visit and a direct question about where the visit took place. Data similar to that presented in this paper on the distribution of visits to physicians in other places, such as company clinics, military clinics, or other types of clinics, are not discussed in this paper, but are available from the authors upon request. In general, the percentage distribution for the other category is similar to that for the doctor's office except that the walk-in category is higher and the percentage with appointments is lower.

Second, many respondents in NMCES reported they had seen medical providers frequently--as much as once a day in the case of serious chronic conditions. In order to reduce the interviewing burden for these repondents, interviewers were allowed to skip the 20 questions on each visit when the respondent volunteered that he had a series of "repeat visits." These are a series of visits for one person in the same round of interviewing, to the same provider, in the same place, for the same condition. In addition, the unit charge for each of the visits in the group of repeat visits had to be the same. In the case of such repeat visits, answers to the 20 questions on the details of each visit were asked for only the first visit in the series, and data collected on the repeat visits include the date of each visit, whether or not the patient had an appointment for all of the remaining visits and the average waiting time to see the provider. A direct question about who initiated the visits and the sources of payment is not asked about repeat visits.

Using the data from the first quarter as an indicator, 11% of the visits have been assigned a value based on the first visit in the series when the information about repeat visits is not contradicted. This assumes that the data about who initiated the repeat visits and the amounts and sources of payment for the visits are the same as for the first visit in the series. This is a reasonable assumption inasmuch as the respondent reported that the series of visits was 1) for the same round of interviewing, 2) to the same provider, 3) in the same place, 4) for the same condition and 5) for the same unit charge.

Under these assumptions, 48.7% of the repeat visits were initiated by the physician, 25.2% were arranged by the patient by calling up for an appointment, none were walk-in visits, and 26% were arranged for by other or unknown means.

The NMCES physicians' practice survey. In order to address supply issues and determine what kinds of patients see what kinds of physicians, the National Medical Care Expenditure Survey also included a 25% sample of physicians named by household respondents. The data on visits used in the logit equations in this paper are based on the visits reported by household respondents whose physician was drawn into the NMCES Physicians' Practice Survey, approximately 25% of all NMCES sample physician visits. The data on visits (e.g., who initiated the visit) has been combined with the data on the patient (e.g., age, color, sex) and the physician (e.g., specialty) to form the analysis file for the logit equations.

Approximately six percent of the sample physicians in the Physicians' Practice Survey were missing answers to the question on how many days a patient would wait for an appointment. These were imputed, based on the reported averages for sample physicians with complete data, by categories of hours worked and specialty.

APPENDIX II

For this particular visit, did (PERSON) have an appointment or walk-in?

> Appointment . . . . . 01(A)
> Walk in . . . . 02(19)

Did the (PROVIDER) tell (PERSON) when to come in during an earlier visit
or did (PERSON) just call up for an appointment?

> Set by provider. . . . 01(19)
> Patient called . . . . 02(B)
> Other. . . . . 03(19)

APPENDIX III

Design Effects and Regression Results

Sampling for NMCES can be characterized as a stratified three-stage area probability design from two independently drawn national area samples. Except for difficulties associated with survey nonresponse and other nonsampling errors, statistically unbiased national and domain estimates can be produced. National general-purpose area samples of the Research Triangle Institute (RTI) and the National Opinion Research Center (NORC) were used in NMCES. The structures of both national samples are similar and thereby compatible.

The first stage in both designs consists of primary sampling units (PSU's) that are counties, parts of counties, or groups of contiguous counties. The second stage consists of secondary sampling units (SSU's) that are census enumeration districts (ED's) or block groups (BG's). Smaller area segments constituted the third stage in both designs from each of which a subsample of households was randomly selected in the final stage of sampling. Combined stage-specific sizes over the two designs were 135 PSU's (covering 108 separate localities), 1,290 SSU's, and 1,290 segments. Sampling specifications required the selection of approximately 13,500 households. (See Cohen, forthcoming, for more details.)

The physicians in the Physicians' Practice Survey represent a sample of the physicians mentioned by the household respondents; thus their weights are calculated on the basis of the joint probability that a particular respondent is selected for inclusion in the survey and that a particular physician is selected by one of the respondents. The first component is the respondent's weight in the household survey. The second component is estimated from a question to the physician which asked the number of unique patients he had seen in his practice during 1977. Both the population weights and the physician weights are post-stratified adjusted. Post-stratification adjustments are made to the individual weights to match Bureau of the Census estimates of the U.S. population by age, race, and sex. Post-stratification adjustments are made to the physician weights to match data from the American Medical Association on the distribution of medical specialties and to match data from the U.S. Drug Enforcement Administration on the geographic distribution of physicians.

Because of the sample design, regression results based on unweighted data assuming a simple random sample may yield biased estimates of the standard errors of the coefficients (Kish and Frankel, 1974). This can lead to t-statistics which are biased high (Shah, Holt, and Folsom, 1977). A computation program (SURREGR) available from Research Triangle Institute, Inc. (Shah, 1976) allows estimates of asymptotically efficient standard errors which account for design effects for least squares estimations. A linear probability model (OLS) and SURREGR estimates are an analog to what we might find if the SURREGR equivalent of the logit model (a logit equation which accounts for design effects), presented in the text, was available. That is, the differences between a linear probability model and a SURREGR equation suggest what differences might be found between the logit model and the SURREGR equivalent of logit. In earlier versions of this paper various models were estimated for slightly different specifications of the logit model presented in the text. The differences between the two models, in terms of the significant variables, indicated that physician density and patient age and race are not significantly related to the dependent variable in statistical terms.

NOTES

[1]Another way to show D is $D = (cP + P_t) q^d$, where P_t = the per-unit time price of output. Now when c is zero, D is equal to $P_t q^d$, suggesting that the physician is still sensitive to the fact that the patient must pay a time price for care, even though the net money price to the patient is zero. In what follows, the model is simplified by dropping $P_t q^d$ without changing the results. We are grateful to Pam Farley for suggesting this multiplicative formulation of the influence of the coinsurance rate on D.

[2]The demand function is the physician's own (firm) demand function; not the average market demand function allocated uniformly among the providers in the area according to the population-physician ratio, as in the Evans and Sloan/Feldman models mentioned. In our model, when R changes, the market share of each physician may not change proportionately. Thus our model does not assume equal market shares.

[3]To be more specific, let the sum of visits demanded without inducement by the jth patient in the ith physician's practice be represented by:

$$q_{ij} = q_{ij} (P^o_{ij}, R_i).$$

The total number of visits demanded for the jth patient, with varying levels of inducement from the ith physician, is:

$$Q_{ij} = q^d_{ij} + q_{ij} (P^o_{ij}, R_i).$$

Summing over the q^d_{id} for the ith physician yields $q^d_j = \sum_i q^d_{ij}$, the number of physician-initiated visits for the ith physician or q^d above.

[4]The second-order conditions require $U_{PP} < 0$ and $U_{PP}U_{q^d q^d} - (U_q d_P)^2 > 0$, which means $U_q d_q d < 0$ and the marginal disutility of initiating visits must be increasing in q^d.

[5]Let $[\cdot] = Y_P = [Pq_P + Q - C_Q q_P]$. If $q^d = 0$, then $Y_P < 0$ by the first-order conditions. If $q^d > 0$, it is still likely that $Y_P < 0$. This can be seen by dividing Y_P by q. Then, $Y_P (1/q) = [Q/q + C_Q E]$, where $E = -P/q(q_P)$, the price elasticity of demand. In order for Y_P to be positive, the number of patient-initiated visits must be very small relative to the total number of visits, or E must be less than one or very nearly one. This seems unlikely, thus Y_P is assumed to be negative.

[6]$U_q d_P = U_{YY}P[\cdot] + U_{QQ}q_P + U_{DD}c^2 Pq^d + U_y + U_{DC} = U_{Pq}d$, assuming symmetric cross-effects.

[7]Sloan and Feldman (1978) and Reinhardt (1977a) discuss this point in detail. In short, the problem with aggregate cross-section results is that the influences are not identified. The number of visits per capita may be higher in higher density areas because consumer demand per capita is higher, not because physicians initiate more visits. By the same token, prices may be higher in such areas because demand is high, and that is why relatively more physicians are drawn there in the first place. As Sloan and Feldman suggest, prices may be higher where physician density is higher because quality and amenities are superior.

[8]$U_q d_c = U_{YY}P[Pq_c - C_Q q_c] + U_{QQ}q_c + U_{DD}cP^2 q^d + U_D P$, assuming a separable utility function.

[9]This assumption may not be too unreasonable. Demand for physician services is probably stochastic and seasonal. Staff may be hired in one time period to work full-time, while the level of demand that prevails in the next time period fluctuates around what was predicted. Waiting time in the physician's office smooths out these fluctuations during the day. Waiting time to get an appointment smooths out these fluctuations over longer periods.

[10]$U_q d_t = U_{YY}P[Pq_t - C_t - C_Q q_t] + U_{QQ}q_t$ and $U_{Pt} = U_{YY} [\cdot] [Pq_t - C_t - C_Q q_t] + U_{QQ}q_P q_t$, assuming separable utility and consumer demand functions.

[11]Education is defined in Table 3 as the education of the patient. Visits for children are not included in the education category.

[12]Physician density is defined as the number of non-federal patient care physicians per 100,000 population in the patient's county of residence.

[13]In the logit model, only those 17 years of age or older are included.

[14]Both this variable and the full money price will be estimated as instruments at a later time.

[15]Mitigating the negative effect of higher income is the possibility that the physician may associate higher income with a reduced financial burden to the patient. This factor is not explicitly included in the model. On the other hand, higher family income suggests that the time price of obtaining care is higher. This reduces demand, increases the disutility the physician receives from demand inducement (if the physician considers the time price to the patient), and confirms the negative sign in the logit equation.

HEALTH, ECONOMICS, AND HEALTH ECONOMICS
J. van der Gaag and M. Perlman (editors)
© North-Holland Publishing Company, 1981

"SUPPLIER-INDUCED DEMAND"
IN A MODEL OF PHYSICIAN BEHAVIOR

Peter Zweifel

INTRODUCTION

Conventional wisdom views the physician as the key figure in the
provision of health care.* Although economists seem to agree ver-
bally, they have treated the private physician as a perfect agent
of his patients. In empirical studies, demand for medical care and
even hospitalization has traditionally been made a function of
patients' characteristics alone, with no reference to the physician,
his objectives, and constraints. Yet there are few instances where
the costs of monitoring an agent are as high as they are for a
patient vis-à-vis his physician.

This paper is an attempt to redress the balance. It describes a
model of private physician behavior where ethical concerns compete
with more material objectives. The next section spells out the elements of the model. There are three decision variables: critical
symptom level (c) determining referral and hospitalization, an implicit wage rate (q), and the average physician-time input per case
treated (t). Using restrictions generated by the assumption of
strong relative risk aversion, the model predicts a reduction in (q)
and an increase of (t) when demand for initial contacts is cur-
tailed, e.g., by a higher coinsurance rate. Since analysts of physician billings only observe the product (q × t), i.e., billings per
case treated, they have come to the conclusion that physicians
indulge in demand creation. In an effort to separate the two components and test the model's implications, sickness fund data are
analyzed using the multiple indicator model of statistical
inference. The final section contains a summary and states a few
conclusions.

THE ELEMENTS OF AN ECONOMIC MODEL OF PHYSICIAN BEHAVIOR

The famous article by Kessel (1958) on physician fee discrimination
contains evidence that income (Y) is an important determinant of

---

*I am indebted to F. Carlevaro (Geneva), M. Grossman (New York), J. P. Newhouse
(Rand), J. Niehans (Bern), J. Ramsey (New York), H. Schneider (Zurich), L. D.
Taylor (Tucson), and P. Tschopp (Geneva) for helpful criticisms and comments.

private physician behavior. But this does not imply that his practice can be viewed as an ordinary business firm. As emphasized by
Sloan (1974), the physician's self-employed status, together with
the restricted substitutability of his time input, call for his
evaluation of business decisions in terms of leisure, too. However
the really distinguishing feature of medical people seems to be a
strong ethical concern (see Arrow, 1963). This idea has not been
incorporated in a formal model, except in the work of Smallwood and
Smith (1975). We therefore propose a utility function of the
general form

$$\bar{U} = E[U(Y,I,L)] \tag{1}$$

E: expectation operator   I: ethical variable (see Eq. 4)
Y: labor income   L: leisure time.

The inclusion of an ethical variable (I) on the same footing as
(Y, L) militates against the view taken by Arrow (1963) and M.S.
Feldstein (1970) that medical choices are constrained by ethical
considerations in an ultimate sense.

Medical associations are rarely able to specify exactly what conduct
constitutes unethical behavior. Hence, ethical concerns are
expected to be violated to a considerable degree if compensation in
terms of income (Y) and leisure (L) is sufficiently large.

Turning to the restrictions, we have

$$Y = qtP \tag{2}$$

where: q = gross price per hour of service, t = average
              treatment time, P = number of patients.

This formulation abstracts entirely from the existence of fee-fixing
contracts between medical associations and health insurers in many
European countries.[1] It also neglects the problem of discrimination
in terms of price (q) and quality (t) among different patient groups.
Rather, emphasis is on a global discrimination against risky cases
that can be referred to a specialist or sent to a hospital.[2]

Specifically in this model, the physician chooses a critical symptom
intensity (c), beyond which he will not accept anyone for treatment.
The number of patients treated is therefore given by

$$P = \int_0^c h(qr, w, s) \times F(s,\bar{s})ds \tag{3}$$

$$0 < h(\cdot) < 1$$

$$0 < s < 1$$

$$h_{(qr)} < 0,$$

$$h_s > 0, \; h_{(qr),s} > 0,$$

where   P: number of patients treated,
             c: critical symptom intensity,
             h: demand for a first contact with physician,
             r: coinsurance rate,
            qr: net price of an hour of physician's time,
             w: other non-health influences on h $(\cdot)$,
             s: symptom level,
             F: number of persons with symptom level (s).

Demand for a first visit is stochastic, depending on the
(nonnormalized) density function $F(s,\bar{s})$, with high frequencies for
low symptom intensities and vice versa. On the other hand, the
probability h $(\cdot)$ of consulting a physician is high for high values
of (s).[3] Since the elasticity of h $(\cdot)$ with respect to net price
per hour of service (qr) is expected to approach zero as (s)
increases, the distribution of potential patients over symptom
levels differs markedly from the population distribution $F(s,\bar{s})$.
(See Lave et al., 1974.) But only potential patients with symptom
level below (c) are treated. All others are relegated in principle.
As a rule, however, potential patients are not just sent home but
referred to some other supplier of medical service.

In particular, a change in (c) indicates, _ceteris paribus_, a changed
tendency of the physician to hospitalize patients.[4] Demand for
admissions to the public hospital is therefore viewed as physician-
initiated and not patient-initiated (contrary to Newhouse and
Phelps, 1976, for example).

Next we give medical ethics (I) operational content. It seems that
physicians everywhere share the belief that fighting disease and
death is the ultimate aim of their activity. This endeavor has a
quantity and a quality component. A physician may try to improve
the chance of survival of as many persons as possible by a given
amount--in the approach taken by Smallwood and Smith (1975), even
the survival of anonymous individuals that the physician has
excluded by setting a nonzero fee count in the target variable.
However, as an agent of his patients, the physician must also be
concerned with the size of his contribution to the health of the
individuals he has accepted for treatment. The following definition
takes both of these aspects into account.

$$I = \int_{0}^{c}[p(s,0) - p(s,t)] \times h(qr,w,s) \times F(s,\bar{s})ds \qquad (4)$$

             p: probability of death within the decision period.

The term in brackets symbolizes the improvement in health afforded
by the input of (t) hours physician's time to an individual with
symptom severity (s). Under the assumption $p_t < 0$ (s < c), the physician can improve the quality of his service by spending more time
per patient on average.[5]

The last restriction is quite simple. If (t) is the amount of time
spent per patient and (P) the number of patients treated within the
decision period, then (t × P) is total working time. Hence, leisure
time is determined by

$$L = T - tP, \tag{5}$$

where   T: total time available.

For ease of reference, the model is presented in full on the facing page, together with a characterization of its variables.

THE NECESSARY CONDITIONS FOR AN OPTIMUM AND THEIR INTERPRETATION

A couple of peculiarities of this model are worth mentioning. First, there is no diagnostic problem. The physician establishes the symptom level of a potential patient the minute he sees him and decides whether or not to refer him to a hospital. In reality the physician may attempt an ambulatory treatment for a while before realizing that he can help a patient better by having him hospitalized.[6] However, we do not expect that letting (s) of a particular patient exceed (c) during the nth instead of the first period would significantly change the implications of the model. Second, the physician also accepts patients with no visible symptoms (s = 0) for treatment. This conforms with informal evidence, reflected, for example, by the popular saying that a physician in his right mind will always retain a rich patient, even if he is perfectly healthy. In a deeper sense, perception of symptom severity (s) may well differ between physician and patient; but again we choose to neglect the difference by using the common symbol (s). Third and most important, only the demand for first visits is under the control of the patients. Given such a first contact, the physician is free to choose his time input (t), subject to his own restrictions only. Patients are assumed to remain indifferent to variations in (t). These variations can take the form of longer or shorter visits or more or less visits per patient. Both cases entail a change in time cost of medical care, with a negative impact on demand (see Acton, 1975, 1976).[7] On the other hand, the fact that a physician is willing to spend more time is often interpreted as an indicator of higher quality. Such an interpretation is quite warranted, given Equation 4 of our model. In sum, the chosen specification of demand may be a sufficient approximation to reality, at least for the limited range of (t) open to physicians themselves, given their own restrictions.

We now turn to the necessary conditions for an optimum. The inequality conditions (0 < c < 1, q > 0, t > 0; L > 0) will be disregarded because it is difficult to envisage a situation where they are binding. Moreover, we view the system expressed in Equation 6 as a pure maximization problem in terms of the primary decision variables (c, q, t). Assuming that an interior solution exists, we have

$$E[U_c] = E[U_Y Y_c]   + E[U_I I_c] + E[U_L L_c] = 0 \tag{7}$$

with $U_Y = \partial U/\partial Y$. The equations derived from (6) are given in Equations 8, 9, and 10.

Model (Equation 6) and Variables

$$U = E[U(Y,I,L)] = \int_0^1 U[Y(\bar{s}), \; I(\bar{s}), \; L(\bar{s})]ds \; \rightarrow \; max. \; S.T. \qquad (6)$$

$$Y = qtP$$

$$P = \int_0^c h(qr, \; w, \; s) \times F(s,\bar{s})ds$$

$$I = \int_0^c [p(s, \; 0) - p(s, \; t)] \times h(qr, \; w, \; s) \times F(s,\bar{s})ds$$

$$L = T - tP$$

Decision variables

c: critical symptom level
q: average fee, defined as an implicit wage rate
t: average time input per patient

Derived decision variables (target variables)

Y: labor income
I: extent of helping
L: leisure time

Exogenous variables

r: coinsurance rate, $0 < r < 1$
w: other non-health influences on h ($\cdot$)
s: symptom level (stochastic)
$\bar{s}$:   parameter characterizing the density function F ($\cdot$); "mean symptom level" (unknown)
T: total time within decision period

Functions

h: demand for a first visit, defined as a probability of seeking care; $0 < h < 1$
p: probability of death, $0 < p < 1$
F: absolute frequency of individuals with symptom level (s) in the population, characterized by $\bar{s}$

$$Y_c = Y_P P_c = qt \times h(qr,w,c) \times F(c) > 0, \tag{8}$$

$$I_c = [p(c,0) - p(c,t)] \times h(qr,w,c) \times F(c) > 0, \text{ and} \tag{9}$$

$$L_c = -tP_c = -t \times h(qr,w,c) \times F(c) < 0. \tag{10}$$

Substitution in (7) and cancellation of terms yields

$$\frac{U_L}{U_Y} = q + \frac{U_I}{U_Y} \left[\frac{p(c,0) - p(c,t)}{t}\right]. \tag{11}$$

The marginal rate of substitution between leisure and income is equal to the wage rate plus a positive term. This positive term is higher the stronger the physician's ethical concern (U_I/U_Y) and the more his activity in fact contributes to the survival of the marginal patients. This holds true for a given value of the parameter ($\bar{s}$); but since the elements of Equation 11 are sign-invariant to changes of ($\bar{s}$), we derive

Proposition 1: Due to professional ethics, a physician will work more than another self-employed individual with a comparable wage rate.

As a matter of fact, physicians in the U.S. consistently report more hours per week and work-weeks per year than dentists, whose wage rate (q) is of comparable magnitude (see Mennemeyer, 1978). The difference in hours per week is much more pronounced, however, possibly due to the simple fact that dentistry is more taxing physically.

The influence of ethical concerns on fee setting has been the object of a continued debate from Kessel (1958), to Arrow (1963), and on to Ruffin and Leigh (1973) and Masson and Wu (1974). In terms of our model, the question hinges on whether U_I is different from zero in the optimum condition

$$E[U_q] = E[U_Y Y_q] + E[U_I I_q] + E[U_L L_q] = 0 \tag{12}$$
$$(-) \qquad (+)$$

For future reference we have

$$Y_q = t(P + qP_q) = tP(1 + e_{P,q}), \tag{13}$$

$$I_q = r \times \int_0^c [p(s,0) - p(s,t)] \times h_{(qr)}F(s)ds < 0, \text{ and} \tag{14}$$

$$L_q = tP_q = -rt \times \int_0^c h_{(qr)}F(s)ds > 0. \tag{15}$$

Here, $e_{p,q}$ stands for the partial elasticity of the number of patients treated with respect to the gross hourly fee (q). The expression (13) has been left unsigned. If ethical concerns are indeed unimportant, the first term in Equation 12 must be negative, implying $Y_q < 0$ and $e_{p,q} < -1$. But most demand studies yield estimates of price elasticity well below one in absolute value (see M.S. Feldstein's 1974 survey).[8] Before concluding that there is a puzzle, a few caveats are in order. First, demand is usually measured by the number of visits. Given the possibility of demand creation by the physician, estimates of price elasticity based on that variable are biased towards zero. Second, the studies included in the survey have used data that are not physician specific. They therefore reflect a demand for medical care when fees of alternative suppliers vary, too. That demand schedule is less elastic than the individual one; hence, the elasticity relevant for a single physician is again underestimated (see Masson and Wu, 1974). Let us consider these arguments in turn.

A recent study by Newhouse and Phelps (1976) distinguishes between first and follow-up visits. In our notation, they estimate $e_{h,qr} = -.11$ (p. 276), with (s) and (w) indeed held constant. The relationship between $e_{p,q}$ and $e_{h,qr}$, with ($\bar{s}$) fixed, is given by

$$e_{p,q} = \frac{r \times \int_0^c h_{(qr)}F(s)ds \times q}{\int_0^c h(qr,w,s)F(s)ds}$$

$$= \int_0^c e_{h,qr}(\cdot,s) \times \frac{h(qr,w,s) \times F(s)ds}{\int_0^c h(qr,w,s) \times F(s)ds} .$$

Hence, $e_{p,q}$ is a weighted average of the state-dependent elasticities $e_{h,qr}(\cdot,s)$, with low values of $e_{h,qr}$ entering with a high weight. The empirical result therefore argues for an even smaller value of $e_{p,q}$. This leaves us with the second question: Is the difference between the industry demand curve and the schedule faced by the individual physician sufficiently great as to bridge the gap between -.1, say, and -1.0? The size of this gap depends on the elasticity of the marginal patient who considers searching for another physician. He may be assumed to react to a money price change as though it were a change of full cost for a nonmarginal patient. Acton (1976, p. 201) derives the following relationship between the two elasticities

$$e_{h,qr} = \frac{qr}{qr+wt} \times e_{h,(qr+wt)} \qquad \text{w: wage rate} \tag{16}$$

(observed)   (effective)

with (t) momentarily denoting search time rather than treatment
time. For an observed elasticity as low as -.1 to be compatible
with an effective marginal elasticity of -1 or more, the share of the
net money price in the total cost of seeking medical care would have
to be no more than 10%. Except for poor urban individuals with (r)
close to zero, such an implication can hardly be reconciled with
reality. We therefore have

Proposition 2: Physician fee-setting is not income-maximizing.
Raising fees would have a positive partial effect on income ($Y_q > 0$).

It should be noted, however, that the available evidence for
Proposition 2 is of a very indirect nature. Granted $Y_q > 0$, it
still does not necessarily follow that professional ethics prevent
price (q) from reacting positively to a demand increase.

The third necessary optimality condition reads

$$E[U_Y Y_t] + E[U_I I_t] + E[U_L L_t] = 0, \text{ involving}$$

$$Y_t = qP > 0 \tag{17}$$

$$I_t = -\int_0^c h(qr,w,s) \times I(s) \times p_t(s,t)ds > 0, \text{ and} \tag{18}$$

$$L_t = -P < 0. \tag{19}$$

After substitution and division by (P), we obtain an expression
similar to (11), in the certainty case:

$$\frac{U_L}{U_Y} = q + \frac{U_I}{U_Y} \left[\frac{-\int_0^c h(qr\cdot w\cdot s) \times F(s) \times p_t(s,t)ds}{P}\right]. \tag{20}$$

Again, the marginal rate of substitution between leisure and income
is equal to the implicit wage rate plus a positive term. Comparison
of Equations 11 and 20 yields the interesting derived optimality
condition

$$\frac{p(c,0) - p(c,t)}{t} = \frac{-\int_0^c h(\cdot) \times F(s) \times p_t(\cdot)ds}{P}. \tag{21}$$

If a physician were observed aiming at this equality, then medical ethics would have a nonnegligible influence on his behavior, i.e., U_I/U_Y differs from zero. By increasing his critical symptom level, the physician can help additional patients--but at a cost. He must draw time away from the rest of his patients. Accordingly, (t) appears in the denominator of the RHS in Equation 21 as an indicator of opportunity costs. The qualitative dimension of helping can be improved by treating patients more intensively. Again, there is the alternative of admitting more patients, symbolized by (P) in the denominator on the RHS of Equation 21. We conclude the interpretation of necessary optimum conditions by noting that the LHS of Equation 21 must be positive as long as $p_t < 0$ for some patients. This implies

Proposition 3: An ethical physician will never choose his critical symptom (c) so high as to have negative impact on the health of his marginal patients.

COMPARATIVE STATICS AND "SUPPLIER-INDUCED DEMAND"

Let us now assume that the demand function for first visits is shifted, e.g., by an increase of the coinsurance rate (r). Differentiating totally the three conditions $E[U_c] = E[U_q] = E[U_t] = 0$, we obtain, for a given value of $(\bar{s})$.

$$\begin{bmatrix} U_{cc} & U_{cq} & U_{ct} \\ U_{cq} & U_{qq} & U_{qt} \\ U_{ct} & U_{qt} & U_{tt} \end{bmatrix} \begin{bmatrix} dc \\ dq \\ dt \end{bmatrix} = - \begin{bmatrix} U_{cr} \\ U_{qr} \\ U_{tr} \end{bmatrix} dr. \qquad (22)$$

The analysis is greatly complicated by the fact that (dr) conceivably influences $U(\cdot)$ through all three channels on the RHS of the above equation system. Moreover, even under the assumption of subjective want-independence ($U_{YI} = U_{YL} = U_{IL} = 0$), U_{cr}, for example, still contains six terms:[9]

$$U_{cr} = U_{YY}Y_cY_r + U_YY_{cr} + U_{II}I_cI_r + U_II_{cr} + U_{LL}L_cL_r + U_LL_{cr}. \qquad (23)$$

The derived decision variables (Y,I,L), depending on the unknown parameter $(\bar{s})$ in $F(s,\bar{s})$, are themselves stochastic. Therefore, the physician has indeed a choice of different prospects occurring with certain probabilities. Due to the independence assumption made above, he considers the (Y), (I), and (L) prospects and their probabilities in isolation when maximizing expected utility. As physicians may safely be considered risk-averse, we obtain from Arrow (1971, pp. 92-93)

$$U_{YY} < 0, \quad U_{II} < 0, \quad U_{LL} < 0. \qquad (24)$$

Arrow (1971) has shown that as (Y) approaches infinity, the coefficient of relative risk-aversion must be greater than one. Hence,

$$\left| \frac{U_{YY}}{U_Y/Y} \right| > 1. \tag{25}$$

Generalizing for (I,L), we derive the following restrictions:

$$\frac{U_Y}{\left| U_{YY} \right|} < Y, \quad \frac{U_I}{\left| U_{II} \right|} < I, \quad \frac{U_L}{\left| U_{LL} \right|} < L. \tag{26}$$

These restrictions, along with some minor additional assumptions, suffice to give the impulse vector the following structure:[10]

$$U_{cr} \gtrless 0, \quad U_{qr} < 0, \quad U_{tr} > 0. \tag{27}$$

Moreover, arguing with an invariance principle as risk aversion goes from zero to infinity, one off-diagonal element of the Hessian matrix may be signed:

$$U_{ct} < 0. \tag{28}$$

For the other off-diagonals, no sign restrictions could be found. To simplify, we therefore posit

$$U_{cq} = U_{qt} = 0. \tag{29}$$

Now we are in a position to examine the implied reactions in terms of the explicit wage rate (q) and the average treatment time (t):

$$\frac{dq}{dr} = \frac{-1}{H} \begin{vmatrix} U_{cc} & U_{cr} & U_{ct} \\ 0 & U_{qr} & 0 \\ U_{ct} & U_{tr} & U_{tt} \end{vmatrix}$$

$$= \frac{-U_{qr}}{H} \begin{vmatrix} U_{cc} & U_{ct} \\ U_{ct} & U_{tt} \end{vmatrix}$$
$$\quad (-) \qquad\qquad (+)$$

$$< 0. \tag{30}$$

Once again, the terms appearing in Equation 30 are sign-invariant to changes in the unknown parameter $(\bar{s})$, related to the distribution of symptoms in the relevant population. Thus we have

Proposition 4:   An increased coinsurance rate induces the physician to lower his implicit wage rate.

The physician does therefore become less expensive. But at least in an insured market with fee fixing agreements, (q) is rarely observed. Rather, the average amount billed per case is monitored. This variable is given by the product (qt). But regarding (t), our model predicts

$$\frac{dt}{dr} = \frac{-1}{|H|} \begin{vmatrix} U_{cc} & 0 & U_{cr} \\ 0 & U_{qq} & U_{qr} \\ U_{ct} & 0 & U_{tr} \end{vmatrix} \tag{31}$$

$$= \underset{(+)}{\frac{-U_{tr}}{|H|}} \underset{(+)}{\begin{vmatrix} U_{cc} & U_{cq} \\ U_{cq} & U_{qq} \end{vmatrix}} - \underset{(-)}{\frac{U_{cr}}{|H|}} \underset{(+)}{\begin{vmatrix} U_{cq} & U_{qq} \\ U_{ct} & U_{qt} \end{vmatrix}} > 0,$$

because U_{tr} dominates U_{cr} and the first minor dominates the second.[11]   We have therefore

Proposition 5:   The reduction in demand for first contacts is partially compensated by longer treatment times.

This is exactly what observers of insured medical markets have dubbed "supplier-induced demand". For insurance data, mirroring the product (qt), masks the possibility that the wage rate (q) may have fallen. But when the physician spends more time with each patient, he will be able to complete more procedures per case. Indeed, the total reaction will be given by

$$e_{(qt)r} = \frac{d}{d\ln r} [\ln q + \ln t] \tag{32}$$

$$= \underset{(-)}{[e_{q,r}} + \underset{(+)}{e_{t,r}]}, \qquad \text{with } e_{(qt)r} = \frac{d(qt)}{dr} \times \frac{qt}{r}.$$

The model predicts $e_{q,r} < 0$, but $e_{t,r} > 0$; the sign of the expression

(32) is therefore indeterminate. Table 1 below gives an overview of
all the predicted impacts of a change (dr), together with some comments on the importance of professional ethics. We may summarize the
comments of Table 1 as follows:

Proposition 6: As far as adjustment to a change of demand for initial visits is concerned, professional ethics will not alter the
direction predicted by income-cum-leisure oriented behavior. It
possibly modifies its speed, much in keeping with the ideology of
"medical autonomy."

Proposition 7: "Supplier-induced demand" appears to be a statistical
artifact. Billings data, compiled by sickness insurance funds, do not
contain direct information about the price relevant for demand, i.e.
the physician's time price.

The reader may compare these conclusions with M.S. Feldstein's
(1970) presumption that professional ethics may account for his
failure to identify reasonable .demand and supply schedules for
physicians' services, or with the belief expressed by Evans (1974)
that a target income model is needed to explain supplier-induced
demand.

FORMULATION OF THE STATISTICAL MODEL

Our data consist of claims submitted in the years 1976 to 1978 to a
major sickness fund active mainly in the region of Bern.[12] In view
of their confidential nature, matching them with data on the characteristics of physicians and their practices was out of the question.
This already precludes testing Propositions 1, 2, 3 as well as 6,
related to professional ethics. There are three different groups of
insured, facing different deductibles; beyond the uninsured amount,
there is a coinsurance rate that asymptotically approaches 10% at the
margin (r = 0.1).[13] When deciding for or against a first contact with
a physician, patients are uncertain as to the total cost of treatment.
Under these circumstances, different deductibles are in principle compared to differences in coinsurance rates (see Keeler, Newhouse and
Phelps, 1977). However, the grouping is also according to income,
and higher income is known to result in a somewhat increased demand
for patient-initiated contacts, as has been shown by Newhouse and
Phelps in their thorough study (1976, Table 2). Therefore, an indicator variable like the share of very well-to-do patients (P3% in
Figure 1) mirrors not only a slightly higher coinsurance rate (r)
but also a patient population with high average income (w_γ).

At the core of Figure 1, the signs of the relationships between
exogenous variables ($\bar{s}$, r, w_γ) and the two endogenous variables
(q, t) show the implications of the behavioral model. For example,
a higher coinsurance rate (r) is predicted to decrease the demand
for first contacts and hence to induce the physician to spend more
time with a patient (t) on average (see also Table 1 above). But
not one of these five theoretical variables is directly observed in
the sickness fund data. There are three measured variables that may
represent average symptom severity ($\bar{s}$) to some degree. In order not

Table 1. Comparative-Static Implications of the Model

Prediction	Verbal description	Discussion, particularly with regard to ethics
$\dfrac{dc}{dr} > 0$	If the marginal coinsurance rate for ambulatory care is increased, the physician will (probably) set his critical symptom level higher. Referrals to specialists and hospitals will become less frequent.	Exceptions only to be expected for physicians with very few referrals in the initial period ($\mid U_{cc} \mid$ minimal). Strong ethics (U_I large relative to U_Y or U_L) tend to reduce the value of dc/dr. They therefore increase the probability of an abnormal reaction. If it is assumed that the adaption period is longer than the observation period, strong ethics would reduce the speed of adjustment.
$\dfrac{dq}{dr} < 0$	If the marginal coinsurance rate is increased, the physician will lower his implicit wage rate.	The model predicts an especially strong adjustment for those physicians charging a high wage rate in the initial period ($\mid U_{qr} \mid$ large). Professional ethics do not modify the result in that U_I may be freely varied without systematic impact on dq/dr.
$\dfrac{dt}{dr} > 0$	If the marginal coinsurance rate is increased, the physician will devote more time to the treatment of a case, on average.	An exception is possible only if there is a behavioral irregularity when the coefficient of relative risk aversion is varied between 0 and infinity. Strong professional ethics reinforce the effect or speed up adjustment.
$\dfrac{d(qt)}{dr} \lessgtr 0$	The sign of this expression is open. It depends on the relative sizes of elasticities $e(q,r) < 0$ and $e(t,r) > 0$.	Since ($q \times t$) must be approximately equal to billings per case, the impression easily arises of "supplier-induced demand" as a reaction to the curtailing of primary demand by the increased coinsurance rate.

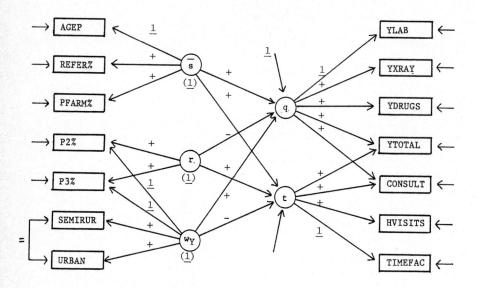

Figure 1. The structural model and the measurement model.

to jeopardize identification of the model, we abstain from using
billing data as indicators of (s̄). Rather, the scanty data characterizing the relevant population are fully used. The first basic
indicator is average age of patients treated (AGEP). Since indicators can be dependable in a relative sense only, a normalization
must be employed. Here, the loading coefficient linking AGEP to (s̄)
is set to one. But this does not imply that AGEP is assumed to be
an infallible indicator of (s̄) because there is still a measurement
error, symbolized by the error pointing to AGEP from the left. The
second indicator is the share of referrals received from other physicians in the total caseload (REFER%). A physician accepting many
referrals is expected to deal with more difficult cases, ceteris
paribus. The variable must be standardized on a per-case basis
because otherwise a low number of referrals received may simply mean
that this particular physician does most of his business with one of
the many other sickness funds. Finally, small farmers and their
employees may be expected to be among the more difficult cases when
they do seek medical care, in spite of their high opportunity costs
in terms of income foregone. Therefore, the percentage of farm-
based patients (PFARM%) is entered as a third indicator of (s̄).

The indicators P2% and P3% tell something about patient income but
also about the respective coinsurance rate, which is highest for P3
patients and higher for P2 than P1 patients. The last two indicators on the LHS of Figure 1 are dummies. In semirural regions
(SEMIRUR), income is usually higher than in rural ones, and it is
highest in urban (URBAN) communities. Here, a continuous variable
(wy) is very imperfectly mirrored by two discrete ones, and measure-

ment error will probably loom large in both. In view of the acute
shortage of indicators for exogenous variables, we simplify the
model by postulating the two error variances to be of equal size.

On the RHS of Figure 1, we find the indicators for the endogenous
variables (q) and (t). By assumption, the physician manipulates
billings per case (YTOTAL) in such a way that (q) and (t) are at
their optimal levels. In particular, the product (q × t) must be
approximately equal to YTOTAL, which explains why there are two
arrows pointing to that variable. A high average claim per patient
can therefore be due to a physician's setting a high implicit wage
rate or spending much time for each case treated. This ambiguity is
precisely what makes it difficult for the sickness fund to monitor
physician performance. In contrast, the number of office visits
(CONSULT) may be thought to be a good indicator of time input.

However, the length of the average visit is not known in the sample,
and it is very easy for a physician to increase his wage rate by
shortening its average duration. A better indicator of (t) might be
home visits per case (HVISITS) because they are time-consuming and
have been traditionally regarded as low-paid. The fee schedule
allows for an adjustment of the basic consultation fee when the
visit turns out to be time-consuming. The frequency with which this
time-factor (TIMEFAC) is billed may indeed mirror the time inten-
siveness of practice. But again, measurement error will be present.
On the other hand, laboratory charges per case treated (YLAB) are
thought to be linked to (q) exclusively because these tasks can be
delegated to auxiliary personnel. Hence, they do not involve physician time. The same holds true of x-ray work (YXRAY) and drugs sold
by the physician himself (YDRUGS).

In sum, the structural model in the center of Figure 1 is supplemented with a measurement model that takes measurement error into
explicit account. Traditional regression analysis cannot handle
these difficulties. Such a system may be estimated using LISREL,
an FIML program developed by Joereskog and Van Thillo (1973). For
details, the reader is referred to that publication. Here we only
note that no general identification rules exist but that a short-
ranked empirical information matrix at the maximum of the likelihood
function is an almost sure sign of underidentification (see Silvey,
1975, pp. 81-82). This test leads to the conclusion that the model
of Figure 1 is not identified. One possible way out of the difficulty is to use the observations of two subsequent years. This
doubles the number of indicators, with the natural exception of the
regional dummies SEMIRUR and URBAN, which remain the same in 1976
and 1977. In order to prevent the number of parameters from
doubling as well, we introduce an invariance hypothesis: The parameters of the structural and the measurement model are to be the
same in both years. Accordingly, the indicator measurements for
1977 are shown but schematically in Figure 2 while the number of
arrows remains unchanged. This discussion may be summed up in the
following proposition.

Proposition 8: Together with an auxiliary hypothesis regarding the
invariance of indicator quality, sickness insurance data allow tests
of Propositions 4, 5, and 7, but not Propositions 1 to 3 and 6,
relating to professional ethics.

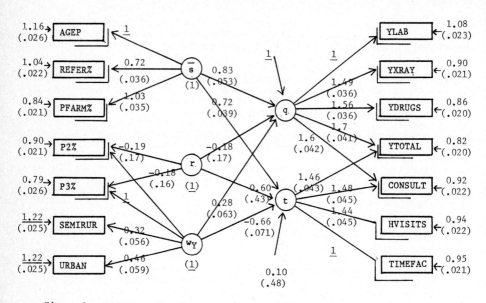

Figure 2. LISREL estimation results, 616 physicians 1976 and 1977.
χ^2 = 9487, with 318 d.f.

ESTIMATION RESULTS

In Figure 2, most of the predictions of the theoretical model are
borne out. Higher average symptom severity ($\bar{s}$) does seem to induce
the physician to set his implicit wage rate higher, with an elasticity of 0.83 (0.053), but also to spend more time with patients, that
elasticity being 0.72 (.039).[14] A higher coinsurance rate has the
predicted negative effect on (q), but lacks statistical significance, as judged by conventional standards.[15] A higher coinsurance
rate also results in a higher average input (t) per patient treated,
subject again to a qualification as to statistical significance
($\hat{e}_{t,r}$ = 0.60 (.43)).

Turning to the income impulse (w_Y), we note that higher income is
associated with shortened time input on the part of the physician.
It is positively associated with the doctor's implicit wage rate
(q), in accordance with the model's implications.

The results relating to the measurement part of the estimation are
not as satisfactory, however. For AGEP, hypothesized to be the
benchmark indicator of mean case severity ($\bar{s}$), has an estimated
"share" of measurement error variance amounting to 1.35 (=1.16^2),
which exceeds standardized total variance (=1). Compared to AGEP,
the share of agricultural patients (PFARM%) appears to be the
superior indicator of ($\bar{s}$), even better than the referral percentage
(REFER%). Most important, both P3% and P2% are estimated to be
negatively related to the mean expected coinsurance rate (r). Both
relationships were predicted to be positive. On the endogenous

side, billings per case (YTOTAL) do approximately reflect the product q × t, with the wage component somewhat overshadowing the time component. Sales of drugs (YDRUGS) appear to be the most dependable indicator of the unobserved physician wage rate, with an estimated error share of 74% (=0.86²) in observed variance.[16] And although the number of consultations per case (CONSULT) is contaminated by (q) as expected, it does contain information about time spent on the patient, with loading coefficient of 1.48 (.045). These conclusions are tentative because the statistical fit of the model is very poor, the calculated chi-square statistic amounting to 9487 with 318 degrees of freedom. But then, this test is probably too severe for a model incorporating measurement error.[17] Summing up, we have

Proposition 9: There is a wage and a time intensity component in the billings data, related to exogenous variables ($\bar{s}$,r,w$_Y$) in accordance with the predictions of the theoretical model.

In order to check the stability of the coefficients, the model was reestimated, but using data for 1977 and 1978. The results are presented in Figure 3. This time, only four of the six elasticities have the signs predicted by the theoretical analaysis. For example, $\hat{e}_{q,r}$ = 1.05 (.12) is a flat contradiction of the model. At the same time P3%, the share of private patients in the total, is now positively related to the coinsurance rate (r), the loading coefficient being 0.22 (.067). Apparently, the data once more do not allow us effectively to separate the influences of patient income and insurance on the decisions of physicians. Unfortunately, the other indicators of (w$_Y$) available, SEMIRUR and URBAN, are of such low quality that measurement error again is estimated to make up for the entire observed variance. On the endogenous side, YDRUGS once more turns out to be a comparatively dependable indicator of the unobservable physician wage rate (q). But billings per total case (YTOTAL) suddenly mirror (q) only, with an unexpected negative loading coefficient on average treatment time (t). Finally, the statistical fit deteriorates significantly, to a chi-square of 12942. There is, at least ex post, a good reason for all this instability. Beginning in July 1978, the insurance fund applied a new fee schedule, designed to discourage "excessive use of medical appliances." This restructuring induced physicians to bill for their time input, making the number of consultations and home calls better indicators of (t). We may therefore formulate

Proposition 10: The introduction of data for the year 1978 brings about important changes in the quality of the endogenous indicators.

Clearly, we must relax the assumption that observations for the year 1978 reflect (q) and (t) in the same way as those for 1977. On the other hand, admitting of two fully different sets of measurement loadings and error variances would lead to underidentification. To guarantee identification, only CONSULT is allowed to have two different measurement error variances in the two years of observation. The results of this seemingly slight relaxation are shown in Figure 4 and are rather impressive. Of the six elasticities, all have the predicted sign, although only three are statistically distinguishable from zero. All the indicators of the exogenous variables have loading coefficients as expected, and the indicators of ($\bar{s}$) form an intuively plausible hierarchy: Given that AGEP is

262 P. Zweifel

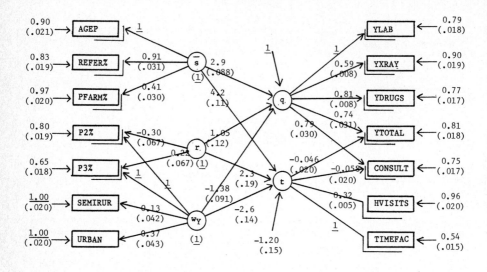

Figure 3. LISREL estimation results, 616 physicians, 1977 and 1978.
χ^2 = 12942, with 318 d.f.

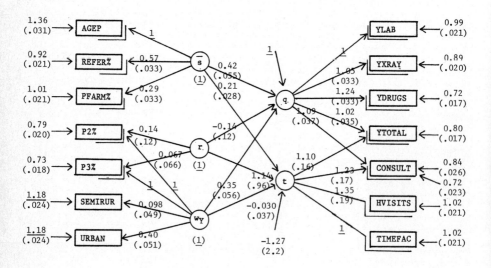

Figure 4. Free measurement error variances in CONSULT, 616 physicians, 1977
and 1978. χ^2 = 12945, with 317 d.f.

the basic indicator, the share of referrals in the total (REFER%) is second with a coefficient of 0.57 (.033), followed by the share of patients with farming background (PFARM%), with 0.29 (.033). Also, the share of middle-class and well-to-do patients, P2% and P3%, can now be interpreted as indicators of the coinsurance rate (r), albeit very weak ones. Concerning the indicators related to the decision variables, YDRUGS retains its prominent position as a wage rate indicator, while YTOTAL can be interpreted as reflecting the wage (q) and the time (t) component about equally, with loading coefficients 1.02 (.035) and 1.10 (.16), respectively. Finally, the estimated measurement error components of the variances of CONSULT do differ: In 1977, it is 71% (=0.84^2), and in 1978, 52% (=0.72^2). The standard error of this difference may be estimated to be 0.035 (=$0.026^2 + 0.023^2)^{1/2}$), so that the hypothesis of a chance variation can be rejected. Only the statistical fit fails to improve.

An important open question remains. Up to this point, we have looked at factors influencing the demand for first contacts, h $(\cdot)$, and have traced their effects through to the decision variables (q) and (t). But no direct evidence has been adduced showing that shifts in the function h $(\cdot)$ do matter. This way of proceeding was adopted because of the lack of indicators relating to h $(\cdot)$. For a high number of patients treated in any given year may be due to the fact that our particular sickness insurance fund looms large in that physician's region. Conversely, a physician having but a few cases on his record may be under great pressure of demand, but arising from members of competing funds. A change in numbers treated, however, or more precisely, in the number of first contacts (DFIRSTC) is an observation directly related to a change dh($\cdot$), i.e. of the probability of seeing a physician, given catchment population. We are therefore able to dispense with the indicators mirroring the arguments of the function h $(\cdot)$, focusing on dh($\cdot$) itself instead. Accordingly, Figure 5 contains but two exogenous variables, (d$\bar{s}$) and (dh). The indicators of (d$\bar{s}$) are the same ones as before, with DAGEP, for example, denoting a change in logarithms. The change of demand for patient-initiated contacts is indicated by three variables measuring changes in the numbers of patients treated, DP1, DP2, and DP3.[18] The best indicator of dh($\cdot$) should be DFIRSTC as defined by the fund, which counts first contacts within a quarter of a year. Nevertheless, it ought to be kept in mind that h($\cdot$) stands for the probability of seeing a physician for the first time within an episode of sickness whose length need not coincide with this three month period. Measurement error is therefore still present.

The estimates presented in Figure 5 tend to confirm the theoretical model again. An increase in average symptom severity does not only have a treatment intensity effect with $e_{dt,ds}$ = 1.14 (.074), but a price effect as well with $e_{dq,ds}$ = 0.38 (.054). This amounts to a "cold" price discrimination by physicians, who undercut the imposed uniformity of the fee schedule. A change in the demand for first contacts has an even more pronounced effect on the implicit wage rate, the estimated elasticity being 0.69 (.052). The effect on time intensity (dt) is about the same and negative, as predicted by the theoretical model. Our a priori judgments concerning the respective qualities of the indicators are also confirmed, as DYDRUGS dominates the other indicators of (dq). The change in billings per case (DYTOTAL) may be interpreted as the approximate

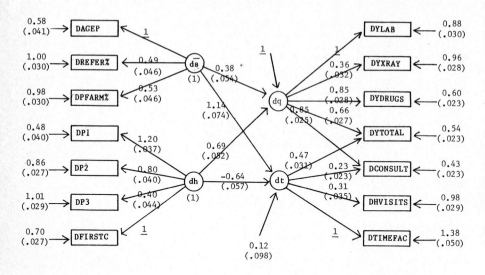

Figure 5. LISREL estimation results, 616 physicians, changes 1977/76.
χ^2 = 3747, with 74 d.f.

sum of the log changes (dq) and (dt), with coefficients 0.66(.027)
and 0.47(.031). What is something of a surprise is the result that
the number of office visits billed (DCONSULT) should mirror the wage
change so much more than the treatment intensity change. The first
estimated coefficient is 0.85 (.025), as high as the one for
DYDRUGS, the second only 0.23 (.023). On the other hand, there does
not seem to be a reasonably dependable indicator of (dt). For 96
(=0.98^2) percent of the variance of DHVISITS is estimated to be due
to measurement error. In the case of DTIMEFAC the implied variance
exceeds the empirical one.

These tests are very weak and preliminary, of course. They do seem
to indicate, however, that curtailing demand for first contacts
induces the physician to adjust his implicit wage rate as well as
the average time intensity of his treatment. A reduction of initial
demand by a 10% hike in the coinsurance rate, say, would be associated with a lowering of the price by 1.4%. At the same time, physicians will tend to increase their time input per case treated by
some 11%, according to the estimates of Figure 4. The wage reduction is transmitted to observed YTOTAL to about 102% and the time
increase to some 110%. As a rough guess, this would make for an
increase of YTOTAL in the order of magnitude of 11% (= -1.4% × 1.02
+ 11% × 1.1), on average. Therefore, observed billings per case
will not decrease. The structure of billings would change, of
course, with somewhat fewer drugs prescribed and more home visits
performed. Held against the impulse, the observed effects are
liable to smack of "induced demand" indeed.

CONCLUSION

We have developed an economic model of private physician behavior that tackles the widely reported phenomenon of "supplier-induced demand." Abstracting from fee-fixing contracts with sickness funds, which are considered largely ineffective, we predict that physicians will decrease their implicit wage rate when the demand for first contacts is curtailed--e.g., by imposing a higher coinsurance rate. But they will also spend more time per case, which tends to obscure the first effect. For what is usually monitored is total billings per case treated, which corresponds to the product of wage rate times time spent on a patient. The model's implications were tested for differences in coinsurance rates and patient incomes. Not all of them were confirmed, possibly because higher incomes and higher coinsurance rates go together in the sample. A second set of estimates relates to changes over time, with physician and practice characteristics held constant. It confirms the demand for initial contacts as a key variable of the model. The estimates generally establish sales of drugs and number of office visits per case as rather dependable indicators of the implicit wage charged by physicians for ambulatory care. Observed changes in total billings may well be positive when demand for initial contacts is reduced, concealing wage rate adjustments physicians in fact make. This will create the impression of "supplier-induced demand," a concept that did not have to be introduced in this model at all.

NOTES

[1]In such fee-fixing contracts, fees are usually set for each major activity, e.g., taking blood pressure. Equation 2 reads

(2a) $Y = f \times a \times P$,

where (f) is the exogenously given fee level, (a) the average number of activities performed, and (P) the number of patients treated. But (a) is linked to time spent per patient by the identity $a \times t_a = t$, with t_a denoting the time an activity takes on average. Hence, we have

(2b) $Y = \dfrac{f}{t_a} \times t \times P$

The ratio (f/t_a) defines an implicit wage rate (q), which is not exogenous because the physician is free to vary t_a by working more or less carefully, talking more or less time with a patient, or delegating certain tasks to his aides.

[2]In Switzerland, as in the majority of European countries, hospitals are predominantly financed by tax money. Only a few private physicians may continue

ment in a hospital; rather, responsibility is handed over to hospital staff when a patient is admitted.

[3]Despite the similarity of notation, h (qr, w, s) is not a density function like $F(s,\bar{s})$. Rather, h (·) acts as a (nonlinear) filter on $F(s,\bar{s})$. In turn, $F(s,\bar{s})$ may be thought of as a Beta function so that $\bar{s}(=\alpha/(\alpha + \beta))$, $0 \leqslant s \leqslant 1$, would stand for the unknown mean symptom intensity prevalent in the population. For details, see Zweifel (1980, Ch. 3).

[4]Although the services of specialists tend to be more expensive than those of general practitioners, the decisive cost differential is between ambulatory and stationary health care. From this viewpoint, little is lost when all private physicians are aggregated into one group.

[5]The difference $[p(s,0) - p(s,t)]$ is positive, at least for $s \leqslant c$. In view of Equation 21 and Proposition 3, this is an optimality condition, not an assumption. Therefore, iatrogenic disease outside the hospital cannot be systematic. As a chance phenomenon, it might stem from an inability to estimate (s) correctly together with the condition $p(s,t) > p(s,0)$ for $s > c$.

[6]In general, the survival probability $[1-p(s,t)]$, and hence (I) itself, should probably be defined in a relative rather than in an absolute sense. As an agent, the physician should evaluate his contribution to health relative to some other source of care, especially the hospital. We have chosen not to reflect this in the notation in order to simplify matters.

[7]It should be noted, however, that Acton defines time cost in terms of travel and waiting times. A change of treatment time (t) is neither necessary nor sufficient for a change of those costs.

[8]M.S. Feldstein (1970) puts emphasis on scientific interest rather than a desire to help. But $[p(s,0)-p(s,t)]$ may easily be given the interpretation of an ignorance reduction due to the treatment of a patient with symptom level (s). This is the same as an information gain. However, to the extent that high symptom cases are also the informative ones, the physician might also raise (c) instead of lowering (q), with comparable effect on leisure (L) but not on income (Y) as sgn $(Y_c) = sgn(Y_q)$.

[9]This is a very strong separability assumption (see Brown and Deaton, 1972, pp. 1165-1166.) However, it is more plausible here than in the context of consumer demand. Physicians are indeed likely to consider (Y), (I), and (L) as three different aspects of their lives, related to each other only by restrictions.

[10]One such assumption is that price (q) does not influence demand for first visits in the neighborhood of the critical symptom level (c). Another is that price reactiveness $h_{(qr)}$ is invariant to changes of (r), implying that the elasticity of demand increases in absolute value with rising (r). For further details, see Zweifel (1980, Ch. 4).

[11]For details, again see Zweifel (1980, Ch. 4).

[12]I am grateful to H. Schmid, director of the "Krankenkasse für den Kanton Bern, KKB," for making these data available.

[13]The deductibles are 30, 50, and 80 Swiss francs per quarter respectively. Beyond billed amounts of 300, 500, and 800 francs per year, the coinsurance rate

is 10% throughout. Since bills amounting to more than 30 but less than 800 francs
make up for some 80% of all billed cases, these differences are likely to be
important.

[14]The figures in parentheses are estimated asymptotic standard errors.

[15]The normality assumption is violated because the dummies SEMIRUR and URBAN
are among the indicators. We neglect this complication for the time being.

[16]Since the latent variables are standardized to unit variance, the indicators
are standardized as well in order to free the loading coefficients from scaling
effects. Hence, estimated measurement error variances may be interpreted as
shares of total observed variances, which are equal to one everywhere. The analyzed matrix is accordingly a correlation rather than a covariance matrix.

[17]The usual standards for evaluating goodness of fit refer to regression analysis. Judged by these standards, but relating them to the explanation of
observed dependent variables only, the results of Figure 2 do not fare badly. For
example, YTOTAL has a total variance of 5.13. The estimated measurement error
variance is 69% (=0.83^2) and the structural error variance is 1 (normalized).
Hence, about 12% (=100 - 69 - 19) of total variance is explained by the model.
But in applications of LISREL, the regressors themselves must be predicted, which
explains why "good" chi-square statistics are conspicuously absent from the
literature. For an extended discussion, see Zweifel (1980, Ch. 7).

[18]Contrary to previous specifications, DP1, DP2, and DP3 are not shares but
(logarithms of) absolute numbers. Hence, there is no summation restriction.

HEALTH MEASUREMENT

HEALTH, ECONOMICS, AND HEALTH ECONOMICS
J. van der Gaag and M. Perlman (editors)
© *North-Holland Publishing Company, 1981*

WELFARE ECONOMICS AND HEALTH STATUS MEASUREMENT

Alan Williams

SETTING THE SCENE*

Welfare economics can variously be interpreted as a search for

(a) some "objective" (i.e., value-free) criterion for measuring improvements in social welfare;

(b) a criterion which satisfies pre-specified conditions of "reasonableness;"

(c) a criterion which commands "general" assent;

(d) the value judgments implicit in any proposed criterion.

The first of these interpretations is now generally recognized to be futile, and most of the action in recent years has been motivated by a search for the second (and to some extent the third) goal. The general conclusion appears to be that it is extremely difficult to devise criteria for social choice which simultaneously satisfy economists' scruples about the nature of the interpersonal comparisons of utility which they are willing to make, survive careful tests for internal consistency from a logical viewpoint, are capable of handling all possible configurations of preferences and choice possibilities, and satisfy individualistic/democratic notions of justice and fairness.

---

*I am grateful to all those colleagues who have offered constructive suggestions in response to an earlier version of this paper, some of which I have managed to incorporate in this revised version. My main debt, however, is to Rachel Rosser, who has shown exemplary patience and persistence in trying to discipline my bolder generalizations by insisting that I pay more regard to what researchers in the field have actually achieved so far in this difficult territory. Finally, I continue to be indebted to the Nuffield Provincial Hospitals Trust, through whose generosity some years ago I was able to take time out from other work to dig more deeply into the whole field of health service planning and evaluation.

This paper does not set out to construct, de novo, a criterion of
social welfare (for the dimension of health) which satisfies all
these desiderata, but instead looks at some existing criteria in
order to elicit any value judgments contained within them (or
implied by them) which are of special relevance from a welfare economics viewpoint. The use of any measure of output implies
valuation as well as description. To identify the value content of
an index the welfare economist has two possible strategies: either
to review all existing indexes and comment on their value implications or to specify a particular context and then explore the feasibility (and implications) of using some existing indexes for the
purpose. This paper adopts the latter strategy, and the specific
context chosen is the following: the benefit measure is to be used
in cost-effectiveness studies in which all changes in resource use
and in production are picked up elsewhere; and the benefit measure
shall not depend on the wealth or "economic" value of the affected
individual.

Before proceeding, this context is worth reflecting on further, if
the subsequent discussion is not to be misunderstood.

When we assume that all changes in real resources associated with
the alternative under investigation have been measured, it is useful
to classify them as:

(a)   changes in resources used in service provision;

(b)   changes in resources used by patients and their helpers;

(c)   changes in gross domestic product.

Item (a) should include all affected services (e.g., local authority
welfare services, ambulance services, primary care services, etc.,
and not just hospital services or whatever service is most closely
involved in the particular option under investigation). Item (b)
must include the value of any time which has opportunity cost, but
to avoid double-counting with what is in the benefit measure itself,
it will concentrate on the value of the patient's time to other
people (as well as including the value of other people's time to
themselves). The patient's own value of own time will not be
included under this head. Item (c) should include non-marketed outputs (such as housewives' services) which do not form part of GDP as
actually measured, but should do so in principle. Note that in each
case it is the "change in" the value of the relevant category of
resource that is to be measured, and this can be positive (hence a
"cost") or negative (hence a "benefit"). Note also that associated
tax and transfer charges are not included, though under a more ambi-
tious rubric they would be separately picked up in a matrix of
distributional consequences, designed to establish the incidence of
the economic costs and benefits, and not simply their nature and
totals, which, for simplicity's sake, are all that will be considered here. Although these "economic" costs and benefits go well
beyond mere GDP calculations, they do deliberately exclude changes
in the health of patients per se.[1] This is because these
"humanitarian" benefits (or costs) are to be the main focus of
discussion in this paper, and left to occupy the "other side" of the
cost-effectiveness account. Thus the dichotomy will not be between

"costs" (= bad changes) and "benefits" (= good changes) but between changes (good and bad) in resources, and changes (good and bad) in health itself.[2]

The benefit measure sought is one which embodies the ethical prin- ciple that any interpersonal comparison of the value of health shall not depend upon the wealth or economic value of the people con- cerned. This reflects not only the ostensible ethic of the medical profession itself, but also the putative political principle on which health services are organized in many countries, and is one of the major reasons why the provision of health services has not been left to the market, but treated more as a "citizen's entitlement" than as part of society's "reward system" (Donabedian, 1971). In that context, measures of the value of health which reflect people's ability to pay will be irrelevant. The interest lies seeing how far we can get in establishing an "uncontaminated" set of values which give as much rein as possible to differences in the relative values they attach to different attributes of health, while pursuing some kind of egalitarian principle between the weight given to one person's valuations compared with another's. This is the central task of the paper. To be of general use, the measure has, in addi- tion, to be a cardinal measure, since in the cost-effectiveness con- text we may need to conduct all the basic mathematical manipulations upon it. The properties of a wide range of extant indexes have been comprehensively reviewed by Rosser (1979), and a regularly updated cumulative annotated bibliography of work in this field (National Center for Health Statistics, Clearinghouse on Health Indexes) has been maintained by the U.S. Department of Health and Human Services since 1972.

The next section of the paper outlines the manner in which one could undertake the measurement of the relative value attached by an indi- vidual to different health states, once one had postulated a "numeraire" health state to act as a unit of value, and a zero- valued state so as to ensure full cardinality. The third section outlines the ethical postulates required to justify various methods of aggregation of these individual valuations in order to derive a community valuation, and their implications are explored. The fourth section shows what happens when the "health status index," so derived, is put back into the cost-effectiveness framework, with the apparent result that the carefully specified egalitarian- humanitarian ethic built into the third section seems suddenly to be undermined by the resource side of the equation. The final section contains some general observations and suggestions for further work.

THE CALCULUS FOR ONE INDIVIDUAL

There are a myriad of ways in which health can be characterized, and, important and controversial though the topic is, I shall here merely assert that for the purposes to which I see this health sta- tus measure being put, measures based simply on presence or absence of disease, or on changes in mortality, are inappropriate. My general position is that the best measure of health for the purpose of economic evaluation must be a "feeling-functional" one, in which

the presumed ideal is a long life in which each individual is able
to undertake the normal pattern of activities free of pain and
distress. Suppose we designate that ability as being "healthy," and
assign it (arbitrarily) the value 1 for a particular individual.
Since "normal" functioning is a socially conditioned notion, this
notion of healthiness may well fall short of "perfect" health, in
the sense of the maximum attainable by anyone, anywhere, ever.
Rather it will have the more modest (and more useful) connotation of
accepting that there is a threshold below which a society considers
someone as "to all intents and purposes" healthy (warts and all, and
although not 100% fit as judged by Olympic standards).

But what lies at the opposite extreme from healthy? The obvious
answer seems to be "dead," but herein lies a hornet's nest of
problems which are not at all easy to resolve. For instance, it
could be argued that the opposite of "painfree ability to conduct
normal activities," is "in very severe pain and totally unable to
conduct normal activities." It may further be asserted that this is
worse than being unconscious (i.e., in no pain but totally unable to
conduct normal activities), and perhaps even worse than being dead
(as witness: the proponents of voluntary euthanasia). There are
two ways of resolving this dilemma in the present context. One is
to constrain individuals to conform to society's view (whatever that
is), by postulating what the worst state is, and assigning that the
value 0. The other is to let each individual choose which is the
worst (i.e., zero-valued) state, and let that be part of the realm
of individual valuation. For the purposes of this exercise, because
it is simpler, it will be postulated that "dead" is the worst state,
which still leaves individuals free to value other states also at
zero if they wish. The other important characteristic of the state
"dead" is that it is, in the jargon of the trade, an "absorbing"
state, i.e., once you are in it, the transition probabilities from
it to any other state are all zero. This will not be true of any
other states, even those which individuals also value at zero.

With these two fixed points to work from, individuals would be asked
to value a large selection of intermediate states, each of which is
a (different) combination of attributes in dimensions such as
pain/distress, physical mobility, capacity for self-care, ability to
play normal social roles, etc. These valuations are usually made in
a context in which it is assumed that:

(a)   each health state is to be thought of as persisting for the
       same length of time;

(b)   the actual length of time must be specified, because it can
       affect the relative valuations of different states;

(c)   the state is to be evaluated for its own intrinsic
       "enjoyability" and not for any instrumental purpose it might
       have in enabling the individual to earn money, etc.;

(d)   all states must be evaluated as if the respondent were in them
       now (and not in earlier or later life);

(e)   no element of prognosis must seep in (e.g., being in any par-
       ticular state now should not be thought to imply anything about

the relative probabilities of being in any particular state in
the future);

(f)   the valuation of each state is independent of the states which
      precede or follow it.

These are very stringent conditions, which make empirical work to
elicit such valuations rather difficult. They are needed in order
to avoid the logistically impossible alternative, which is to present subjects with all possible future time profiles of health
states, and then to get them to value each profile as a whole
relatively to each other profile as a whole.

Even in the more limited exercise there are difficulties at both
theoretical and technical levels, which begin with the selection of
the dimensions of health, which must emerge from empirical investigation in which respondents are permitted to reveal their own
constructs of health. In the foregoing discussion the results of
this process were prejudged (on the basis of work already done) to
lead to the dimensions mentioned. The choice of valuation technique
is a second important area, where the strategic choice is between
behavioral and psychometric techniques. The former are largely
observational, and therefore "realistic," but uncontrolled, multi-
factorial, and difficult to purge of "wealth effects." Psychometric
methods therefore seem to predominate in this kind of work, the precise method being determined partly by the kind of measure required
(e.g., interval or ratio scale, etc.). It is important, however, to
ensure that what you get is what you set out to get, whether
people's valuations are internally consistent, or different methods
(e.g., category rating, magnitude estimation, or equivalence
assessment) are consistent with each other when applied to the same
subjects, or respondents seem equally able to respond to each. It
is not sufficient simply to apply statistical tests of correlation
to establish such concordance, because one also needs the more
pragmatic test of whether, where they differ, these differences are
crucial in their consequences for actions in the field, or whether
they make no significant difference as to what people do. Current
testing is deficient in this latter respect.

The kinds of measurements on which economists can draw for this purpose are epitomized in the work of investigators such as Patrick,
Bush, and Chen (1973), Card, Rusenkiewicz, and Phillips (1977),
Rosser and Kind (1978) and Torrance (1976) though none of them would
probably accept my specific formulation. I have deliberately
steered away from the technical and practical problems of conducting
this kind of work. In this connection, see Johnson and Huber
(1977), which also includes an extensive bibliography. I have
instead concentrated on eliciting the underlying value judgments,
because it is important that these be recognized if the work is to
be used in an ethically appropriate context.

THE PROCESS OF AGGREGATION AND ITS IMPLICATIONS

In an exercise of this kind an aggregation rule designed to elicit

the community's relative valuation of different health states must
of necessity imply an ethical postulate, and cannot be regarded as a
mere computational device. In the foregoing section, individual
valuations were constrained in such a way that one unit period of
time (say a year) in the state "healthy" was to be valued at 1, and
being dead was to be of zero value (from the viewpoint of our
earthly existence, at any rate). We now have to make a heroic leap
and postulate some relationship between Individual A's one year of
health (or death) and Individual B's one year of health (or death).

The simplest postulate consistent with the egalitarian-humanitarian
ethic is that a year of healthy life is to be regarded as of equal
intrinsic value to everyone, irrespective of age, sex, etc. This is
equivalent to regarding one year of healthy life expectation as a
"numeraire" commodity, exchangeable on a one-for-one basis within
the community, but with individuals free to establish their own
relative values of all other health states (except dead) which they
might experience. This seems to be the commonest aggregation rule,
and is explicitly adopted in the work of Patrick, Bush, and Chen
(1973) and Torrance (1976). This rule implies that an extra ten
years of healthy life for one individual are of equal social value
to one extra year of healthy life for each of ten different individuals. A second, more complicated postulate would be to argue that
an additional year of healthy life expectation is to be regarded as
of differential intrinsic value according to the age, and/or sex of
the beneficiary. Thus if we established as the numeraire "one year
of healthy life for a man aged 40," we would need to elicit the
values placed by all the individuals in the community on the value
of one year of healthy life at each other age for each sex.

It seems to me to be a weakness of the existing work on health
indexes that a disproportionate amount of attention has been paid to
the eliciting of relative values from individuals, and to comparison
of these relativities between individuals, but very little to eliciting people's views about how the valuation of one person should be
weighed with those of another in order to reach a set of "social"
values. The reason for this relative neglect is probably that most
such indexes have been designed for purposes other than planning or
resource-allocation. (See, for example, Thouez, 1979.) Those that
have had this latter orientation, have tended to add (or average)
data in a rather unreflective way (as shown by Culyer, 1978a), and a
common escape route in the more theoretical literature, as Whitmore
(1973) has observed, is simply to postulate that everyone has the
same utility index (an assumption I am here seeking to avoid).

On whichever basis it is decided to proceed, the derivation of a
scale for the whole community requires only one further step, viz.,
defining the relevant community. This could, in principle, range
from all humanity (including generations as yet unborn), to a
small number of people living in one small geographical area at some
specific time, for whom some health-related choice has to be made
between alternative uses of a given amount of resources. This
"choice of community" is an issue that I intend to duck in this
paper, since it is essentially a political decision which does not
affect the essence of the argument, but only the precise form in
which it would be applied in a given situation. It might mean, for
instance, that for purposes of health service planning at national

level, it would be thought advantageous to elicit the valuations of
a large random sample of the entire citizenry (or at least that subset eligible to vote). Adopting an entirely different approach, it
might be argued that "proxy" or "representative" or "expert" valuers
might be chosen as the respondents, on some such grounds, respectively, as the following: "proxies" might be required for infants
and very young children, for the mentally ill and handicapped, and
other non-competent subgroups; "representatives" might be required
through the political process because of the practical difficulties
of organizing the frequent redrawing of large samples of the population for direct consultation on these matters; and "experts" might
be required because the issues involved are so complex that only
people with the right training, experience and intellectual skills
could respond properly. (Although I have views on these matters,
they are set aside here as separable from the main theme.)

Having come this far, the final step is aggregation itself. The
simplest (and commonest) procedure is to take each health state in
turn and add up the score assigned to it by each of the N individuals, and take the average as the community's valuation of that
health state. What emerges may not coincide with the actual
valuations of any particular individual, of course, and it is a
fascinating exercise in its own right to investigate what are the
correlates of any significant deviation from the average, e.g.,
whether they are associated in any systematic way with the
respondent's age, sex, family circumstances, political or religious
beliefs, educational level, occupation, recent or current
experience of illess, etc. (See, for example, Rosser and Kind,
1978.) It has frequently been suggested in casual conversation
(though I have not found an example in the literature) that distributional equity dictates that it is better for many people to get a
little than for a few people to get a lot (i.e., contradicting the
notion that one person getting ten years' additional life expenditure
is the same as ten people getting one each). To pick up that ethical postulate we would have to take (say) the logarithm or the
square root of the "quantity" of benefit gained by each individual,
and then work with that transformed value in the subsequent
analysis.

There remain only three further matters for discussion before this
"tariff" of values is ready to be fed back into the framework of a
cost-effectiveness study in order to see how it would be used. The
first of these concerns whether "time preference" does or should
exist, and if so, whether it is for each individual or for the community to choose the precise discount rate to be applied in order to
give effect to it. The argument for individuals each applying their
own discount rate is essentially that there may be great variation
in private time preference rates for health states across the community, and a valuation scheme which only allowed individuals to
compare health states at a point in time, but not between present
and future periods, would be seriously defective. The coun-
ter-argument is based on the observation that because it is possible,
at the margin, to transform health into wealth, and vice versa, at
any point in time, and since the "wealth" is (ideally) allocated
through time with reference to the rate of social time preference,
then it would be inconsistent to apply a different rate of discount
to "health" from that being applied to "wealth." I incline to the
latter view.

This leads on to the second consequential matter, which is the
respondents' attitudes to "risk," and whether the "certainty"
approach employed here is not seriously defective because it fails
to elicit risk-aversity. A similar line of argument to that in the
preceding paragraph can be employed here. The "risks" concern the
likelihood that an individual will be in one state rather than
another, and this is a matter on which others are likely to be more
knowledgeable than the individual is, and one about which, for the
community as a whole, there may be virtually no uncertainty whatever
(e.g., over age/sex specific death rates). Since the decisions on
which this "tariff" of community valuation of health states is to
bear are ones which will typically involve choices for largish
populations, the uncertainty is more relevant to distributional
issues than to those addressed here. It therefore seems quite
defensible to take advantage of the considerable simplification
facilitated by valuing the states as if they were certain, but
generating the probability distribution of states separately.

The third and final consequential matter is the fear that, once
respondents realize how their responses are going to be used, they
will engage in some kind of "false signalling" in order to manipu-
late the outcome to their own advantage. For instance, if someone
is already (chronically) in a particular health state, then it might
be thought advantageous for that person to undervalue that state
(i.e., declare a value lower than the "real" one) in the hope that
this will help draw more resources into any activity which would
move him into a better health state (and it certainly would help to
do that in the circumstances postulated, although only to a very
small extent if the total population of respondents is fairly
large). But the danger to the individual with this kind of false
signalling is that it automatically entails the respondent under-
valuing the difference between his current state and various worse
states, so that he or she might find resources drawn away from activities which would prevent a worsening of his or her situation. It
does therefore seem to be a rather risky business. Moreover, it is
generally very difficult for individuals to be at all sure which
health states they will be in, even in the immediate future, which
adds yet another deterrent to false signalling. All in all, it does
not seem to be serious danger.

ON MIXING SUGAR AND SAND

Suppose we now have a set of relative values for different health
states, on a scale 0 to 1, which can be used as the building blocks
for constructing a time profile of expected future health states and
the impact of a treatment upon that profile. The difference between
the two profiles is the value of the treatment in humanitarian
terms, best described as expected years of life expectation adjusted
for health quality. These will then be aggregated according to
whichever principles were deemed appropriate in the light of the
considerations set out earlier. When this is juxtaposed with the
resource cost data mentioned earlier, it would be possible to say
that treatment A "costs" 10,000y and yields health benefits of
1000z, while B "costs" 7500y and yields benefits of 1500z and C

costs 500y and yields benefits of 25z (where y is a unit of money
value and z is the numeraire health state). Thus each unit improvement in health costs 10 with A, 5 with B, and 20 with C, so if
resources are limited and there are constant returns to scale in
each case, then the priorities for new investment would be, first,
treatment B, then A, then C. (In reality it is likely that as the
scale of provision increases, each successive increase in capacity
will result in less suitable patients being treated, so costs per
achieved unit of health improvement will actually be increasing.)

But now we come to some further problems. Suppose that the reason
why treatment B "costs" only 7500 is that (a) it typically gets
highly paid patients back to work quickly, (b) the associated GDP
benefits have been "netted out," and (c) had this not been so the
costs would have been much higher, say 30,000. Suppose the other
two treatments were for the chronically mentally handicapped and the
very elderly, respectively, and generated no GDP benefits whatever.
It now seems that, despite our humanitarian-egalitarian principles,
priorities are still being affected by the very things we were
trying to shut out, for without the GDP benefits treatment B would
have cost 20 per unit of health benefit achieved, and would have
been given the lowest priority instead of the highest. Was it all
worthwhile? Did we labor so mightily merely to bring forth a mouse?

The root of the problem is that we have two valuation systems
operating side by side. In the nonhealth sector we have valuations
"contaminated" by unequal ability to pay, whereas in the health sector we wanted a set of "decontaminated" values. But which of these
should we use to measure the opportunity cost of the resources used
in the health sector? So long as the society thinks it right that
nonhealth benefits should be valued, relatively to each other, by
the "contaminated" set of values, then there is no valid argument
for excluding the GDP benefits once you include benefits in the form
of savings of service costs. So the question at issue is whether
any of the resource costs should influence priorities in the health
sector. If it is held that they should not, then it will be
impossible to guarantee the maximization of health benefits for any
given level of resource use. If it is held that they should, then
all elements of resource use will exercise an influence, and we
shall have to face up to the consequence that it is in society's
interests to give some precedence in matters of health care to those
members of the society whose activities others value most highly.
Not to do so seems perversely masochistic.

This brings us to the final critical issue, viz., just how much
weight should be given to the "economic" as opposed to the
"humanitarian" benefits? This is another way of posing the
question, "How much precedence should be given to those whose activities others value most highly?" It will also determine,
indirectly, what fraction of the community's resources are devoted
to the health sector. So far I have shied away from the question of
money valuation of health benefits, but now it has inescapably to be
faced, and there is no easy answer to it. It would be self-
defeating if, at this stage, each individual's money valuation of a
unit change in health were elicited from his or her own behavior
when confronted with situations in which money had to be sacrificed
to improve health, since such values would be "contaminated" with

the wealth and income inequalities whose effects we are trying to
neutralize. It might be argued that this would be less of a problem
if each individual's marginal valuations of "units" of health,
derived in this way, were somehow averaged, and that average then
applied to every unit improvement in health, no matter who got it.
But although these individual marginal rates of substitution between
health and all other goods may be a useful guide to the approximate
magnitude of the corresponding social marginal rate of substitution,
ultimately the latter has to be a community-wide decision, just as
with the choice of a social rate of time preference. It brings us
back squarely to the issues raised in the literature on the value of
life (recently surveyed by Mooney, 1977).

This should not be interpreted as meaning that the earlier exercise
was fruitless, however, because a different set of relative
valuations of quality and quantity of life will almost certainly
emerge from the calculus compared with the "economic" calculus.
Moreover, if units of health are valued very highly at the margin,
the "resource" element in the calculation will carry correspondingly
little weight. Thus a very "humanitarian" health system will select
a different set of patients from one more concerned with resource
savings (i.e., non-health benefits). It might be speculated that
the economic side of the equation will have more weight in communities where the overall standard of living is close to sub-
sistence levels, whereas the more humanitarian side of the equation
will have more weight where a community can afford to carry a significant proportion of "unproductive" people. It should be noted,
moreover, that this issue is distinct from the one about how differently the humanitarian benefits should themselves be valued
(i.e., whether a person's income and wealth should influence the
weight given to that person's views in that part of the calculus).
Since the GDP consequences and the level of income will be highly
correlated, if humanitarian benefits are weighted by such influences, this will tend to augment the influence of economic considerations on priorities in health care.

CONCLUSIONS

I have tried to work through, and expose, all the important ethical
considerations underlying the computation of a health index which
seeks to estimate, by psychometric methods, an individual's relative
valuations of different health states, and then to fuse these into a
set of social valuations over the same set of health states, in a
manner suitable for use in cost-effectiveness studies. I have
imposed on the "fusion" process an additional requirement, namely
that it must be ethically appropriate, by which I mean that in my
selected context the social valuations which emerge must not be
vulnerable to influence from the distribution of income and wealth
across respondents.

There obviously remains plenty of work to be done in developing and
refining the approach here outlined. Tight and widely applicable
descriptions of key health states need to be established as the
basic building blocks. Epidemiological and other clinical research

needs to be so designed as to measure the course of each patient's
condition in terms of these states, so that we slowly build up a
clear picture of the relative effectiveness of various interventions
in fairly standardized terms. All this is needed before valuation
can be brought to bear but in the meantime the testing of the
valuation process itself can continue, and the rival methods carefully appraised for their sensitivity, reliability, and accep-
tability. The applied welfare economists could, at the same time,
be assisting in this task, while the theoretical welfare economists
could be grappling with the dilemmas of principle posed by this
approach, both internally, and when it is put back into the context
of an economic evaluation which values resources on a different
basis.

It seems to me a potentially rich field for economists, especially
in view of the fact that practitioners (and researchers) in the
health care field are (and will be) using very crude, and often
quite inappropriate, proxies to fill the vacuum caused by the
absence of theoretically satisfactory ways of measuring levels of
health.[3]   There are doubtless some who would argue that since our
interests and expertise lie primarily in assessing money valuations
as elicited from market or quasi-market data, then if that is not
what people want, they should look elsewhere for help. I believe
this latter view to be misguided, and, if widely adopted, it will
exclude economists from exercising their analytical skills over
large areas of social policy where the ethic of the market (and consequently the market as a source of information about valuations) is
rejected. That would be a great waste of our talents. I sometimes
fear that things are worse still, and that the way in which the
welfare economics of social choice has developed recently, with
almost exclusive concentration on the second of the four tasks set
out at the beginning of this paper, may have already so inhibited
and emasculated the subject that the third and fourth tasks are no
longer considered even legitimate, and to practise them (and especially to go so far as to set about estimating interpersonal comparisons of cardinal utility) puts one beyond the pale. If so, so
be it, but those who thereby find themselves in exile will at least
be able to take comfort in the thought that though their light may
be dim, it shines where the world is darkest.

NOTES

[1]"Patients" here means whoever are the subjects of the study. Since some
"treatments" are given to one person in order to improve the health of another
person, the latter may be "patients" as well as the former.

[2]For a fuller discussion of this way of looking at things, see Drummond
(1980).

[3]The contents of the joint publication by the World Health Organization and
the International Epidemiological Association (1979), called Measurement of
Levels of Health, bear adequate testimony to the diversity of approach and content
that represents the current state of "best practice" in this field.

HEALTH, ECONOMICS, AND HEALTH ECONOMICS
J. van der Gaag and M. Perlman (editors)
© North-Holland Publishing Company, 1981

A NEW HEALTH STATUS INDEX FOR CHILDREN

Barbara Wolfe
Jacques van der Gaag

INTRODUCTION

This paper is primarily an attempt to use a latent variable technique to measure health status in a system of health care demand
equations.* The structural model we will develop contains both
causal equations and a set of health indicators, or need measures.
More specifically: the need measures, such as days ill, activity
limitations, subjective health rating and particular disease categories, are specified to be proportional to an overall health-status
measure, which in turn is assumed to be a function of the age and
sex of the child and a number of household characteristics. The
need measures then enter the utilization equations indirectly
through the overall health status measure. The endogenous overall
health status measure can be estimated for each observation in the
sample. In principle, this measure can be used for health-care
planning purposes, for improving the geographical distribution of
health-care services and for improving the equity of health-care
utilization.

A good deal of previous research in health-related fields has been
plagued by the lack of appropriate measure(s) of health status.
Volumes have been written on indices (e.g. Berg, 1973) searching for
the appropriate measure. Such measures would facilitate health
planning, demand analysis, production-function work and distributional work. It may be that measures of health status are best
designed for the specific purpose at hand--in our example for utilization analysis. The purpose may dictate whether a single or
multiple measure is better suited; for example, utilization of mental health-care providers may require an index other than a broad-
based health measure. For many purposes (such as health-care
planning or the study of the production of health) a single measure
which provides an overall view of health is clearly attractive.

---

*This research was supported in part by funds granted to the Institute for
Research on Poverty at the University of Wisconsin-Madison by the Department of
Health and Human Services pursuant to the Economic Opportunity Act of 1964. The
authors wish to thank members of the Rochester Child Health Study Project for
making the data available.

A STRUCTURAL MODEL OF HEALTH-CARE UTILIZATION FOR CHILDREN

Structural Versus Reduced Form Models

The literature (see Hyman, 1971, and M. S. Feldstein, 1974, for
overviews) dealing with the explanation of differences in health-
care utilization--among individuals, between regions or over time--
usually employs a regression model, with health-care utilization as
the dependent variable and a set of other variables as exogenous
explanatory variables.

An important weakness of such an approach can probably be best
illustrated in the following example:

Let us assume we are interested in the income elasticity of health-
care demand, and we estimate:

$$D = \alpha + \beta Y + \delta'Z$$

where D = the demand for health care

   Y = income

   Z = a vector of other variables

   α, β and δ' are parameters.

If we find β to be positive, we conclude that health care is a
"normal" good; but if β turns out to be negative, or close to zero,
alternative explanations are suggested. For instance: income is
positively related to health, and healthier people seek less health
care. The addition of measures of health status to utilization
equations is one way partially to remedy this problem.[1] However,
satisfactory health measures that measure that component of
someone's health status relevant for health-care utilization are
generally not available, or the number necessary to measure health
status would be large, and the different measures would be highly
correlated.

Recently a number of authors have suggested a way to overcome the
ambiguity in these types of analysis based on reduced form
equations. They specify a health-care demand model as:

$$H^* = \gamma'X$$
$$D = \alpha + \beta Y + \delta'Z + \mu H^*$$

where H* = "health," a unobservable variable (as indicated by the
      asterisk*)

   X = a vector of variables relevant for the "production" of
        health^2

μ and γ are parameters.

If measures of income (or income-related variables) are included in
X, β can unambiguously be interpreted as the income effect on
health-care demand. And from estimates of μ and γ the impact of
income on health can be derived. Of course we do not have to
restrict ourselves to analyzing the role of income. Many other
variables may have an impact <u>both</u> on health and on health-care utilization. Thus, the quality and usefulness of health-care demand
analysis can be improved if structural models are used that explicitly deal with this complication.

We develop a structural model of children's health-care utilization
in which health status and permanent income are unobservables.
Figure 1 gives a simplified pictorial presentation of the model.
Socioeconomic factors ("predisposing variables") are determinants of
health. These factors include age, sex, family size, and race. We
have seven imperfect measures of health (need variables) to serve as
indicators of the unobservable overall health status. Each of these
indicators is specified to be proportional to the overall measure of
health status.

Utilization is used as another indicator of health status.
Utilization, however, is also determined by enabling variables, such
as income, health insurance and the availability of care.

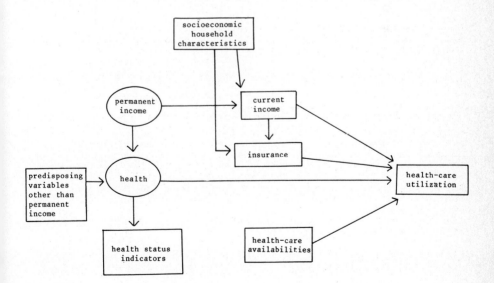

Figure 1. Simplified scheme of the health-care utilization model.

Permanent income (unobservable), representing the continuing socio-economic level influencing someone's health, is estimated using a quasi-earnings function. Current income serves as an indicator for permanent income. It is also the relevant income variable in the utilization equations, as it represents the income flow during the period of analysis.

Health insurance is treated as endogenous in the model, thus shedding more light on the complicated role income plays in the utilization of health care. However, we avoided the complication of having health insurance be influenced by health status. This is probably less restricted than it seems, since we restrict our analyses to observations on children of age 1-17 only.

This restricted sample has the further advantage that we do not have to deal with the possible simultaneity between health and income. Two caveats regarding the model should be mentioned in advance. First, the model puts some severe restrictions on the data. For example: since age only enters the utilization equations through the variable health, the age-utilization profiles are the same in each demand equation, apart from a multiplicative constant. Our analyzing data only on children between the ages of 1 and 17 may make this restriction less severe, but does not eliminate it.

Second, we do not specify health to be influenced by health-care utilization. Such an extension of the model calls for a dynamic model, in which present health status is influenced by past utilization, in order to avoid reversed causality problems.

Thus, this paper is but the first stage in a larger effort to estimate health-status measures from health-care demand models.

A total of seventeen equations compose the model: one for health status, seven for the health indicators, three insurance equations, four health-care demand equations, one quasi-earnings function and an indicator equation for income.

In the next sections we will present these equations in more detail.

Factors Affecting Children's Health-Care Utilization

Grossman has developed an economic model of the demand for health. The main feature of his model is that it explicitly recognizes that "what consumers demand when they purchase medical services are not these services per se but rather good health" (Grossman, 1972a, xiii). His theoretical model, which emphasizes the investment aspect of medical care utilization, has formed the basis for a large number of empirical studies, showing the importance of this distinction for modelling the demand for health care and for the interpretation of the estimation results.

Starting from a different angle, Andersen (1968) developed a framework within which health-care utilization can be studied. Both

Table 1. Enabling Variables

Symbol	Definition	Mean	Variance
LINC	Log of total family income	4.97	.37
	Proxy variables for health-care availability:		
HOSP	Travel time to nearest hospital, in minutes	11.36	38.34
HMO	Travel time to nearest HMO-clinic	11.54	72.20
XHMO	Travel time to nearest non-HMO-clinic	14.65	64.65
PHYS	Physician/population ratio[a]	.08	.01
	Dummy variables for health-care insurance:		
INSHMO	= 1 if insured for HMO-clinic; = 0 elsewhere	.07	.07
INSPRIV	= 1 if private insurance; = 0 elsewhere	.89	.10
MCAID	= 1 if covered by Medicaid; = 0 elsewhere	.08	.08

[a]The physician/population ratio is the number of family doctors per 1000 population in the census tract, plus a weighted sum of these ratios for all other census tracts. As weights we used the travel time, in 15-minute intervals, squared.

approaches lead to similar empirical work (see Andersen et al., 1975).

We will adopt Andersen's stratification of the data to ease the exposition of our model. Our estimation results will be discussed with reference to Grossman's and related work.

Enabling variables. The set of enabling variables include all variables that represent financial or other barriers for the utilization of health services: income, prices, insurance, and the availability of services as measured by travel time, distance, etc. Unfortunately, no prices of health-care services are available in the data. However, since we limit our empirical work to one SMSA, we do not expect this to be a large limiting factor. Measures of the enabling variables that are included in our model are given in Table 1, together with some summary statistics.

Acknowledging the fact that many of the variables that enter the demand equations for health care will also have an impact on the demand for health insurance, we treat the three insurance variables as endogenous in our model.

The insurance variables available include only type of insurance, rather than depth of coverage. We distinguish between private insurance, HMO and Medicaid coverage. To the extent insurance purchase is voluntary, it is likely to be determined by factors

Table 2. Household Variables Explaining Health Insurance

Symbol	Definition	Mean	Variance
LINC	Log of total family income in 00's	5.00	.33
	A linear spline in income:		
INC	Total family income (in 00's)	169	4096.30
INC-P.A.	Maximum (income-public assistance eligibility level, 0)		
INC-M.A.	Maximum (income-medical assistance eligibility level, 0)		
	Mother's employment status:		
MFULL	= 1 if mother works full-time; = 0 elsewhere	.21	.17
MPART	= 1 if mother works part-time; = 0 elsewhere	.20	.16
	Other parental variables:		
NOTMAR	= 1 if single parent; = 0 elsewhere	.13	.11
MSCHOOL	Years of schooling completed by mother	12.65	6.69
MOCC	Bogue socioeconomic index of mother's occupation	49.29	58.47
FOCC	Bogue socioeconomic index of father's occupation	49.20	461.92
	= 0 if father not present		
MAGE	Mother's years of age	35.79	65.92
	Race of household head:		
NWHITE	= 0 if white; = 1 elsewhere	.13	.11
	Children:		
NSIB	Total number of children in the household	2.54	1.46
	Welfare recipient:		
WELF	= 1 if household receives support = 0 elsewhere	.15	.13

related to expected medical care utilization in addition to the price of insurance; Medicaid is somewhat different since a family must meet certain criteria to be eligible.

Work-related variables are included in the health insurance demand equations to reflect the "price" of insurance; most insurance is group insurance, purchased or received as fringe benefits through an employer. Thus, we expect a mother's working to add to the availability of insurance packages which reduces the cost and thus has a positive association with private insurance and HMO insurance. Occupational variables are less clear since we expect low status occupations but also self-employed occupations to have less insurance available.

Higher income permits the purchase of more insurance, so a positive association with income is expected. More education is thought to be associated with a longer time horizon, which may suggest more insurance purchases.

In terms of expected utilization, age may represent greater need and thus be associated with greater probability of insurance purchase.[3] Greater family size, particularly given the standard package of rates for insurance, is likely to show a positive relationship. Not being married may either reduce the numbers who would use insurance and so decrease the probability of insurance purchase, or it may represent less availability (only 1 worker). In either case a negative effect of not being married is expected. Nonwhites are likely to have less insurance than whites, either because of limited availability through employment, historic patterns of less availability of medical care reducing expected utilization, or perhaps through norms regarding insurance. If some of the income is received in the form of welfare or child support, private insurance purchases are expected to be less.

The Medicaid demand equation is one that combines eligibility criteria--income, marital status, family size--with price proxies for private insurance. Income is included as a linear spline reflecting eligibility criteria; the first slope measures income up to the public assistance level, the second, income up to the medical assistance level, and the last, income above these levels. The eligibility levels are matched to families on the basis of family size (Menchik, 1977, p. 174). We expect the first two slopes to be negative and the last flat, so that those above the medical assistance level show no association with Medicaid. The first two slopes should indicate decreasing probability of Medicaid coverage as income increases, reflecting the transitory component of the income measure. Children in families without a father are most likely to receive welfare--and also Medicaid, so the expected sign is positive. Mother's working may both reduce welfare and Medicaid but also increase the availability of private insurance, so the coefficients should be negative.

In a short-hand notation we write the demand equations for health insurance as follows:

$$n_{1i} = \gamma'_{1i} \, \xi_1 + \varepsilon_{1i} \qquad i = 1,3 \qquad\qquad (1)$$

with $\eta_1 = (\eta_{11}, \eta_{12}, \eta_{13})$ a (3x1) vector of insurance demand
      (INSHMO, INSPRIV, MCAID; see Table 1);

ξ_1 a (15x1) vector of exogenous variables (see Table 2; a
     constant term is added);

γ_{1i} a (15x1) vector of parameters, $i = 1,3$, some of which are <u>a
      priori</u> set equal to zero; and

ε_{1i} a disturbance term, $i = 1,3$.

<u>Predisposing variables</u>. The set of predisposing variables contains
those variables that show a clear relationship with health-care utilization (e.g., age, sex), but are themselves no reason for seeking
care. Clearly the impact of these variables on health-care utilization is indirect, via the variable health. Consequently we specify
the following relationship between health and a set of predisposing
variables.

$$\eta_2^* = \beta_1 \, \eta_3^* + \gamma_2' \xi_2 + \varepsilon_2 \qquad\qquad (2)$$

where η_2^* is the unobservable variable health (HEALTH*)

η_3^* is an unobservable predisposing variable ("permanent
     income," to be discussed below)

ξ_2 is (12x1) vector of the other predisposing variables (to
    be discussed below; see also Table 3)

β_1 is a parameter and

γ_2 is (12x1) vector of parameters, and

ε_2 is a disturbance term.

This equation has a twofold interpretation. First, it can be
viewed as a demand equation for health. For example: since
someone's health status influences the time available in the market
place, the demand for good health will generally increase with
someone's wage rate.

Second, Equation 2 can be interpreted as a production function of
health. For instance: the efficiency of the production of good
health will differ at different age levels.

Even in our restricted sample (children of age 1-17 only) a clear
distinction between both interpretations cannot be made. It is
unlikely that a child's demand for health care is a function of his
or her price of market time, but parents have a major impact on a
child's demand for health. This suggests that in families with
severe time constraints (e.g., two-earner households), or with
expensive market time (high wage rates) the demand for a child's
health will be relatively high. On the other hand, if a parent's

time does enter the production function of a child's health, one
would expect relatively little time devoted to production of child's
health in these families. So in some cases no unambiguous prediction of the explanatory variables on HEALTH* can be given.
Regardless of which interpretation one wants to give to this
equation, the variable HEALTH* can readily be interpreted as a
child's health status, and we will make use of this in the final
section.

The exogenous variables that enter the health equation are listed in
Table 3. The first variables entering the HEALTH* equation represent the employment status of the mother. As indicated above, the
expected impact of a working mother on a child's health cannot be
predicted unambiguously. Generally, however, a negative or non-
significant relationship is found (Edwards and Grossman, 1979a).
Mother's schooling is expected to be positively related to a child's
health. More education is expected to lead to both greater demand
for a child's health and more efficiency in producing it. The
number of children in the household generally shows a negative
impact on health-care utilization, but its effect on a child's
health is unknown. To the extent the economic model of fertility is
relevant, the expected effect is negative, since parents can substitute quality (health status) for quantity (number of children:
Becker and Lewis, 1973).

We include a dummy variable representing a low age of the mother
(less than 19 years) when the child was born. Following Edwards
and Grossman (1978) we expect this to have a negative impact on
health. Age and sex and race of the child are also represented by
dummy variables. So is marital status. Since all the children are
beyond infancy, age is likely to be generally insignificant. Based
on the literature, we expect nonwhites to have poorer health.
Following infant mortality differences, we expect girls to be
healthier. Finally, we expect children of currently married parents
to be healthier, reflecting either greater resource availability
(time) or perhaps less previous family strife.

An important variable entering the production (or demand) function of children's health is income, or, more generally, economic
well-being of the households. Current observed income is in this
case not an appropriate measure of economic well-being, because of
possibly large, transitory components. We therefore estimated a
quasi-earnings function that, apart from variables representing the
parents' employment status and schooling, includes the variable
homeownership, to represent a household's "permanent" economic well-
being. In all households in the sample the mother is present. The
variables related to the father interact with a dummy variable equal
to 1.0 if the father is present and equal to 0.0 otherwise.
Observed income serves as an indicator for permanent income. So we
have:

$$\eta_3^* = \gamma_3' \xi_3 \qquad\qquad (3)$$

$$\eta_4 = 1.0\ \eta_3^* + \varepsilon_4$$

Table 3. Exogenous Predisposing Variables

Symbol	Definition	Mean	Variance
MSCHOOL	Years of schooling completed by mother	12.48	6.87
NSIB	Total number of children in household	3.09	1.83
	Race of household head:		
NWHITE	= 0 if white; = 1 elsewhere	.14	.12
	Mother's employment status:		
MFULL	= 1 if mother works full-time; = 0 elsewhere	.19	.15
MPART	= 1 if mother works part-time; = 0 elsewhere	.19	.16
	Low mother's age:		
LMAGE	= 1 if age of mother below 19 when child was born; = 0 elsewhere	.07	.07
	Age of child:		
AGE4	= 1 if age 1-4; = 0 elsewhere	.27	.20
AGE1015	= 1 if age 10-15; = 0 elsewhere	.30	.21
AGE1617	= 1 if age 16-17; = 0 elsewhere	.08	.08
	Sex of child:		
SEX	= 1 if female; = 0 if male	.49	.25
	Marital status of mother:		
NEVMAR	= 1 if never married; = 0 elsewhere	.02	.01
PREVMAR	= 1 if previously married; = 0 elsewhere	.11	.10

with η_3^* an index of the household's economic well-being ("permanent income")

η_4 observed household income

ξ_3 a (10x1) vector of exogenous variables entering the quasi-earnings function (see Table 4),

γ_3 a (10x1) vector of parameters, and

ε_4 a disturbance term ("transitory income").

Need variables. The data set available has a large number of health measures on children which can be used as proxies for a child's need for health care. Table 5 gives definitions and summary statistics of these measures.

Usually measures like the ones listed are added to health-care utilization equations "to control for health status". However, to the extent that these health measures are themselves a function of age, sex, income, etc., this approach is unsatisfactory.

Instead of specifying for each measure a function that explains their variation among the children, we treat the need variables as indicators of the overall health measure specified in Equation 2. More precisely, we assume that, apart from a random measurement error, each need variable is proportional to a child's overall health status.

$$\eta_{5i} = \beta_{2i}\eta_2^* + \varepsilon_{5i} \qquad i = 1,7 \qquad\qquad (4)$$

with η_{5i} a need variable $i = 1,7$ (see Table 5)

β_{2i} a parameter, $i = 1,7$, and

ε_{5i} a disturbance term, $i = 1,7$.

Demand equations. In a model with latent variables, the unobservable variables are completely determined by their causes and indicators. As we have seen above, as causes of the latent variable health, we use the set of predisposing variables.

As indicators of a child's health status we use two sets of variables. First, we use the need variables as indicators of a child's health, measured with error (Equation 4). Second, we will use the utilization of health-care facilities as indicators of a child's health status. In other words, we specify a child's use of health-care facilities as a function of his or her health (η_2) and the set of enabling variables: insurance, η_1, income, η_4 and availability, ξ_4. We finally include a variable representing a household's attitude with respect to seeking professional medical care. This variable is the average number of doctor visits by the

Table 4. Exogenous Variables Entering the Quasi-Earnings Function

Symbol	Definition	Mean	Variance
	Employment status father:		
FFULLT	= 1 if father works full-time	.79	.16
	= 0 elsewhere (including father not present)		
FPART	= 1 if father works part-time	.01	.01
	= 0 elsewhere (including father not present)		
FOCC	Bogue socioeconomic index of father's occupation	48.46	476.90
	= 0 if father not present		
	Mother's employment status:		
MFULLT	= 1 if mother works full-time; = 0 elsewhere	.19	.15
MPART	= 1 if mother works part-time; = 0 elsewhere	.19	.16
	Other parental variables:		
FSCHOOL	Years of schooling completed by father	11.77	28.16
	= 0 if father not present		
MSCHOOL	Years of schooling completed by mother	12.48	6.87
HOME	= 1 if owned home; = 0 elsewhere	.83	.14
MAGE	Years of age of mother	35.67	50.38
	Race of household head:		
NWHITE	= 0 if white; = elsewhere	.14	.12

Table 5. Need Variables

Symbol	Definition	Mean	Variance
HRATE	Parents' rating of child's health (1 = excellent; 2 = good; 3 = fair; 4 = poor)	1.47	.40
DAYSILL	Days ill during past year	5.10	88.70
DAYSBED	Days in bed during past year	2.39	19.62
	Presence of several health distortions:		
LIMIT	= 1 if child has physical limitations; = 0 elsewhere	.02	.02
MAJOR	= 1 if child has some health distortion other than LIMIT; = 0 elsewhere	.53	.25
PROBLEM	= 1 if parents report a problem with the child's behavior; = 0 elsewhere	.13	.12
ALLERG	= 1 if child has an allergy; = 0 elsewhere	.23	.18

Table 6. Health-Care Utilization

Symbol	Definition	Mean	Variance
HOSPVS	Number of visits to a hospital outpatient clinic	.12	.47
HCVS	Number of visits to a health center or nonhospital clinic	.27	.91
SCHOVS	Number of contacts with the school physician	.08	.08
PRIVVS	Number of visits at a private practice	1.4	3.17

parents in the previous year (AVPR; mean 2.29, variance 6.4).
So we have:

$$\eta_{6i} = \beta'_{3i}\eta_1 + \beta_{4i}\eta_2^* + \beta_{5i}\eta_4 + \gamma'_{4i}\xi_4 + \varepsilon_{4i} \qquad i = 1,4 \qquad (5)$$

with $\eta_6 = (\eta_{61}, \eta_{62}, \eta_{63}, \eta_{64})$ a (4x1) vector of health-care utilization variables (HOSPVS, HCVS, SCHOVS, PRIVVS; see Table
6) and

ξ_4 = a (6x1) vector of four availability measures (as described
in Table 1), AVPR, and a constant term.

β_{4i} and β_{5i} are parameters, $i = 1,4$,

β_{3i} and γ_{4i} are respectively (3x1) and (6x1) vectors of parameters, $i = 1,4$, some of which are a priori set equal to
zero, and

ε_{4i} is a disturbance term, $i = 1,4$.

Availability is matched on an equation-by-equation basis: in the
first equation, explaining the number of visits to a hospital outpatient clinic, the availability of care is measured as the travel
time to the nearest hospital. In the second equation, explaining
visits to health centers, the distances to the nearest HMO clinic
and non-HMO clinic are added as availability measures.

To the last two equations, dealing with visits to the school doctor and to a private physician respectively, the physician population ratio is added.

In all but one of the cases we assume a positive impact on utilization from the availability of health care facilities. The exception is in the third equation where we expect an ample supply of
physicians to be a substitute for medical care provided at schools.

In the estimation, one parameter β is set equal to -1.0 (for health
in the equation for private visits) to standardize the health index,
that is, a one-unit increase in HEALTH* will correspond to one visit
less to a private practice.

We assume all disturbances to be normally distributed and independent across equations.

The data used to estimate this model stem from the Rochester
Community Child Health Studies, Child Health Survey, 1975. It is a
very rich data source, limited to one county containing a large city
and the surrounding area. Observations on 675 households with 1589
children are used in this study. Data from this survey are more
fully described in Wolfe (1980).

ESTIMATION RESULTS

Maximum likelihood estimates of the entire model can be obtained using the assumption that the disturbance terms are normally distributed (e.g., see Jöreskog and Sörbom, 1978). However, in order to reduce the amount of computer time needed to find an optimum for such an extensive model, we estimated the three insurance equations separately by least squares on 675 household observations. We then obtained maximum likelihood estimates of the parameters in the remaining 14 equations using observations of the 1,589 children. Since the insurance module is recursive to the rest of the model, all parameter estimates presented are consistent.

The estimation results of Equations 1, 2, 3 and 5 are given in Table 7.

The Demand for Health Insurance

Most of the signs of the estimates for private insurance are as expected: positive for income, mother working, mother's schooling and mother's age; negative for being nonwhite and not being currently married. The negative coefficient on family size is puzzling; perhaps rather than being a factor reflecting expected utilization, it primarily represents greater demands on income. The negative signs on occupational prestige after controlling for income suggest it is likely to pertain to self-employed professionals who face higher prices.

The estimation results of the HMO insurance equation show little, perhaps because few families have such insurance. Older families are less likely to have HMO coverage, perhaps reflecting tastes or greater experience with the traditional fee-for-service arrangements. The insignificance of income is at first glance surprising. We expect a positive sign reflecting ability to purchase more insurance. The explanation may be that those with lower income wish for more extensive coverage, with everything paid for; the location of HMO facilities or the stronger preference of high-income families to use traditional fee-for-service care may also be behind this result.

The Medicaid equation contains all the expected signs. The income spline suggests a small reduction (-0.1) in probability of coverage as income increases to the public assistance level. Beyond this income level and up to the medical assistance level, we observe a further reduction (-.03), and, as expected, beyond that level no further association is observed (-.01 -.02 + .03 = 0.0). Nonwhites, larger families and those with single parents are more likely to have Medicaid coverage (the last two variables are related to eligibility criteria). Finally, labor force participation reduces the probability of Medicaid coverage, possibly because of greater availability of private insurance.

Table 7. Estimation Results

Dependent Variables	Equations (1)			Equation (2)	Equation (3)
	INSPRIV	INSHMO	MCAID	HEALTH*	PINC*
Independent Variables:					
PINC*				-.24	
INC	.23	-.01 NS			
MFULL	.12	.03 NS	-.08	-.04	.33
MPART	.05	.03	-.03	-.09	- .03 NS
FFULT					.83
FPART					.84
MSCHOOL	.01	-.01 NS		.02	.12
Linear Inc. Spline:					
INC			-.01 NS		
INC-Public Asst.			-.02		
INC-Medical Asst.			.03		
WELF	.01	-.05 NS	.14		
FSCHOOL					.07
MOCC	-.003	-.00 NS			
FOCC	-.003	-.00 NS			.01
HOME					.30
MAGE	.001	-.004			.03
NWHITE	-.10	-.09 NS	.03	-.13	.07 NS
NSIB	-.02 NS	.01 NS	.08	-.03	
LMAGE				.04 NS	
AGE4				-.09	
AGE1015				.02 NS	
AGE1617				-.02 NS	
SEX				-.07	
NOTMAR	-.24	-.01 NS	.17		
NEVMAR				-.43	1.09
PREVMAR				-.23	1.17
CONSTANT	-.23	.41	.31		

	Equations (5)			
	HOSPVS	HCVS	SCHOVS	PRIVVS
INSHMO	-.11	.70	-.02	- .60
INSPRIV	-.13	-.25	-.03 NS	.03 NS
MCAID	.14	.50	-.02	- .70
HEALTH*	-.30	-.47	.07	-1.00
AVPR	.01 NS	.01 NS	.00 NS	- .00 NS
INC	-.10	-.08	.02	.41
HOSP	.01 NS			
HMO		-.01 NS		
XHMO		-.01		
PHYS			-.04	- .37
CONSTANT	.35	.32	.11	-1.48

Coefficients marked NS are not significant at 5% level.

The Demand for Health Care

Most variables behave as predicted in our demand equations. For
example, the type of insurance seems to be very important with
respect to the type of health care chosen: those with HMO insurance
tend to go to health clinics and not to a private practice, etc. It
is less obvious, however, that, given the type of health insurance,
income has an important direct impact both on the choice and on the
total amount of health care: the results suggest that an increase
in income, ceteris paribus, will result in an important increase in
the number of visits to a private physician, and a slight decrease
in the visits to a hospital outpatient clinic or HMO clinic.

A child's health status has the expected negative impact on health-
care utilization, i.e., better health results in less utilization,
except for school doctor visits. Perhaps this measure of health-care
utilization is not an adequate indicator of health status, given the
mostly preventive character of care provided at schools (check-ups,
immunization). Also, the average number of visits to a school doctor is very small (Table 6). The impact of the availability of care
on a child's demand for health-care is generally as expected but
small.

We finally mention that our measure of attitude towards seeking
medical care (AVPR) never has a significant impact on children's
health-care demand. This is not too surprising, since AVPR is an
imperfect measure of parental attitudes toward seeking medical care.
It is influenced by other factors, and parents' attitudes may differ
regarding appropriate care for children compared to care for themselves.

Children's Health

The focus of this study is on the measurement of a child's health
status. Since the method we employed is relatively new, the con-
gruence of our results with the ones obtained using more conventional methods does shed some light on the validity of our approach.
A child's health is specified as a function of a number of predisposing variables. Most of them show the expected significant
influences on health. If the mother in the household is employed,
we observe a negative impact on a child's health, perhaps reflecting
less time input. (Edwards and Grossman, 1978, found a similar negative impact only for health measures related to nutrition.) Perhaps
surprisingly, this impact is larger for part-time working mothers
than for full-time workers. Possibly full-time working mothers find
more adequate substitutes to take care of their children than part-
time working mothers.

Mother's schooling has, ceteris paribus, a positive effect on a
child's health. This result is consistent with the analysis of
others including Shakotko (1980).

Permanent income (PINC*) shows an important negative effect on
health. The latter is not surprising--similar results have been

found for adults (Auster et al.). It has been argued that
variables associated with higher income, such as better nutrition
and better housing, result in better health. However Edwards and
Grossman (1978, 1979a) found little association between income and
a number of dimensions of child health, but for certain health
measures--blood pressure, allergies and tension--they found a negative effect similar to the one reported here. For the sample used
here, simple correlations between the seven need variables and both
log income and median income show negative correlations for DAYSBED,
LIMIT, MAJOR and ALLERGY. And, in a simplified version of the model
using median income of the census tract as a proxy for economic status, the results showed a similar significant negative effect between health and income. These results from our model using an
estimate of permanent income as the explanatory variable in the
health equation may indicate either a belief that medical care can
be purchased to "repair" the damage from consumption of high priced
'junk' food, or, as suggested by Edwards and Grossman's findings and
found by Haggerty et al. (1975), using earlier data from this survey, they may indicate an association between income and the new
morbidity. New morbidity incorporates health problems other than
traditional physical health problems such as acute diseases. It
includes the presence of allergies, behavioral problems and mental
health distortions. The negative relation between income and health
cannot simply be explained by assuming that better schooled parents
(in higher income classes) can better detect health distortions,
since mother's schooling also enters the health equation. The negative income effect thus calls for a closer look at the causal relationship between children's health and the economic status of the
household.

Apart from PINC*, two other variables play an important role with
respect to HEALTH*: NEVMAR and PREVMAR.[4] These reflect a time
constraint so we expect a negative effect. The child of a mother
who has never been married has, ceteris paribus, .43 units less
HEALTH* than the child of a married woman. This corresponds with
.43 x 1.00 = .43 more visits to the private doctor (on an average of
1.4), .43 x .30 = .13 more visits to a hospital clinic (average .12)
and .43 x .47 = .20 more visits to a HMO clinic (average .27). If
the mother has been previously married, the effects are similar, but
smaller.

We finally mention the negative coefficient of NWHITE with respect
to HEALTH*, and that the effect of the variable SEX is, contrary to
our expectations, negative. The result with respect to race
contrasts somewhat with Edwards and Grossman's results. They find
significant differences by race which are more robust than for
income. However, the direction of racial differences depended on
the particular health measure used. The results here are more
general since we link race to an overall health status measure.
Thus, the predisposing variables, in general, performed as expected.

Another source of validation is through the correlations between one
latent variable health and the observed health measures. Recall
that HEALTH* as specified in our model has seven need measures as
indictors, as specified in Equation 4. We now present the estimation results of these equations (Table 8). Each column represents
one equation.

Table 8. Estimation Results of Equation (4)

	HEALTH*
HRATE	-1.17
DAYSILL	-4.45
DAYSBED	-2.08
LIMIT	- .02
MAJOR	- .43
PROBLEM	- .11
ALLERGY	- .19

We see that if HEALTH* goes up, HRATE decreases (the lowest rating: 1 = excellent health) and so does the numbers of days ill or days in bed, and the probability of having one or another health distortion.

Our new health measure thus relates to all conventional need variables as expected. Again, we believe this evidence supports the usefulness and validity of our methodology.

DISCUSSION

In the previous sections we developed a structural model for children's health-care utilization. Because of the structure of the model we also obtained an overall index for a child's health status. This single health measure has a number of advantages over the measures usually employed (like the need variables in this paper): it gives clear policy implications in identifying which socioeconomic groups have lower health status; it can serve as an outcome measure for the utilization of health services; it is a broad measure that incorporates multidimensional aspects of health, including the physical, the mental and the behavioral; and it is an operational measure that incorporates the effects of socioeconomic variables and capitalizes on the impact of health on health care utilization. Thus, it fits well into the call for an index that permits the evaluation of the effectiveness of health service delivery systems. It can be used on an individual level, for instance, to predict the health status changes likely to result (ceteris paribus) from demographic changes such as reduced fertility or increased labor force participation of mothers. Similarly, it can be useful in predicting health-care utilization as a result of such changes.

It can also be used on an aggregate or population level to compare populations such as racial and/or income groups. It moves beyond the work of Levine and Yett (Berg, 1973), since it directly relates to socioeconomic factors of health-care utilization, as well as to more direct measures of health status.

Our index incorporates a number of the measures of health status used in scales developed for the Health Insurance Study (HIS) currently being conducted by the Rand Corporation for the Department of Health and Human Services (Eisen et al., 1979). For example, the measures used to assess physical health rely largely on items similar to LIMIT in our scale. The HIS measure, however, contains more detail on the nature of the limitation. An additional HIS scale tries to capture mental health. We capture this in a single combined item--PROBLEM--which includes behavioral or school problems. Finally, the HIS general health rating is similar to the self-rating measure used in this study. The HIS scales are a simple algebraic sum of scores of items which satisfy certain scaling criteria. Again, the index we have developed goes beyond this work since it is weighted by and directly relates to both health-care utilization and socioeconomic factors. The HIS measures are more comprehensive, however.

To give an indication of the potential usefulness of this method, we computed the health status of various socioeconoic groups using our results.

In Table 9 we see that no clear income gradient can be observed: the negative impact of PINC*, as estimated in the model, seems to be offset by related positive effects of, for instance, mother's schooling. However, when we make a comparison across neighborhoods, we see a U-shaped relation with income (as measured by the median income of the neighborhood): the children in neighborhoods with a medium income between $10,000 and $15,000 are on average the healthiest.

There are important differences in health status if children are grouped by race, sex, marital status of the mother, family size or age. Nonwhite children, on average, are less healthy than white children. Children living with parents who are currently married are generally healthier than those living in alternative settings.

A number of caveats are in order. As stated before, the model puts some severe restrictions on the data. These restrictions are the direct results of the specification of the equations. The estimation results may prove quite sensitive to changes in these specifications, and consequently more research is needed regarding the stability of our results.

The need measures employed were chosen for the sole reason that they were available; the addition of more extensive measures of mental health would have been desirable. Furthermore, the data were reported by parents, and were not collaborated by medical authorities. In addition, all data are collected in one relatively small geographical area only, so our results should not be generalized to all children in the U.S.

Finally it should be mentioned that, since many of the endogenous variables are restricted either to be positive (health care utilization) or to take the values 1 or 0 (some need variables), the assumption of independent normally distributed disturbance terms may be violated.

Table 9. Health Status by Socio-Economic Group

	Mean	Standard Deviation	Number of Observations
Total sample	-1.20	.15	1587
Household income <4000	-1.15	.23	50
4000-8000	-1.23	.16	131
8000-12000	-1.17	.17	258
12000-16000	-1.14	.14	389
16000-20000	-1.18	.13	325
>2000	-1.26	.13	434
Median income of neighborhood <7000	-1.37	.08	18
7000-10000	-1.22	.19	236
10000-12000	-1.18	.16	283
12000-15000	-1.16	.14	658
15000-18000	-1.24	.12	239
>18000	-1.25	.13	153
Marital status: previously married	-1.43	.08	173
never married	-1.26	.14	23
married	-1.19	.15	1391
Number of siblings: 0-1	-1.17	.15	601
2-3	-1.20	.15	763
>4	-1.25	.16	223
Race: white	-1.18	.14	1368
nonwhite	-1.34	.13	219
Sex: male	-1.16	.15	812
female	-1.23	.15	775
Age: 1-4	-1.23	.17	294
5-9	-1.18	.15	575
10-15	-1.19	.15	587
16+	-1.24	.14	131

Despite these caveats, we believe our approach is a useful one both to study health-care utilization and to obtain a comprehensive index for the health status of children. A single index has the following clear advantages: it permits evaluation of the differences in health status among subgroups of the population; it permits evaluation of the quality of health services; and it offers the possibility that it may lead to the discovery of underlying relationships. By using weights, the multidimensionality of health status can be incorporated. Previous work by van de Ven and van der Gaag (1979) and Lee (1979) suggests that this type of approach can be usefully employed to study health-care utilization and the health status of adults. The evidence presented here makes the approach seem like a useful one for studying health status and health-care utilization among children. Clearly extensions to all age groups and to more comprehensive data bases would be necessary for many policy purposes.

NOTES

[1]An additional problem arises if health and income are determined simultaneously.

[2]See the next section for a further explanation of this.

[3]Ideally one would like to include a health status measure here. However, since health-care insurance is generally purchased by a household, this calls for a "household health status index". Since the construction of individual health indices is problematic enough, we use a number of proxy variables.

[4]The estimation results of the PINC* equation are generally as expected. The large positive effects of NEVMAR and PREVMAR are on first sight surprising, but they should be looked at in combination with the effects of the variables FFULLT, FPART, FSCHOOL and FOCC. These four variables are all set to be zero if no father is present. So, if we compare a two-parent household with a full-time working father with 12 years of schooling and occupational status 48, and a fatherless household (NEVMAR), the average difference in log income in our sample is $+1.09 - (.83 - .07 \times 12 - .01 \times 48) = -.49$.

HEALTH, ECONOMICS, AND HEALTH ECONOMICS
J. van der Gaag and M. Perlman (editors)
© *North-Holland Publishing Company, 1981*

AN EXPLORATION OF THE DYNAMIC RELATIONSHIP BETWEEN
HEALTH AND COGNITIVE DEVELOPMENT IN ADOLESCENCE

Robert A. Shakotko
Linda N. Edwards
Michael Grossman

Recent studies of children have documented the existence of a relationship between health and cognitive development, reporting typically that good health is associated with higher levels of cognitive
development (Edwards and Grossman, 1979b, and the references cited
therein).[*] This association may arise from causality running in one
or both directions. Poor health may impede cognitive development in
diverse ways. Children who had excessively low birth weights may
experience defective brain functioning and abnormally low IQ's
throughout their lives. Children who are frequently sick or who are
undernourished may be less able to benefit from school instruction
because they are either absent from school or lethargic and passive
when present. A similar comment can be made about children with
vision or hearing problems. Causality runs in the other direction
when more intelligent children and adolescents are better able to
manage or avoid health problems. Such children can better
understand and follow instructions, and they may be more conscien-
tious about taking prescribed medicine or following a specified
treatment. In addition, they may better appreciate the importance
of eating a nutritious diet and act appropriately.

While existing studies of childhood document this association between health and cognitive development, they do not provide much
evidence concerning the direction of causality. This is because
they rely almost exclusively on cross-sectional data. The use of
cross-sectional data does not necessarily preclude the investigation
of causality, of course, but in the present context the underlying
theory does not yield enough prior restrictions to allow one to
address this issue. Another stumbling block that arises when one
tries to unravel the complicated health—cognitive development relationship with cross-sectional data is the impossibility of holding
constant certain unmeasurable genetic factors which may be correlated with both health and cognitive development.

*Research for this paper was supported by grants from the Ford Foundation, the
Robert Wood Johnson Foundation, and the National Center for Health Services
Research (PHS Grant No. 1 R01 HS02917) to the National Bureau of Economic
Research. We are indebted to Ann Colle for research assistance and to Anthony
Cassese and Lee Lillard for their comments on an earlier draft. This is a revi-
sion of a paper presented at the fifty-fourth annual conference of the Western
Economic Association, Las Vegas, Nevada, June 1979.

A partial remedy for these problems lies with the use of longitudinal data. With such data it is possible directly to model and estimate the dynamic relationship between health and cognitive
development. Causality· is probed by examining which attribute of
children is statistically prior to the other. For example, if it is
found that early health status influences later IQ but that early IQ
does not influence later health status, it is concluded that health
affects IQ but not vice versa. (This notion of causality is akin to
that of Granger, 1969.) The problem of separating out the impact of
unmeasured genetic factors is not so readily dealt with, but it may
have less damaging consequences when longitudinal as opposed to
cross-sectional data are used.

In this paper we investigate the relationship between health and
cognitive development using a longitudinal data set compiled from
two nationally representative cross-sections of children: Cycles II
and III of the Health Examination Survey (HES). Cycle II samples
7,119 noninstitutionalized children aged 6 to 11 years in the 1963-65
period; and Cycle III samples 6,768 noninstitutionalized youths
aged 12 to 17 years in the 1966-70 period. There are 2,177 children
common to both cycles, and they were examined in both periods.
These 2,177 children constitute the sample on which our longitudinal
analysis is based. For these 2,177 children we have measures of
health and cognitive development in both periods (childhood and
adolescence) and an array of family background variables taken from
the first period.

Two multivariate equations are estimated with these data. The first
relates adolescent health to childhood health, childhood cognitive
development, and family background; and the second relates adolescent cognitive development to childhood cognitive development,
childhood health, and family background. Thus, the resulting estimates will enable us to compare the effect of prior health on
current cognitive development with the effect of prior cognitive
development on current health. As a byproduct, these equations provide sharper estimates of the environmental as opposed to
genetically related impacts of selected family background variables
on children's health and cognitive development.

SOME THEORETICAL CONSIDERATIONS

The general type of model estimated here can be represented by the
following equation

$$y_{i,t} = A\ y_{i,t-1} + B\ x_{i,t-1} + \varepsilon_{i,t} \tag{1}$$

where $y_{i,t}$ represents a vector of health and cognitive development
measures in period t for individual i, $x_{i,t}$ is a vector of economic
and background variables for that individual in period t, and A and
B are matrices of coefficients.[1] The variables in $x_{i,t}$ are those
that determine the quantity and productivity of the various inputs
in the health and cognitive development production functions:

family income, parents' educational attainment, family size, and the prices of medical care, schooling and nutrition.[2] Some of these variables vary through time and some are assumed to be constant in all periods. In the special case where $y_{i,t}$ is a dichotomous measure (when it denotes the presence or absence of a particular illness, for example), Equation 1 can be directly interpreted as a transition probability function; it gives the probability that individual i has a given health status in time t conditional on his health status in time t-1 and on the values of the other predetermined variables in t-1.

Estimation of this type of model improves on existing cross-sectional analysis of causality because it explicitly treats the time sequence of changes in health and cognitive development. Briefly, this approach, suggested by Granger (1969), relies on a temporal ordering of events: a variable x is said to cause y if predictions of y conditional on lagged values of both y and x are statistically superior to predictions conditional on lagged values of y alone. In this setting, causality between cognitive development and health can be discovered by examining the coefficients of childhood health in the adolescent cognitive development equation and the coefficients of childhood cognitive development in the adolescent health equation.

The problem raised by omitted genetic factors is less tractable. Nevertheless, if such factors can be assumed to operate once and for all by determining the "endowed" levels of health or cognitive development $[y_{i,0}]$, past values of these variables will fully embody and control for all genetic effects. Under this assumption, the fact that one cannot directly measure genetic factors does not mar the above analysis of causality. Even as restrictive an assumption as this, however, cannot rescue cross-sectional work because cross-sectional data do not typically include past values of the dependent variable.[3]

An additional implication of this assumption is that the estimated impacts of the various family background measures and of early health or IQ represent true environmental (as opposed to genetic) effects. That is, they represent effects that operate through the parents' demand for health or cognitive development inputs or through the degree of productive efficiency. This is in contrast to estimates generated from cross-sectional data. In the latter case, the relationship between parents' educational attainment and children's IQ, for example, reflects both an environmental effect (more highly educated mothers do a better job of educating their children) and a genetic effect (more highly educated mothers have on average greater native intelligence, which is passed genetically to their children). When it is assumed that early health or cognitive development fully embodies the genetic contribution, family background variables will reflect only environmental influences.

Admittedly, this assumption concerning genetic impacts is very restrictive. With data like ours, however, which cover only two points in time, it is impossible to partition the effect of the unobservable genetic factors from other time-invariant factors without making some fairly restrictive assumptions. We choose to make this particular assumption for the balance of this paper

because it has the advantage of permitting us to use single-equation
estimation techniques, a not insignificant consideration with a data
set as large as this one.[4]

To illustrate better the exact nature of this assumption and its
necessity, we present the following simplified two-period formulation, of which our model is a special case (the i's are
suppressed for simplicity):

$$H_1 = a_1 GH + b_1 E + \varepsilon_1 \tag{2a}$$

$$H_2 = a_2 GH + b_2 E + c_2 H_1 + d_2 Q_1 + \varepsilon_2 \tag{2b}$$

$$Q_1 = \alpha_1 GQ + \beta_1 E + \varepsilon_1' \tag{3a}$$

$$Q_2 = \alpha_2 GQ + \beta_2 E + \gamma_2 Q_1 + \delta_2 H_1 + \varepsilon_2' \tag{3b}$$

In this two-period model H_t represents health, Q_t represents cognitive development, GH represents the time-invariant genetic health
endowment, GQ represents the time-invariant cognitive endowment, and
E represents a time-invariant background variable. Since GH and GQ
are unobserved, we write H_2 and Q_2 in terms of the predetermined
values of H and Q (assuming a_1 and α_1 do not equal zero):

$$H_2 = \left[\frac{a_2}{a_1} + c_2\right] H_1 + b_2 \left[1 - \frac{a_2}{a_1} \frac{b_1}{b_2}\right] E \tag{2c}$$

$$+ d_2 Q_1 + \left[\varepsilon_2 - \frac{a_2}{a_1} \varepsilon_1\right]$$

$$Q_2 = \left[\frac{\alpha_2}{\alpha_1} + \gamma_2\right] Q_1 + \beta_2 \left[1 - \frac{\alpha_2}{\alpha_1} \frac{\beta_1}{\beta_2}\right] E \tag{3c}$$

$$+ \delta_2 H_1 + \left[\varepsilon_2' - \frac{\alpha_2}{\alpha_1} \varepsilon_1'\right].$$

In the context of this model, the assumption of no direct genetic
effects after the first period is equivalent to fixing a_2 and α_2 at
zero. When these are not zero, one cannot determine directions of

causality because the error terms in the equations are correlated with the explanatory variables and this correlation leads to biased estimates of both d_2 and δ_2. Nor can one obtain unbiased estimates of pure environmental effects, because the reduced form coefficients of the background variable (E) and of the lagged dependent variable (Q_1 or H_1) embody both genetic (a_1 and a_2 or α_1 and α_2) and environmental (b_2, c_2 or β_2, γ_2) impacts.[5]

EMPIRICAL IMPLEMENTATION

The Data

Equations 2 and 3b are estimated (under the assumptions that $a_2 = 0$ and $\alpha_2 = 0$) using the longitudinal sample compiled from Cycles II and III of the HES. Both cycles are described in detail in NCHS (1967a and 1969, respectively). Ninety-nine percent of the youths in the longitudinal sample are between the ages of 12 and 15 years at the time of Cycle III, and the remaining 1% are 16 years old.

The HES data include medical histories of each youth provided by the parent, information on family socioeconomic characteristics, birth certificate information, and a school report with data on school performance and classroom behavior provided by teachers or other school officials. Most important, there are objective measures of health from detailed physical examinations and scores on psychological (including IQ and achievement) tests. The physical examinations were given to the children and youths by pediatricians and dentists, and the IQ and achievement tests were administered by psychologists, all of whom were employed by the Public Health Service at the time of each cycle of the HES.

This paper uses only data for white adolescents who at the time of the Cycle II exam lived with either both of their parents or with their mothers only. Black adolescents are excluded from the empirical analysis because Edwards and Grossman (1979b, 1980, and forthcoming) have found significant race differences in slope coefficients in cross-sectional research using Cycles II and III. Separate estimates for black adolescents are not presented because the black sample is too small to allow for reliable coefficient estimates. Our working sample also excludes observations for which data are missing.[6] The final sample size is 1,434.

The health and cognitive development measures are described below. In labeling these measures, we denote those that refer to childhood (from Cycle II) by the number 1 at the end of the variable name, and those that refer to adolescence (from Cycle III) by the number 2.

Measurement of Cognitive Development

Two measures of cognitive development are used: an IQ measure derived from two subtests of the Wechsler Intelligence Scale for Children (WISC1, WISC2), and a school achievement measure derived

from the reading and arithmetic subtests of the Wide Range
Achievement Test (WRAT1, WRAT2). Both measures are scaled to have
means of 100 and standard deviations of 15 for each age-group (four-
month cohorts are used for WISC and six-month cohorts are used for
WRAT).[7] WISC is a common IQ test, similar to (and highly correlated with results from) the Stanford-Binet IQ test (NCHS, 1972).
The full test consists of twelve subtests, but only two of these--
vocabulary and block design--were administered in the HES. IQ estimates based on these two subtests are highly correlated with those
based on all twelve subtests (NCHS, 1972). Similarly, a test score
based on the reading and arithmetic subtests of Wide Range
Achievement Test have been found to be highly correlated with the
full test and with other conventional achievement tests (NCHS,
1967b).

Measurement of Health

The measures of childhood and adolescent health are: the periodontal index (APERI1, APERI2); obesity (OBESE1, OBESE2); the presence
of one or more significant abnormalities as reported by the examining physician (ABN1, ABN2); high diastolic blood pressure (HDBP1,
HDBP2); the parent's assessment of the youth's overall health
(PFGHEALTH1, PFGHEALTH2); and excessive school absence for health
reasons during the past six months (SCHABS1, SCHABS2). These six
measures are negative correlates of good health, and with the exception of the periodontal index, they are all dichotomous variables.
Detailed definitions of these health measures (as well as the cognitive development measures) appear in Table 1. All but two of the
measures--APERI and ABN--are adequately explained by the table.
Additional discussion of APERI and ABN follows.

The periodontal index (APERI1, APERI2) is a good overall indicator of
oral health as well as a positive correlate of nutrition (Russell,
1956). It is obtained from an examination of the gums surrounding
each tooth and is scored in such a way that a higher value reflects
poorer oral health.[8] Because the periodontal index has marked age
and sex trends, our measure is computed as the difference between
the adolescent's (or child's) actual index and the mean index for
his or her age-sex group, divided by the standard deviation for that
age-sex group. Oral health is one of the few aspects of health for
which a well-defined continuous index has been constructed.

Significant abnormalities (ABN1, ABN2) are defined to be heart
disease; neurological, muscular, or joint conditions; other major
diseases; and in Cycle III only, otitis media. This minor difference between the definitions of ABN1 and ABN2 will have little
impact on our results because otitis media constitutes only a small
percentage (about 1%) of all reported abnormalities in Cycle III.

In choosing these six particular health measures, our overriding
consideration was diversity.[9] Indeed, it is the well-known multidimensional nature of health that led us to study a set of measures
rather than a single composite index. Diversity is desired not only
with respect to the systems of the body covered, but also with
regard to the degree to which the health conditions can be affected

by environmental influences. For example, both obesity and the
periodontal index are greatly affected by life-style and preventive
medical care. In the case of either of these measures, therefore,
one would expect to observe a significant impact of family
background variables. On the other hand, health problems like high
blood pressure and significant abnormalities may not be responsive
to family or medical intervention. Such measures may, however, have
an impact on other aspects of health or on cognitive development.
Subjective health measures like the parents' assessment of the
child's health or school absenteeism have the advantage of
reflecting people's perceptions about their health. But, at the
same time, they may depend on the socioeconomic status of the
family. For example, parents with low levels of income and
schooling may be dissatisfied with many aspects of their lives
including the health of their offspring. (This type of reporting
bias is largely controlled for in our analysis, however, because we
hold constant both a group of socioeconomic variables and the lagged
value of the subjective measure.) A secondary criterion used in
choosing the health measures was prevalence. In particular, we
avoided health problems like abnormal hearing that have a relatively
low prevalence in this cohort.

Measurement of Other Variables

In addition to lagged (i.e., childhood) cognitive and health development, each equation includes the set of family and youth characteristics defined in Appendix 1. All family and youth
characteristics are taken from Cycle II (except for the variable
INTERVAL which measures the elapsed time between the child's two
examinations). The child's age as of the Cycle II exam and/or his
sex are also included when the dependent variable is not age-and/or
sex-adjusted (that is, for ABN, PFGHEALTH, SCHABS, WISC, and
WRAT).[10]

The rationale for including each of these youth and family characteristics variables has been discussed extensively elsewhere
(Edwards and Grossman, 1979b, 1980, and forthcoming) and will not be
treated here. In the empirical section we discuss the effects of
only the most important family background variables: mother's
schooling (MEDUCAT), father's schooling (FEDUCAT), and family income
(FINC). We view parents' schooling as representing the parents'
efficiency in the production of their offspring's health and cognitive development, and family income as representing the family's
command over resources.

EMPIRICAL RESULTS

The results of the estimation of ordinary least squares multiple
regression equations for the dependent variables WISC2, WRAT2,
APERI2, ABN2, HDBP2, PFGHEALTH2, OBESE2, and SCHABS2 are discussed in
this section. (The regression equations are available on request.)
Since the six adolescent health measures are negative correlates of

Table 1. Definitions of Health and Cognitive Development Measures

Variable Name	Sample[a] Mean	Sample Standard Deviation	Definition[b]
A. Cognitive Development Measures			
WISC1[c] WISC2c	103.508 104.513	13.924 13.998	Youth's IQ as measured by vocabulary and block design subtests of the Wechsler Intelligence Scale for Children, standardized by the mean and standard deviation of four-month age cohorts, in Cycles II and III, respectively. (Source: 4)
WRAT1[c] WRAT2[c]	103.568 104.112	12.017 13.563	Youth's school achievement as measured by the reading and arithmetic subtests of the Wide Range Achievement Test, standardized by the mean and standard deviation of six month age cohorts, in Cycles II and III, respectively. (Source: 4)
B. Health Measures			
APERI1[c] APERI2[c]	-.055 -.138	.792 .852	Periodontal Index, standardized by the mean and standard deviation for one-year age-sex cohorts, in Cycles II and III, respectively. (Source: 3)
ABN1 ABN2	.096 .188	.294 .391	Dummy variables that equal one if the physician finds a significant abnormality in examining the youth, in Cycles II and III, respectively. (Source: 3)
HDBP1 HDBP2	.054 .054	.226 .227	Dummy variables that equal one if youth's average diastolic blood pressure is greater than the 95th percentile for the youth's age and sex class, in Cycles II and III, respectively. (Source: 3)

Table 1 (continued)

Variable Name	Sample[a] Mean	Sample Standard Deviation	Definition[b]
OBESE1	.110	.312	Dummy variables that equal one if
OBESE2	.094	.292	youth's weight is greater than the 90th percentile for youth's age, sex, and height class, in Cycles II and III, respectively. (Source: 3)
PFGHEALTH1	.441	.497	Dummy variables that equal one if
PFGHEALTH2	.272	.445	parental assessment of youth's health is poor, fair, or good in Cycles II and III, respectively. Variable equals zero if assessment is very good in Cycle II and very good or excellent in Cycle III; there is no excellent category in Cycle II. (Source: 1)
SCHABS1	.033	.178	Dummy variables that equal one if
SCHABS2[d]	.054	.221	youth has been excessively absent from school for health reasons during the past six months, in Cycles II and III, respectively. (Source: 5)
SCHABSUK1	.068	.252	Dummy variation that equals one if information about school absence in Cycle II is not available (see footnote 6). (Source: 5)

Source: Data from the Health Examination Survey, Cycles II and III.

[a]The means and standard deviations are for the sample of 1,434 white youths described in the text.

[b]The sources are the following: 1 = parents, 2 = birth certificate, 3 = physical examination, 4 = psychological examination, 5 = school form.

[c]The means of the cognitive development measures are not equal to 100, and the means of the periodontal indexes are not zero because standardizations were done using the entire Cycle II or Cycle III sample rather than the subsample reported here.

[d]The mean and standard deviation are based on a subsample of 1,321 youths for whom the school form was available.

Table 2. Regression Coefficients of Lagged Health and Lagged Cognitive Development

Current \ Lagged	WISC1	WRAT1	APERI1	ABN1	HDBP1	PFGHEALTH1	OBESE1	SCHABS1
WISC2	.603 (27.35)	.231 (9.47)	-.164 (-0.54)	-1.619 (-2.15)	-1.791 (-1.82)	.388 (0.84)	.946 (1.33)	-.650 (-0.53)
WRAT2	.192 (9.79)	.728 (33.52)	-.073 (-0.27)	-.204 (-0.30)	-.740 (-0.85)	-.341 (-0.82)	.421 (0.66)	-.699 (-0.64)
APERI2	-.004 (-2.25)	-.005 (-2.35)	.340 (12.16)	-.005 (-0.07)	-.195 (-2.15)	.039 (0.90)	.114 (1.73)	.146 (1.28)
ABN2	-.001 (0.98)	-.002 (-2.00)	.020 (1.41)	.146 (4.16)	.042 (0.91)	.001 (0.03)	.049 (1.47)	.064 (1.11)
HDBP2	-.001 (-1.11)	-.0003 (-0.51)	-.003 (-0.41)	.030 (1.47)	.169 (6.38)	-.010 (-0.78)	.096 (4.97)	.033 (1.00)
PFGHEALTH2	-.001 (-0.92)	-.003 (-2.76)	.019 (1.22)	.139 (0.37)	.043 (0.86)	.243 (10.43)	.019 (0.52)	.096 (1.54)
OBESE2	.0001 (0.08)	-.001 (-1.45)	-.014 (-1.60)	-.020 (-0.91)	.013 (0.43)	-.016 (-1.15)	.512 (24.28)	.007 (0.18)
SCHABS2	.0002 (0.34)	-.001 (-1.78)	.004 (0.49)	.011 (0.49)	.009 (0.34)	.045 (3.45)	.020 (1.03)	.159 (4.60)

Source: Data from the Health Examination Survey, Cycles II and III.

Note: t-ratios are in parentheses. The critical t-ratios at the 5 percent level of significance are 1.64 for a one-tailed test and 1.96 for a two-tailed test.

good health, negative (positive) effects of family background and
lagged cognitive development in the health equations reflect factors
associated with better (poorer) health outcomes. Alternatively,
positive coefficients of lagged health in the current health
equations signify that poor health in childhood is associated with
poor health in adolescence. Finally, negative coefficients of
lagged health in the current cognitive development equations mean
that poor health in childhood reduces cognitive development in adolescence.

Although five of the eight dependent variables are dichotomous, the
method of estimation is ordinary least squares. Preliminary
investigation revealed almost no differences between ordinary least
squares estimates and dichotomous logit estimates. Given the size
of our sample and the minimal improvement in the accuracy of the
estimates, we decided to rely on OLS estimation. When the dependent
variable is dichotomous, the estimated equation can be interpreted
as a linear probability function.

Causal Priorness

In order to address the issue of the direction of causality between
health and cognitive development, we present in Table 2 an 8 x 8
matrix of lagged coefficients from the eight equations. The off-
diagonal elements of the matrix provide information with regard to
mutual feedback between health and cognitive development, mutual
feedback between various health conditions, and mutual feedback between IQ (WISC) and achievement (WRAT). The elements on the main
diagonal of the matrix are the own-lagged effects, or the regression
coefficients of the lagged dependent variable.

We begin by looking at the own-lagged effects. The size of the own-
lagged coefficients are an indication of the persistence of each
health condition. For example, if the coefficient of the lagged
dependent variable is close to one, this signifies that the health
condition (or the stochastic process governing the occurrence of
that condition) has a relatively low frequency and is slow to
change. Coefficients close to zero indicate a higher frequency process. For slowly changing conditions one would expect to find that
other explanatory variables (besides the lagged dependent variable)
will not have such large effects as they would for conditions that
are more readily altered. When the dependent variable is dichotomous, the own-lagged coefficient can be directly interpreted as the
degree of persistence in the particular aspect of health in
question: in this case the lagged coefficient is the difference
between the expected conditional probability of an adolescent health
condition, given that the same condition was present in childhood,
and the conditional probability given that the condition was absent
in childhood. Each of the eight own-lagged effects is positive and
statistically significant at all conventional levels of
confidence.[11] The coefficients range from a high of .73 in the case
of WRAT to a low of .15 in the case of ABN.[12] Among the dichotomous
variables, obesity is the most persistent: obese children have
approximately 50 percentage point higher probabilities of being
obese adolescents than do non-obese children.

The cross-lagged effects, however, appearing off the diagonal in
Table 2, are the primary focus of this paper. From these coefficients, it appears that causality runs more strongly from cognitive development to health than vice versa. When the two cognitive
development measures are the dependent variables, only two of the
six health measures (ABN1 and HDBP1) have significant impacts on
WISC2; and none have significant impacts on WRAT2 (the latter statement holds whether the statistical test is done on each health
variable separately or on the set of six). In the two cases where
there is a significant impact, the effect is as expected, with
poorer health being associated with lower values of WISC2. When the
health measures are the dependent variables, one or both of the
cognitive development measures have significant impacts for four of
the six health measures: APERI2, ABN2, SCHABS2, and PFGHEALTH2
(these results hold whether the statistical test is done on WISC1
and WRAT1 separately or together). In all four cases, higher
levels of WISC1 or WRAT1 are associated with better health. To
conclude, while these off-diagonal elements affirm a two-way relationship between health and cognitive development, the link from
cognitive development to health appears to be the stronger one.

Several other interesting relationships are evident in Table 2.
There is evidence of mutual feedbacks between IQ and achievement:
childhood achievement has a significant impact on adolescent IQ even
when childhood IQ is held constant; and childhood IQ has a significant impact on adolescent achievement when childhood achievement is
held constant. There are also dependencies between some of the
health measures: obesity in childhood is related to poorer oral
health and high blood pressure in adolescence,[13] and a parental
rating of health in childhood as poor, fair, or good (as opposed to
very good) is associated with excessive school absence due to
illness in adolescence. Finally, there is one seemingly "perverse"
and statistically significant relationship in the table: high blood
pressure in childhood is associated with better oral health in
adolescence, although this may be due to excessive consumption of
dairy products.

Family Background Effects

A secondary objective of this paper is to obtain better estimates of
the impacts of environmental factors on health and cognitive development. The three environmental measures we focus on are mother's
schooling (MEDUCAT), father's schooling (FEDUCAT), and family income
(FINC).

Coefficients of these three variables in the adolescent health and
cognitive development functions are shown in Table 3. Two types of
estimates are reported. Those in the first three columns, labeled
cross-sectional coefficients, are taken from multiple regressions
that control for all of the family and youth characteristics listed
in Appendix 1 but exclude all lagged (childhood) cognitive
development and health measures. The estimates in the last three
columns, labeled "dynamic" coefficients, are taken from multiple
regressions that include all lagged cognitive development and health
measures in addition to the family and youth characteristics. The

first set of estimates shows background effects as typically computed in a cross-section. The second set shows background effects
estimated in a dynamic context which controls for initial levels of
cognitive development and health. As we argued in the first section, the "dynamic" estimates are free of genetic bias if genetic
effects are fully embodied in the early health and cognitive development measures.[14] Under this assumption, then, the "dynamic"
coefficients represent the pure contribution of the home environment
to cognitive development and health outcomes in the interval between
Cycles II and III.

Let us consider first the impacts of the three family background
variables on cognitive development. In the cross-section estimates,
all six family background coefficients are positive and statistically significant, and they tend to remain significant when the
lagged variables are included. The magnitudes of the "dynamic"
family background effects are, however, much smaller than the magnitudes of the cross-sectional effects. To be precise, the ratios of
"dynamic" coefficients to the corresponding cross-sectional coefficients range from .15 in the case of mother's schooling in the
WISC2 equation to .47 in the case of family income in the same
equation.

In the case of adolescent health, the difference between cross-
section and dynamic family background estimates is less dramatic.
First, fewer of the cross-section estimates themselves show significant impacts: only mother's educational attainment is a consistently important variable (except when ABN2 is the dependent
variable). Father's educational attainment has significant positive
health impacts for the periodontal index and the subjective health
rating, and family income is significant in determining only the
subjective health rating. All of the statistically significant
background effects are reduced in absolute value when childhood
health and cognitive development are included in the equations. The
ratios of the "dynamic" coefficients to the corresponding cross-
sectional coefficients range from .14 in the case of family income in
the PFGHEALTH2 equation to .80 in the case of mother's schooling in
the SCHABS2 equation. Moreover, there are only three statistically
significant dynamic coefficients: those belonging to mother's
schooling in the APERI2, PFGHEALTH2, and SCHABS2 equations.

A clear message in Table 3 is that the "dynamic" estimates of family
background effects on cognitive development and health are much
smaller than the corresponding cross-sectional estimates. The
important point here, however, is not that the "dynamic" estimates
of background effects are smaller than the cross-sectional estimates. This decline is to be expected if our procedure does in fact
remove many of the genetic effects otherwise embodied in the family
background variables.[15] The main point, rather, is that after
removing the genetic component from the family background variables,
family background--especially mother's education--remains an important determinant of cognitive development and of some aspects of
health. This finding is strong evidence that the family environment
plays an important role in the overall development of adolescents.

An interesting sidelight to the discussion of family background
effects is found in a comparison of the results for cognitive deve-

Table 3. Regression Coefficients of Parent's Schooling and Family Income

Independent Variable / Dependent Variable	Cross-Section Coefficients			Dynamic Coefficients		
	MEDUCAT	FEDUCAT	FINC	MEDUCAT	FEDUCAT	FINC
WISC2	.986 (6.19)	.904 (6.80)	.288 (3.33)	.146 (1.32)	.207 (2.24)	.135 (2.27)
WRAT2	.942 (6.03)	.805 (6.18)	.271 (3.20)	.177 (1.79)	.136 (1.65)	.103 (1.94)
APERI2	-.039 (-3.67)	-.019 (-2.17)	0.005 (-0.91)	-.023 (-2.25)	-.006 (-0.75)	.0001 (0.00)
ABN2	-.002 (-0.36)	-.005 (-1.26)	.004 (1.60)	.003 (0.51)	-.003 (-0.65)	.005 (1.83)
HDBP2	-.005 (-1.84)	.002 (0.66)	-.001 (-0.33)	-.003 (-0.89)	.003 (1.07)	-.001 (-0.53)
PFGHEALTH2	-.015 (-2.71)	-.012 (-2.47)	-.007 (-2.21)	-.009 (-1.69)	-.006 (-1.23)	-.001 (-0.47)
OBESE2	-.012 (-3.19)	.00002 (0.00)	.001 (0.55)	-.005 (-1.42)	.001 (0.53)	.0004 (0.21)
SCHABS2	-.010 (-3.11)	.003 (1.09)	-.002 (-1.32)	-.008 (-2.46)	.004 (1.35)	-.001 (-0.66)

Source: Data from the Health Examination Survey, Cycles II and III.

Note: t-ratios are in parentheses. The critical t-ratios at the 5% level of significance are 1.64 for a one-tailed test and 1.96 for a two-tailed test. The cross-sectional coefficients are taken from multiple regressions that contain all family and youth characteristics. The dynamic coefficients are taken from multiple regressions that contain all variables.

lopment versus health. First, regardless of which set of estimates
is used, family background variables as a group are less likely to
have significant impacts on adolescent health than on adolescent
cognitive development. Second, according to the "dynamic" estimates, either one year of additional educational attainment for either
parent or one thousand additional dollars of family income are associated with roughly the same increase in WISC2 or WRAT2. For the
health measures, however, the "dynamic" estimates show that mother's
educational attainment tends to have a larger impact than the other
variables, and it is frequently the only statistically significant
background variable. Taken together, these points suggest that
there is more "home production" of health than of cognitive develop-
ment--at least in the period between childhood and adolescence.

SUMMARY AND IMPLICATIONS

Our exploration of the dynamic relationship between health and
cognitive development in adolescence has generated two important
results. First, there is feedback both from health to cognitive
development and from cognitive development to health, but the latter
of these relationships is stronger. Second, estimates of family
background effects taken from the dynamic model--which can be
assumed to be less influenced by genetic factors--are smaller than
their cross-sectional counterparts, but some still remain statistically significant.

The first finding calls attention to the existence of a continuing
interaction between health and cognitive development over the life
cycle. Since an individual's cognitive development (measured by IQ
or achievement tests) is an important determinant of the number of
years of formal schooling that he ultimately completes (see Grossman,
1975), our findings may be viewed as the early forerunner of the
positive impact of schooling on good health for adults in the United
States reported by Grossman (1975), Shakotko (1977), and others.

The second finding suggests that nurture "matters" in cognitive
development and health outcomes. All three background variables are
important contributors to cognitive development, but mother's
schooling is singled out as the crucial component of the home
environment in adolescent health outcomes. This is an especially
strong result because, in the words of Keniston and the Carnegie
Council on Children, "Doctors do not provide the bulk of health care
for children; families do" (1977, p. 179). Since the mother typically spends more time in household production than the father, her
characteristics should be the dominant factor in outcomes that are
determined to a large extent in the home. The importance of
mother's schooling in obesity and oral health is notable because
these are outcomes that are neither irreversible or self-limiting.
Instead, they can be modified by inputs of dental care, medical
care, proper diet, and parents' time.

The two findings interact with each other. Cognitive development in
childhood has a positive effect on health in adolescence, and cognitive development in childhood is positively related to parents'

schooling and family income. Both findings imply that the health of adults is heavily dependent upon their home environment as youths. They also imply that public policies aimed at children's and adolescents' health must try to offset the problems encountered by offspring of mothers with low levels of schooling. In particular, they should try to improve the skills of uneducated mothers in their capacity as the main providers of health care for their offspring.

APPENDIX 1

Family and Youth Characteristics[a]

Variable Name	Sample[b] Mean	Sample Standard Deviation	Definition[c]
FEDUCAT[d]	11.310	3.355	Years of formal schooling completed by father
MEDUCAT	11.216	2.704	Years of formal schooling completed by mother
FINC	8.060	4.607	Continuous family income (in thousands of dollars) computed by assigning mid-points to the following closed income intervals, $250 to the lowest interval, and $20,000 to the highest interval. The closed income classes are:
			$500 - $999 $1,000 - $1,999 $2,000 - $2,999 $3,000 - $3,999 $4,000 - $4,999 $5,000 - $6,999 $7,000 - $9,999 $10,000 - $14,999
LESS20	3.700	1.813	Number of persons in the household 20 years of age or less
MWORKFT MWORKPT	.149 .149	.356 .356	Dummy variables that equal one if the mother works full-time or part-time, respectively; omitted class is mother does not work
NEAST MWEST SOUTH	.265 .315 .203	.442 .465 .402	Dummy variables that equal one if youth lives in Northeast, Midwest, or South, respectively; omitted class is residence in West

APPENDIX 1 (continued)

Variable Name	Sample[b] Mean	Sample Standard Deviation	Definition[c]
URB1	.189	.392	Dummy variables that equal one if
URB2	.126	.331	youth lives in an urban area with
URB3	.200	.400	a population of 3 million or more
NURB	.140	.347	(URB1); in an urban area with a
			population between 1 million and
			3 million (URB2); in an urban area
			with a population less than 1
			million (URB3); or in a non-rural
			and non-urbanized area (NURB);
			omitted class is residence in a
			rural area
LIGHTA	.008	.091	Dummy variable that equals one if youth's birth weight was under 2,000 grams (under 4.4 pounds) (Source: 2)
LIGHTB	.054	.227	Dummy variable that equals one if youth's birth weight was equal to or greater than 2,000 grams but under 2,500 grams (under 5.5 pounds) (Source: 2)
BWUK	.138	.345	Dummy variable that equals one if youth's birth weight is unknown (Source: 2)
FYPH	.068	.252	Dummy variable that equals one if parental assessment of child's health at one year was poor or fair and zero if it was good
BFED	.302	.459	Dummy variable that equals one if the child was breast fed
LMAG	.057	.231	Dummy variable that equals one if the mother was less than 20 years old at birth of youth
HMAG	.119	.324	Dummy variable that equals one if mother was more than 35 years old at birth of youth
NOFATH	.047	.213	Dummy variable that equals one if youth lives with mother only
FIRST	.292	.455	Dummy variable that equals one if youth is the first born child in the family

APPENDIX 1 (continued)

Variable Name	Sample[b] Mean	Sample Standard Deviation	Definition[c]
TWIN	.028	.165	Dummy variable that equals one if youth is a twin
FLANG	.110	.312	Dummy variable that equals one if a foreign language is spoken in the home
MALE	.522	.500	Dummy variable that equals one if youth is a male
AGE	9.712	1.042	Age of youth
INTERVAL	42.327	6.404	Number of months between the physical examinations given for the Cycle II survey and the Cycle III survey (Source: 3)

Source: Health Examination Survey, Cycles II and III.

[a]All family and youth characteristics are from Cycle II unless otherwise stated.

[b]The means and standard deviations are for the sample of 1,434 white youths desribed in the text.

[c]Source for all is 1, parents, unless otherwise indicated; 2 = birth certificate; 3 = physical examination.

[d]For youths who were not currently living with their father, father's education was coded at the mean of the sample for which father's education was reported.

NOTES

[1]This is a reduced form equation derived by solving a system of equations that include a family utility function (with the health and cognitive development of each child in each period as arguments), a children's health production function, a production function for children's cognitive development, and a wealth constraint. Note that at any point in time, t, both $y_{i,t-1}$ and $x_{i,t-1}$ are predetermined variables.

[2]A detailed discussion of the types of variables included in $x_{i,t}$ can be found in Edwards and Grossman (1979b and 1980).

[3]One technique that has been used in cross-sectional analysis is to include indicators of the unobserved variable. These indicators, which are not themselves part of the original cross-section specification, are taken to be instruments for the unobserved variable. An example is the inclusion of test scores as a proxy for ability in earnings equations. Investigators generally acknowledge that this is a second-best procedure because it introduces an errors-in-variables bias which may be nearly as large as the original omitted-variables bias (Griliches, 1974).

[4]See Shakotko (1979) for an alternative model formulated in the spirit of the ability-bias problem as described, for example, by Griliches (1977). While relaxing the restrictive assumption in the present paper regarding genetic embodiment, Shakotko requires an alternative set of restrictions in order to identify and estimate a factor structure.

[5]Since H_1 is correlated with the error term in Equation 2c, the coefficient of Q_1 in this equation is biased unless the partial correlation between Q_1 and H_1 with E held constant is zero. This is extremely unlikely because GQ and GH are bound to be related, probably, in a positive manner. The same comment applies to the coefficient of H_1 in Equation 3c. Note that if the partial correlation between E and H_1 or between E and Q_1 is non-zero, ordinary least squares estimates of the reduced form environmental parameters, given by the coefficients of E in 2c or 3c, are biased.

[6]We did not, however, exclude observations from the analysis if data were missing for the school absenteeism variables (SCHABS1, SCHABS2) and birth-weight variables (LIGHTA, LIGHTB). Information on school absenteeism is taken from the school form completed by the child's school. This form is missing for roughly 7% of the sample. Since excessive absence due to illness is the only variable taken from this form, a dummy variable that identifies youths with missing Cycle II school forms (SCHABSUK1) is included in all regression equations as an independent variable. Youths without a Cycle III school form are eliminated from the empirical analysis only when SCHABS2 is the dependent variable. Birth weight is taken from the child's birth certificate, which is missing for 14% of the sample. Since birth weight is the only variable taken from the birth certificate, we do not delete these observations, but rather we include a dummy variable that identifies youths with missing birth certificates (BWUK) in the regression equations.

[7]Although these and other test scores have been widely criticized, they are used here and elsewhere because they are so readily obtainable and because they are roughly comparable across diverse populations. WISC and WRAT are adjusted for

sex as well as for age in some studies, but the variables used here are not
sex-adjusted.

[8]Kelly and Sanchez (1972, pp. 1-2) describe the periodontal index as follows:

> Every tooth in the mouth...is scored according to the presence
> or absence of manifest signs of periodontal disease. When a
> portion of the free gingiva is inflamed, a score of 1 is
> recorded. When completely circumscribed by inflammation, teeth
> are scored 2. Teeth with frank periodontal pockets are scored
> 6 when their masticatory function is unimpaired and 8 when it
> is impaired. The arithmetic average of all scores is the
> individual's [periodontal index], which ranges from a low of
> 0.0 [no inflammation or periodontal pockets] to a high of 8.0
> [all teeth with pockets and impaired function].

[9]The choice of appropriate measures of health in childhood and adolescence is
discussed in detail in Edwards and Grossman (1979b, 1980, and forthcoming).

[10]The periodontal index and the two cognitive development measures are continuous variables. In these cases we have experimented with the raw score as the
dependent variable in a multiple regression that includes in the set of explanatory variables age in Cycle II, the square of age, the time interval between the
Cycle II and III examinations, the square of the interval, the product of age and
the interval, and a dummy variable for male adolescents. The results obtained
(not shown) with respect to family background, lagged health, and lagged cognitive
development effects are similar to those reported in the third section.

[11]Statements concerning statistical significance in the text refer to the 5%
level in a one-tailed test, except when the direction of the effect is unclear on
a priori grounds or when the estimated effect has the "wrong sign." In the latter
cases two-tailed tests are used.

[12]If the dynamic processes that we study have the same structures over time
and if cross-lagged effects are ignored, they all have stable long-run solutions.
To be specific, if $H_t = aH_{t-1} + bE$, the long-run solution, obtained by setting $H_t = H_{t-1}$, is $H_t = (b/1-a) E$. This is a stable solution when a is positive and smaller
than one.

[13]This finding is consistent with cross-sectional results reported by the
National Heart, Lung, and Blood Institute's Task Force (1977). The Task Force
points out that obesity is a risk factor in the incidence of high blood pressure
in adolescents.

[14]Some evidence supporting the validity of this assumption appears in the
regression results. In particular, the coefficients of birth weight, mother's age
at the birth of the youth, and parental assessment of the youth's health in the
first year of his life are almost never statistically significant. These
variables are proxy measures of the genetic endowment. If they had had large
significant impacts in the dynamic equations, this would have thrown into question
the validity of our assumption.

[15]Even if the family background variables had no genetic components, we would still expect the "dynamic" coefficients to be smaller than the cross-sectional coefficients, because the "dynamic" estimates represent short-run effects in the sense that they hold constant the lagged values of health and cognitive development. Since these lagged values themselves depend on family background, the cumulative or long-run impacts of family background are likely to exceed the "dynamic" or short-run impacts. To be precise, if cross-lagged effects are ignored, a full representation of the dynamic health process that we study is (ignoring stochastic terms):

$$H_1 = \alpha GH + b_1 E, \text{ and}$$

$$H_t = a_t H_{t-1} + b_t E, \quad t=2,\ldots,n.$$

Solving recursively, one obtains

$$H_t = \left[\alpha \prod_{i=1}^{t} a_i \right] GH + \left[b_t + \sum_{i=1}^{t-1} b_i \prod_{j=t-1}^{i} a_j \right] E.$$

The parameter of E in the above equation is the cumulative environmental effect. If the b_i all have the same sign, the long-run parameter unambiguously exceeds b_t in absolute value. Of course, the long-run parameter estimate may be larger or smaller than the cross-sectional estimate if GH is omitted from the equation.

STRUCTURE OF THE MARKET
FOR HEALTH CARE

HEALTH, ECONOMICS, AND HEALTH ECONOMICS
J. van der Gaag and M. Perlman (editors)
© North-Holland Publishing Company, 1981

INCOMPLETE VERTICAL INTEGRATION: THE DISTINCTIVE STRUCTURE
OF THE HEALTH-CARE INDUSTRY

R. G. Evans

The traditional analysis of market structure in a particular
industry presupposes a bilateral relationship between two classes of
independent transactors, the producers (or suppliers) of a particular set of commodities, and the buyers (or consumers). The set
of exchange relationships between these two is the market, although
the exact location of the boundaries of this set is frequently
problematical. Industries may be defined in terms of specific kinds
of commodities produced, or specific firms, while the markets in
which they transact may be more or less broadly defined in time and
space; but overlapping of category boundaries is usually unavoidable. Since commodities form a continuum, particularly when
viewed as bundles of characteristics, and time and space come in
discrete blocks only in official statistics, any definition of a
market or an industry has an arbitrary element.

The health-care industry and its marketplaces share these general
problems of boundaries and definitions: Which set of economic activities constitutes health care, and what is the appropriate cate-
gorization of subindustries? But the structure of resource
allocation processes in the health care industry differs from that
in others; it is a blend of administrative or "command" and market
mechanisms, with the mix varying considerably across countries.
Thus a focus on "market" structure alone would be incomplete and
misleading even where markets are still much in evidence (e.g., the
United States). In other countries such a limitation would ignore
most, or all, of the processes whereby resources are actually
allocated.[1]

Furthermore, the health-care industry also presents a structural
feature of a quite different level of complexity. Health-care
markets are not, in general, adequately characterized by the
interactions of pairs of transactors; rather, they reflect multi-
lateral transactions among participants whose degree of independence
is limited and variable across jurisdictions. Managerial and
entrepreneurial functions are in effect shared among different firms
on the supply side. Hospitals and pharmacies, for example, do not
deal directly with patients. Their relations are mediated by physicians, who admit patients to hospitals and direct their treatment
there, and who prescribe the drugs which pharmacies are to supply.
Such submarkets as hospital care, physicians' services, and
prescription drugs display a form of incomplete vertical integration
which makes it inaccurate to describe (and misleading to analyze)

any one of them as a simple, bilateral relationship between consumers and a more or less homogeneous class of supplier.[2]

This central feature, of incomplete vertical integration among different forms of transactors, extends beyond care suppliers. The
governmental function of regulation, or establishing a "web of
rules" for economic activity, is common in all industries. In
health care, however, regulation is not only more extensive than in
most other industries, but is qualitatively different. Its oldest
and most characteristic form is the delegation of public authority
to certain classes of providers to govern their own conduct and that
of certain other providers. This integration of suppliers with the
regulatory authority is a fundamental structural feature with important consequences for conduct and performance--a feature not captured by structural analyses which focus only on bilateral
supplier-consumer relations.

The pervasiveness of insurance, public or private, likewise significantly modifies market structure. Efforts to capture its influence
solely through its impact on consumer choices miss the most significant effects. Even in the United States, the special case of
insurance sold at arm's length by private, for-profit firms independent of the health-care industry is not the dominant form, though
many "demand" analyses implicitly treat it as universal. In fact,
most health insurance is provided by governments and in conjunction
with some form of direct regulation. Provider-sponsored or provider-
dominated plans formerly supplied a significant proportion in
Canada, and still do in the United States (Blue Cross/Blue Shield).
There a growing share is provided in conjunction with private,
direct-delivery systems. Thus in practice the provision of health
insurance is directly linked, in most jurisdictions, with one of the
other transactors in the health-care market. And, as is well known,
the particular pattern of linkage has very significant effects on
the conduct and performance of the health-care industry.

This paper will sketch the more common forms of linkages among the
minimal number of classes of transactors in the health-care market.
Different patterns of linkage give rise to different patterns of
conduct that can be observed within alternative delivery systems and
that constitute the "stylized facts" of operations of the health-
care industry under different structures. These in turn lead
directly to questions of performance evaluation, which is
necessarily somewhat more subtle than in more conventional
industries. Finally some observations about appropriate policy, and
its possibility, will be based on these evaluations.

CHARACTERISTIC PATTERNS OF INTEGRATION

Exploration of linkage patterns in health care seems to require at
least five different classes of transactors, in contrast to the
customary two. These are (1) consumers, (2) first-line providers,
contacted directly by consumers, (3) second-line providers, whose
output is either used by consumers under the direction of first-line
providers, or is supplied as intermediate products to first-line or

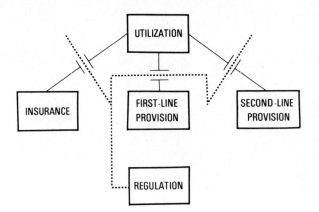

Figure 1. Hypothetical free market model: free choice among independent transactors. ⊣ ⊢ Arm's-length market exchange relationship, independent transactors. ------ regulatory environment structuring a market relationship.

other second-line providers, (4) governments, and (5) suppliers of insurance or purchasers of risk associated with health-care use.

These categories do not precisely coincide with the usual partitioning of health care into the subindustries of physicians' services, hospital care, drugs, etc. A pharmacy, for example, is a first-line supplier of OTC drugs but supplies Rx drugs only in response to a patient's compliance with a physician's order. A hospital might operate an emergency ward or an outpatient department as a first-line service. Patients are admitted from these to inpatient wards only on order of a physician, but if the physician is a salaried member of the hospital staff the line between physician and hospital is tenuous at best. Specialist physicians in referral practice represent an ambiguous middle ground between first- and second-line suppliers: at what point does the consultant take over the patient? Practice varies in different systems. Thus the split between first- and second-line depends on the directness of the supplier-consumer or provider-patient relation, not necessarily on the identity of the institution or the nature of the service. This logic underlies grouping hospitals with drug and medical equipment manufacturers, for example, because although they are organized very differently, and indeed the last two supply products to the first, the output of all three flows to the ultimate user under the direction of a first-line provider.

A Hypothetical Free Market Model

The linkage among transactors, incomplete vertical integration, is reflected in the transfer of functions from one transactor to another. This transfer can best be seen relative to a hypothetical model of health care organization (Figure 1) where each class of transactor deals independently and at arm's length with some or all

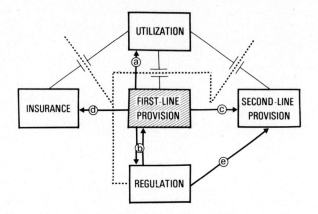

Figure 2. Fully professional model: all transactions directly
influenced/controlled by first-line providers.
     Direct administrative influence or control; ▨ ▧ primary location of admin-
istrative power – two or more imply institutionalized conflict; a agency –
direct influence of providers over utilization; b self-regulation – providers
collectively regulate individuals; c prescriptive power – first-line providers
direct hospital, Rx use; d providers directly influence insurance function, by
control (II) or collective negotiation (III, IV?); e Government regulates and
subsidizes hospitals and (some) other second-line provision – under first-line
direction; for other symbols, see Figure 1.

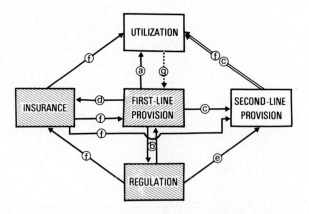

     Figure 3. Universal public health insurance (Canada) model: public (via
insurance) and professional influence coexist or conflict. f Direct public
control of insurance, and thereby providers; g Patient influence on provider
behavior – non-market; for other symbols, see Figures 1 and 2.

of the others, none exerting any control over the others except
through price signals.

Government, of course, would be the exception, in that its function
is to define and maintain property rights (in the broadest sense)
through orders backed up by a monopoly of coercive power, but it
would confine its activity to such orders, and would issue them in
pursuit of some general or external interest, not in response to the
interests of any one class of transactors. In Figure 1, government
regulates markets by defining and enforcing contracts and policing
fraud, but (assuming property to be defined) imposes no direct
orders on market participants.

In this Arcadia, consumers decide upon the level and mix of health-
care services to be used by responding to price information from
suppliers, income (or factor endowment and market) constraints, and
exogenously determined "tastes." Fluctuations in health status--a
cold or a perforated appendix--would be represented as changes in
"tastes" for health care leading to increased demand at current
prices/incomes; congenital problems would presumably represent long-
run taste differentials. But information from the health-care
system itself would be restricted to price quotes. Knowledge of the
characteristics of new products presumably becomes available through
some independent channel.

Producers make the key production decisions about the mix of inputs
to use and how much to produce, in response to production function
information and factor and product prices (or, if markets are imperfectly competitive, product demand and factor supply curves). But
each firm chooses its techniques of production and sets price and
output independently, subject only to the information and
constraints embodied in market prices. No one firm directly inter-
venes in another's choices. Government may intervene, but is
strictly exogenous to producers, and does not itself produce.
Insurance companies exist to formulate and sell a variety of claims
contracts that are contingent on health status, or more commonly its
imperfect signal, health-care use, but do not intervene in any other
market except through the structure and price of contracts offered.
Consumers' use of care will depend on their insurance status, and
thus their choice of contracts and their subsequent use patterns are
interdependent. But insurers and providers of care have no dealings
with each other.

Non-market Linkages Among Transactors

Of course, there is not now and never has been such an Arcadia in
health-care delivery. In fact, the range and richness of nonprice
interactions among different classes of transactors yields an
embarrassment of analytic opportunity. But perhaps the most fundamental linkages, certainly those with the longest history and the
greatest similarity across otherwise different health-care systems,
are those among patients, first-line providers, and government.

These linkages are expressed in the twin concepts of "agency" and
"self-government," both of which involve the transfer of economic
functions from their "normal" holders to the first-line providers.
Patient/consumers permit providers to act as their agents in making
consumption choices, with respect both to the output of second-line
providers and to the agents' own first-line services.[3] Utilization
decisions are the outcome of joint decision-making, in which the
relative influence of provider and consumer varies by type of decision. The provider has integrated forward into the consumer role,
acting as both provider and consumer, thus significantly increasing
the information, and changing the objectives, reflected in utilization outcomes. Hence it is, in general, misleading to identify
measured utilization of health care with "demand" in its economic
sense of consumer choices responding only to price information.

There remains, of course, a "demand" in the conventional economic
sense for treatment of episodes of illness, with first contacts initiated by patients in response to, inter alia, price information.
With a few exceptions, however, economic analyses have equated
measured utilization with points on a demand curve. This appears to
require either that utilization patterns (and costs) in any illness
episode subsequent to the initial contact are uniquely defined and
known to the user before contact is initiated, or that consumers
retain full discretion over follow-on treatment and receive only
service price information (and offers) from physicians as the case
unfolds. Such assumptions appear aggressively counterfactual, yet
without them a large part of the health-care demand literature in
economics rests on misspecified models.

The issue is often obscured by the level of aggregation of analysis--
medical or, worse, health care being treated as a homogeneous commodity so that the episodic structure is suppressed. Empirical
studies which use "visits" or "patient days" as quantity measures
further compound the problem since such concepts are heterogeneous
across providers (and especially jurisdictions) and are seriously
incomplete descriptors of utilization. Further, both heterogeneity
and incompleteness are endogenous to the market setting--they are
price-sensitive. The impact of fee schedule structures on practice
patterns is widely observed.

The clinical literature on utilization, in contrast to the economic,
tends to focus very narrowly on specific procedures or conditions
and to assume a dominant role for the physician acting from
"Hippocratic," if not always perfectly informed, motives. Its
richer information base frequently permits more reliable causal
inferences; but generalizing such inferences requires strong aggregation assumptions which are frequently implausible. Furthermore,
it is clear that the integration between first-line providers and
consumers is incomplete and that the professional maintains personal
objectives which may conflict with those of the consumer. The
essence of professionalism is the internalization and management of
this conflict of interest.

Paralleling the transfer from patient/consumer to provider, regulatory functions are delegated by the state to first-line providers

collectively, in the form of rights to self-government. Individual
providers are required to belong to professional organizations which
regulate their conduct, deploying the full coercive power of the
state. Although this delegation is in principle subject to review,
traditionally and still in most jurisdictions the professional organization functions to a significant extent as a private government,
enjoying considerable independence in its limited area.

In an important analysis of this parallelism, Tuohy and Wolfson
(1977) have shown that self-government is essentially an agency
relation in which the providers collectively undertake to act in the
interests of the state, for the same reasons of informational asymmetry that lead to agency relations between individual providers and
consumers.[4]   Further, they argue persuasively that these relationships are self-supporting, and must exist at both levels or
neither. Self-government is a political privilege received to support the individual agency relation, and loses its raison d'être if
the latter decays, but without self-government individual agency is
also threatened.

These two forms of functional delegation represent fundamental
structural features of the health-care market. The conduct of firms
is directly influenced, rather than merely induced by traditional
structural features such as the number and size distributions of
firms, or their concentration in particular geographic or other submarkets. Similarly, structural issues, such as product characteristics and differentiability, or buyer information and demand
elasticity, are all subsumed in the individual seller's capacity to
exercise the ultimate "advertising" power--to make the consumption
decision on the buyer's behalf.[5]

The treatment of self-government in formal economic analysis has
focused primarily, not on agency, but on the potential for monopoly
behavior created by entry barriers. Implicitly, the argument that
the profession functions as a monopoly requires us to treat all self-
government as a costly error of public policy. Costs of monopoly
are evaluated in the context of consumer demand curves, a fact which
requires that social welfare functions respect consumer sovereignty.
But if this standard were relevant, professions as legal entities
need not and should not exist. If, however, professionalization is
"needed" to remedy imperfect consumer information, the conventional
monopoly critique based on ill-informed demand curves may be
irrelevant. In most jurisdictions, moreover, the restrictions over
entry to the professions have been reasserted by governments and are
no longer, if they ever were, in the hands of providers. Entry to
the professions is now a part of public educational (or even
immigration) policy. What we observe are "structurally competitive"
industries, with large numbers of firms and relatively rapid, though
not at all free, entry. What is missing is competitive conduct, and
it is the self-government over conduct which remains critical.
Restrictions vary by jurisdiction and by profession, but in general
they extend to how firms may be organized (corporate or
noncorporate), who may own the firm (it is considered "unethical"
for a professional to be employed by a nonprofessional), what production processes may or may not be used (in particular what may be
delegated to other professionals) and, where relevant, what pricing
behavior is permissible. These restrictions are mutually rein-

forcing, and are supported by absolutely restricted access to particular service markets. Indeed, access to markets, not to an
occupational role, is the crucial entry barrier. The key structural
feature is that such access is open only to firms owned by and
deploying the services of members of particular occupations; such
"professionalized" natural persons (unlike corporations or entrepreneurs from other backgrounds) are much more sensitive to both formal
and informal methods of conduct control. A focus on entry control
implicitly assumes that once entry is achieved professionals/firms
behave like "ordinary," unregulated profit-maximizing entities, ame-
nable to the usual forms of analysis, and thus ignores the critical
direct impact of collective self-regulation on firm conduct.

Linkages to Second-Line Providers

The largest components of the health-care system, in terms of expenditure and employment, are not the first-line providers but the
hospitals, drug manufacturers, and equipment makers whose output is
directed by the first-line group. The triangular relation of physician, patient, and hospital has been particularly difficult to
handle analytically; economic models range from ignoring the physician and assuming that patients buy hospital services directly, to
suppressing the hospital as an independent transactor and treating
it as an extended physician's office. More recent thinking has
moved back toward realism, and suggests that a hospital be thought
of as two firms, not one, interacting in a single institution, and
transacting as much politically or bureaucratically as economically.
No explicit prices or markets govern internal hospital allocation
processes, but no single authority relation exists either.[6]

What is clear, however, is that a number of the "managerial" decisions in hospitals (what to produce, and how) are made by physicians
who, at least in a North American setting, are not employees of the
organization. Many of the functions of the hospital as a firm
(i.e., decisions on output at a given price and on mode of production) have been delegated to first-line providers. But in the
longer run a hospital can reassert these functions as it makes its
capital and staff decisions (though these, too, are influenced by
physicians) and can also influence physician practices. Indeed, a
hospital with a salaried staff can be thought of as having
integrated forward into medical practice--a salaried physician is a
factor input, not a firm.

Thus the boundary between physicians and hospitals which demarcates
separate firms can be very fuzzy. In North America, full integration in either direction is still relatively rare. The pattern of
incomplete vertical integration which characterizes the
patient/provider (agency) and provider/state (self-government) relations emerges here as well. Physicians do not in general own and
manage hospitals, though private hospitals and particularly special
purpose facilities (e.g., surgical centers) seem to be expanding in
the United States. Some hospitals have large house staffs, but private physicians still bring in the patients. Moreover integration
patterns differ significantly across national boundaries, making
generalization hazardous. In Canada, the hospital can be thought of

as three firms, not two, for provincial governments exercise very
significant management powers by determining annual operating
budgets and (separately) capital allocation. Here the state has
taken over a number of functions of the hospital "firm" directly,
not merely by regulation, although for a variety of political
reasons it chooses not to own and operate the hospitals. But it is
questionable whether a hospital per se still exercises enough
entrepreneurial functions to be considered a firm, after one allows
for the decisions delegated to (or taken over by) physicians on one
side and government on the other. In the U.K., integration appears
to have gone so far that hospitals can no longer be treated as independent firms. In the United States, hospitals as separate firms
seem to be still in existence, but it is unclear, when one tries to
describe the conduct of the hospital industry, whose conduct is
being observed and whose objectives are being sought. The firm as a
category in economic analysis does not necessarily correspond either
to a legal entity or to a physical/organizational structure, though
each may be called "hospital." Hence the unsatisfactory state of
hospital modelling. The other second-line providers appear much
more distinct in their relations with the rest of the health-care
system. Manufacturers of drugs and medical equipment are organized
as private, strictly for-profit firms with highly differentiated
products, and though extensively regulated by government have
control over their own entrepreneurial functions. Their markets,
however, are rather peculiar. Drug manufacturers sell to patients
through physicians; equipment manufacturers sell to hospitals and,
to a lesser extent, to physicians who supply patients. The ultimate
user of services does not generally make the utilization decision;
accordingly, the very large marketing effort of such second-line
suppliers is aimed at the first line. Drugs are marketed to
physicians; equipment to hospital medical staffs. The extent and
sophistication of this marketing effort can be thought of as a
structural feature, in that physicians' perceptions of optimal technique are altered by second-line suppliers. Thus manufacturers
integrate forward into patterns of output mix and volume by reaching
through the agency role of the first-line provider. It is unclear
at what point this process ceases to be most usefully regarded as
advertising and becomes rather an absorption either of the
supplier's function of choosing technique or the consumer's function
of choosing what to use. - But although the agency role of the first-
line provider, with its inherent conflict of interest, is supported
by a variety of "ethical" constraints intended to ensure that
patients' interests will be incorporated into providers' objectives,
no such agency role binds the for-profit suppliers at the next
level. Profit-maximizing leaves no room for agency. This places
further strain on the agency role of the first-line provider, whose
attempts to balance personal and patient interests are subjected to
very deliberate and sophisticated pressures designed to shift his
preferences and perceptions in the direction of more use of specific
second-line products or services. Thus agency at one level must
limit opportunism at two.

What is however interesting is the relatively limited extent to
which first-line providers have integrated backward into pharmacy
ownership or drug supply (repackaging companies). Such integration
is regarded as "unethical," though it is not clear why the conflict
of interest for a physician prescribing his own drugs is more
severe than that in prescribing his own diagnostic or therapeutic
services, or admitting to his own hospital. How this boundary has

been maintained might be an interesting question. One may speculate
that the restrictions on patterns of firm organization at the first-
line level have inhibited the growth of firms large enough to be
able to surmount the scale barriers to direct drug or equipment firm
ownership and control, or for that matter to direct hospital
ownership, but that explanation seems incomplete.

The widest range of variation across jurisdictions seems to be in
the patterns of government and insurance integration with the rest
of the health-care system. In Canada, government has completely
taken over hospital and medical insurance, and plays a significant
role in pharmaceutical and a growing role in dental insurance. This
control of insurance is a critical lever in controlling current
operations and capital formation in the hospital sector; it is thus
the vehicle for partial integration of government into second-line
supply. Government also engages in first-line supply in such traditional areas as public health and immunization, services in remote
areas, and (in Saskatchewan) dental care for children. In the U.K.,
government seems likewise to have absorbed the insurance function
almost completely, and to have gone much farther into the management
of second-line and first-line supply. In the United States, in
contrast, government has taken over only a part of the insurance
function, principally the unprofitable components (insurance for the
poor and elderly) which private firms did not want. It appears,
from comparing U.S. and Canadian experience, that partial takeover
of the insurance function by government does not permit it to reach
through to providers in the same way that full takeover does. The
ability of governments to influence hospital budget/capital investment decisions or physician price formation directly through the
payments process is not in proportion to its share of funding when
funding sources are multiple and diverse. Hence the apparent
failure of hospital cost-control efforts in the United States
(Pearson and Abernethy, 1980). Overall health-care costs in that
country rose from 7.1% of GNP in 1970/71 to 9.1% in 1977/78. In
Canada, where public hospital and medical insurance became universal
in 1971, the 7.3% figure of that year fell to 6.7% in 1974, rose to
7.1% in 1976, and has remained at 7.0% in 1977 and 1978.

But integration of transactors through the insurance mechanism can
go in several other directions. Many of the early health insurance
plans were sponsored and directed by physician or hospital
organizations; they served as ways of increasing the flow of
payments into the health-care industry, enabling it to raise effective prices and/or outputs, as well as redistributing costs. Thus
first- and second-line providers integrated backwards into
insurance. The initiative to integrate can come from the insuring
agency; Goldberg and Greenberg (1977) have documented early and
recent efforts by U.S. insurers to influence patterns of behavior
among providers.[7] The salient feature of their discussion, however,
is that the attempts were complete failures. On the other hand, the
successes of Health Maintenance Organizations in the United States,
and the philosophy most recently expressed by Enthoven (1978) in the
"Consumer Choice Health Plan," are based on much more extensive forward integration of the insuring organization into delivery, for
instance, by establishing exclusive contracts with closed-panel physician groups and owning its own hospitals. A generalization of
this approach seems to depend on extensive entry by competitive,
for-profit firms combining service and insurance, but this leaves
open the _very_ thorny question of how to care for the identifiable

high-risk patients, while preserving patient choice of firm.
Indeed, forward integration by the insurer per se, as envisioned by
Enthoven, represents a departure from historical HMO experience, in
which the insurance function was a vehicle through which other
groups (employers, unions, physicians with unconventional views)
tried to influence the delivery process.

The consequences of choosing one or the other route are very different. It is extensively documented that the forward integration
of the seller of insurance into care (HMOs) leads to very different
levels and patterns of service utilization and costs, from those
generated when sellers of services integrate backwards into
insurance (Blue Cross/Blue Shield Plans) or when government takes
over the insurance function (as in Canada), regardless in each case
of the out-of-pocket costs, if any, borne by patients. The U.S.
literature on utilization differences between subscribers to closed-
panel insurance plans and to arm's-length (private) or provider-
dominated plans emphasizes the importance of provider organization
and objectives in influencing utilization levels. As Figure 4
below indicates, the "competitive HMO" organizational structure
emphasizes the agency role of first-line suppliers and suppresses
the "market" between users and suppliers. It is thus built on
assumptions about resource-allocative processes quite different from
those underlying the arguments for arm's-length private insurance
with large deductibles and coinsurance, which rest on the structure
of Figure 1. The distinction is blurred by a common rhetoric about
private enterprise versus the state.

A Fully Professionalized Model of Health Care

Alternative ways of organizing the production and delivery of health
services can be represented as alternative patterns of vertical
integration among the five basic classes of transactors, starting
from the hypothetical, freely competitive market of Figure 1. In
contrast to that abstraction, Figure 2 presents an idealized case of
"private enterprise" medicine as viewed by first-line providers
(self-employed physicians).

In Figure 2 the underlying market structure of Figure 1 persists,
but its resource-allocation functions have been supplemented or
supplanted by direct administrative or legal controls emanating from
the first-line providers. "Markets" remain as revenue-raising
institutions. Utilization now depends on doctors' orders--the
agency role of the physician. The profession collectively exercises
regulatory functions over its individual members and would-be members. Insurance plans are either administered by providers (the
"Blue" model, nonprofit and provider-trusteed) or if private, are
restricted in the contracts they may offer. Short-run outputs of
hospitals or pharmacies are directed by physicians; longer-run
hospital decisions are influenced by medical staffs and physician
trustees or owners. Government regulates and subsidizes hospitals,
but under professional direction.

This extensive concentration of functions serves two objectives. It
enables first-line providers to increase the resource and rent flows
into the industry, and to concentrate the rental flows so they come

out in one place. But further, the deployment of professional
authority seems to be an objective for its own sake, an end rather
than a means, and this too is maximized in the "private enterprise"
structure of Figure 2. The policy objectives of first-line suppliers
are thus clearly furthered by this structure; what is less clear is
why so much external economic analysis has accepted, largely by
default, efforts by industry spokesmen to portray the structure of
Figure 2 as a set of freely competitive private marketplaces along
the lines of the hypothetical Figure 1. Such efforts seem intended,
inter alia, to discourage direct public intervention.

Universal Public Health Insurance

The public administration of universal health insurance, with negotiated fees and/or budgets, creates quite a different pattern of
structural linkages, as can be seen in Figure 3. Government now
integrates forward to control (be) the insurer, and all markets
disappear. The contrast with 2 is more apparent than real, for
much of the resource-allocation function of markets in 1 had already
been preempted by administrative mechanisms in 2. Under 3, however,
the costs of care are raised via taxes, as in Canada, rather than
via direct charges or insurance premiums in pseudo-markets as in
the U.S.

The integrated regulator-insurer now negotiates fees directly with
first-line providers, controls hospitals through budgets as well as
regulation, and determines the terms of the insurance "contract"
with users. Utilization is influenced both by "doctor's orders" and
by direct rationing through the hospital system. Patients' preferences have some direct influence on providers, but not through
any market.

The sources of conflict in this Canadian-style model are obvious.
Self-government, agency, and direct control over hospitals' short-
run output decisions remain with physicians, while government uses
the insurance mechanism to control the availability of hospital services and to influence physicians' incomes and (to a limited extent)
practice behavior. The structure thus embodies points of continuing
struggle over both resources and rents. In this context physician
and hospital efforts to reopen "markets," for instance by direct
charges to patients, are quite explicitly efforts to acquire new
sources of finance and thus extend their own discretionary power--
not to share it with users.

The Consumer Choice Health Plan

Figure 4 represents quite a different polar case. Here as in 3 the
insurer is the vehicle for control over physicians and hospitals.
Figure 4 represents both as employed or directly administered by the
insurer, but one could also envision markets between insurers, physicians, and hospitals. Users transact only with insurers, in
markets minimally regulated, as in Figure 1, by the state. In practice, however, it turns out that enforcing performance by insurers
of a rather complex (and partially implicit) forward contract is a
serious regulatory problem.

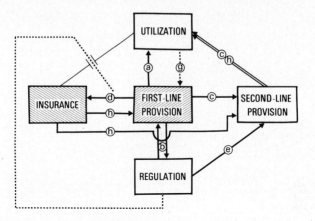

Figure 4. HMO or consumer choice health plan model: competitive insurers influence or control all other suppliers. h Direct influence (ownership or control) of independent insurers on providers; for other symbols, see Figures 1-3.

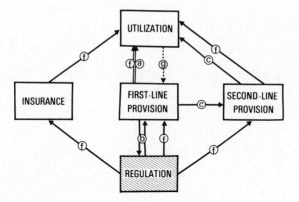

Figure 5. Public delivery ("socialized") model: government consolidates all insurers and suppliers. For symbols, see Figures 1-3.

The self-government and public regulation/subsidy of hospitals remain, as does physician influence on short-run hospital decisions. The key shift from 3 to 4 is that the user/insurer market substitutes for the state in driving the resource allocation process. Whether political or market processes will come closer to some sort of social optimum is an interesting and critical issue. Of course, powers of self-government must be limited to prevent the first-line providers from taking over or suppressing the "activist" insurers through that route, a pattern common in U.S. history, and with some Canadian parallels. And the fee negotiation between public insurer

and collective profession has been replaced by separate contracts
between competitive insurers and physicians as individuals or
groups. Thus, depending on the self-regulatory structure, physician
influence might be significantly less in Figure 4 than in Figure 3.

A Public Delivery, "Socialized" Model

Finally, Figure 5 suggests what a truly "socialized medicine" model
might look like: government ownership and control of hospitals,
medical practices, and the insurance function. Clearly, the sources
of conflict in 3 disappear and the bureaucrat's life becomes
simpler. It is hard to reconcile truly "socialized" medicine with
any concept of self-government. Comparison of 3 and 5 should indicate the structural difference between "socialized medicine" and
nationalized health insurance on the Canadian model or indeed most
others.

PERFORMANCE CRITERIA - PROBLEMS OF DEFINITION

Different structural forms lead to different patterns of conduct
and performance. And the general performance criteria applicable to
the health-care industry and its components are the same that one
would apply to any other industry. The industry can be evaluated by
criteria of allocative efficiency (are its products, at the margin,
valued more than the products of the next best resource use?), technical efficiency (are particular patterns of output produced at
minimum resource cost?), income distribution effects (does the
industry generate patterns of economic rent, and if so are these
distributional effects more or less in line with social
objectives?), and technical progress (is the industry advancing in
its capacity to offer new outputs or to produce existing ones at
lower resource cost?). In the case of health care, however, most
societies express additional redistributional objectives, relating
to equality of access to care and to the distribution of the burdens
of illness and care, which are in principle (but not, it seems, in
practice) separable from the evaluation of industry performance
itself.

The distinction between allocative and technical efficiency criteria, however, presupposes a well-defined end product. Yet in fact
most health care is merely intermediate production, regrettables,
whose consumption is anticipated to improve or maintain health. The
marginal utility to the user of most health care, holding health
status constant, is negative. And services can be hierarchically
ordered, so that specific services are intermediate to production of
more comprehensive packages. A diagnostic test is intermediate to a
spell of hospitalization, which is part of the treatment of an episode of illness, which in turn improves (or prevents deterioration
of) health. Thus one can evaluate diagnostic test activity in terms
of the allocative efficiency of test production, or the technical
efficiency of hospital-care production. Or, more generally, the

allocative efficiency of resource use in the pattern and level of health-care production can also be considered as the technical efficiency of health production.[8]

This, after all, is the basic source of the informational asymmetry between supplier and consumer which gives rise to the agency relationship. Consumers may indeed be the best judges of the value to them of health, a utility-function question, but they obviously are not and cannot be the best judges of the technical, production-function questions surrounding the contribution of health care to health. And health, unfortunately, is not a traded commodity.

The performance of the health-care industry is frequently and widely criticized on both allocative and technical efficiency grounds. It is essential to distinguish, however, several quite different performance critiques which imply different structure/conduct origins. The broad literature, most of it medical or epidemiological, on "unnecessary servicing" focuses on the provision of health care which has little or no (or even negative) impact on health status, such as unnecessary surgery, diagnostic testing, periodic screening or examinations without sickness, drug use, and unnecessarily prolonged hospital stays, and of which the quantitative implications, both in resource costs and in potential negative health outcomes, are large. Illich (1976), though rather polemical, reflects an extensive clinical literature. The assumption behind the criticism is that health care derives its utility at the individual or social level from its impact on health status--only uninformed consumers use inefficacious care, and they would not do so if they knew--so efficacy is a proxy for social value. The overallocation of resources to unnecessary care is a reflection of supplier conduct; it results from the structural characteristics of the supply side, in particular the agency influence over the consumer/patient, the provider's direct economic interest in volume of output, and the absence of any systematic mechanism to feed improved information on efficacy back to a fragmented and highly independent group of suppliers. It is not that suppliers deliberately choose to provide inefficacious or harmful services, but rather, that the structural pattern induces selective sensitivity to new information. The organization of first- and second-line suppliers is such as to encourage expansion of activity, and acceptance of information which supports this expansion. Information which discourages or discredits economically profitable and professionally satisfying activity is much harder to "hear."

Alternative patterns of vertical integration then are of great importance, insofar as they provide different channels for and incentives to the spread of resource-using or resource-curtailing information. When insurance providers integrate forward into supply they may or may not have (depending on insurance market structure) incentives to reduce unnecessary servicing by attempting to influence providers directly. Governments, in this role, clearly do. Insurance sellers who also supply a full line of services, the HMO model of Figure 4, appear to have had considerable success in restricting inefficient overallocation of resources to health care; arm's-length insurers have not. Governmental experience is similar. Canadian provinces have been relatively successful in controlling real resource inputs in the hospital sector, where they have signi-

ficant management authority; much less so in modifying patterns of
physician care except where these depend on hospital access. The
U.K. government has apparently been more successful. The potential
for system-wide generalization of the U.S. experience with improved
allocative efficiency from forward integration of competitive
insurers, vis-à-vis the alternative of government integration, is
still an open issue.

Two things seem clear, however. First, as long as the insurance
structure is controlled by providers (backward-linked) either
directly, as in Blue Cross/Blue Shield, or indirectly, through the
influence that providers collectively can bring to bear on individual insurers in a fragmented, arm's-length insurance market
(whether or not wholly private), then no significant improvement can
be made in allocative efficiency. Second, efforts to deal with
excessive utilization through manipulating the incentives aimed at
consumers will be ineffectual, as theirs is not the relevant conduct
to be modified by new information.

This is a critical point, and depends inter alia on the identification of allocative inefficiency with overprovision of inefficacious services. There is a more traditional strand of economic
literature which defines overprovision, quite independently of efficacy, in terms of consumer willingness to use at particular prices.
The marginal social value of care is identified with marginal private values as reflected in (assumed) consumer choices in response
to out-of-pocket costs. In this view, insurance (of any sort)
lowers out-of-pocket costs and induces consumers to "overuse" care,
in the sense that its marginal value to them is below its true marginal resource cost. This view totally ignores the information issue,
and identifies use with consumer choice; it has the awkward consequence that society "loses" when snake oil is regulated off the
market. More generally, it cannot deal with the very detailed
structure of supply-side regulation in health care, and either
ignores its existence (assuming prices equal to long-run constant
marginal cost) or dismisses it as a policy error to be corrected
where possible. Nor does this view cope with the variety of allocative results which emerge from alternative systems of organizing
insurance.

The allocative and technical criteria blur into each other as we
move from the wholly unnecessary episode of care (the tonsillectomy,
e.g., technically inefficient health production) to the unnecessary
laboratory test (technically inefficient production of one part of a
hospital episode that is possibly quite necessary). One moves from
the observation of "things which shouldn't have been done" to "things
which should have been done differently/with less resource use,"
depending on how "things" are defined. But we reach a central core
of technical efficiency questions in the patterns of use of health
manpower. An extensive literature in all the main branches of the
first-line subindustry, and to a lesser extent in the second, documents the technical inefficiency of the production of services independently of the allocative or efficacy question of whether they
should have been supplied at all.[9] This pattern, in turn, is

easily traceable to the conduct of the firms supplying such
services--choice of non-cost-minimizing points on the production
function--and to the structures of the relevant markets which both
permit and encourage them to do so.

FROM STRUCTURE TO PEFORMANCE--THE CONDUCT LINKAGES

The integration of providers into government roles enables them
collectively to influence structure and conduct in important
respects. Historically, economists have focused on the use of this
power to create entry barriers, and indeed its earlier manifesta-
tions were in the form of reduced access to professions and control
of numbers. Further, of course, it is definitionally true that
supernormal rents cannot persist and be protected without entry
barriers.

As noted above, however, control on entry to professional occupations has in most jurisdictions reverted to the state. Entry,
though far from free, has been relatively rapid for many years.
Moreover, the analysis of entry processes requires consideration of
the role and objectives of training institutions, especially univer-
sities, for whom a crude set of objectives would include high rates
of entry and overqualified entrants (they sell qualifications), with
maximum government subsidy of training, and subsequent regulatory
protection of human capital values to ensure future markets. The
important uses of self-government are now to restrict access to service markets to firms controlled by members of particular professions, and to control the conduct of those members so that even
in a structurally competitive environment where there is rapid entry
and a large number of firms, price-competitive behavior can be
suppressed and rents protected (even if more widely shared).

Such protection requires restriction of output-expanding technologies. Individual firms run by a solo practitioner, in dentistry, pharmacy, or many branches of medicine (family practice,
obstetrics, anesthesia) can now expand their output per "peak
professional" by up to several hundred percent, with corresponding
increases in net income or reductions in prices, by deploying
well-known and tested types of auxiliary workers who are potentially
in very elastic supply. When 80% - 90% of the work of a general
dentist can be performed to or above professional quality standards
by a high school graduate with 20 months' training, the potential
exists for dramatic expansions in output per firm and for reductions
in unit costs of about 40% (Evans and Williamson, 1978). These
could trigger competition destructive both of the value of existing
human capital and of currently capitalized rents. By using state
authority to ban the use of such technologies, the profession
collectively ensures that each individual firm faces a steeply
rising marginal cost curve (the supply of professional own time) and
hence is discouraged from initiating a price-cutting, competitive
strategy to expand the market share. This, rather than restrictions

on price advertising per se, seems to be the critical control mechanism in protecting rents. Thus the erosion in the power of all professions to control price advertising which is taking place in the
United States (and possibly Canada, though the legal rearguard may
succeed in keeping the substance while abandoning the shadow of
control) will not likely generate any significant change in competitive behavior unless regulatory power over technology is
dismantled as well.[10]

Even that may not be enough. "Conscious parallelism" is very powerful among firms all owned and managed by members of the same profession, acutely conscious of their mutual interdependence, their
heavy investment in industry-specific human capital, and their low
opportunity costs outside the industry. In such circumstances the
"conjectural variations" in other firms' behavior are quite easy
for each firm to define, and their consequences are equally clear.
Add a relatively price-inelastic market demand curve arising from
insurance or consumer perceptions of "need", and the expected payoff
to an individual competitive strategy becomes very low. Since, in
addition, agency confers the power to induce utilization, and do
even more "good," when supply expands through rising
provider/population ratios, firms are unlikely to be driven to the
abyss of price competition unless capacity expands explosively.

Of course, firms owned and managed by nonprofessionals, simply
hiring their services, would take a very different view. The human
capital of providers would then become a cost of production, to be
minimized, not the principal earning asset of the practice, to be
conserved and maximized. Dental practices owned by the Hudson's Bay
Company might conduct themselves very differently in the output
market--and even have an interest in changing the locus of regulatory
power. But here again, conduct of professionals is controlled, in
that they may not be employed by nonprofessionals in the supply of
professional services. All firms in the product market must be
owned/managed by an owner of human capital with much to lose if competition breaks out.

Thus improvement of technical efficiency in service production by
reducing the present substantial and costly overuse of human capital appears to require significant change, either in the control of
providers over regulation of their own conduct--de-integration in our
terms--or a shift in the patterns of vertical integration to
separate management and professional roles. Direct government
supply is one possibility: the Saskatchewan Dental Service uses 16
dentists, among a staff of several hundred dental nurses and auxi-
liaries, to provide almost all the services needed by 90% of the
province's children. Costs per child are correspondingly low,
access much improved, and quality of care is as good as or better
than the private system. But government takeover of supply merely
creates the possibility of more efficient input use--it is far from
a guarantee. Integrated insurance and care-supply firms--HMOs--have
some of the same potential, but they are still severely restricted
by professional self-government. Yet whether one attempts to deal
with the technical efficiency problem through increased reliance on
markets, or more direct public intervention, it appears clear that
the current structure of linkage between professions and government
must be significantly modified.

THE LIMITED ROLE OF PRICES

The discussion of allocative and technical efficiency has largely disregarded the role of prices, on the ground that in the health-care industry prices perform primarily an income distributional function. There is still a lively economic literature on the hypothetical resource allocation role of prices in modifying consumer behavior, but providers and reimbursers discuss them almost exclusively in income distribution terms. The numerous "demand," and associated insurance impact and burden, studies are all in the context of arm's-length models of the Figure 1 type, and give rather diverse results--not surprising if the model is misspecified.

The emphasis on income distribution is partly due to the almost universal insulation of users of care from all or most of its cost, but this universal phenomenon is in turn rooted in the special characteristics of health care as a commodity. Insofar as prices do play an allocative role, their influence is on provider choices of what to recommend to their patients, and there does seem to be support for the view that relative rates of reimbursement per unit time affect (though do not fully determine) providers' choices of the mix and volume of services to recommend and provide. The literature analyzing this phenomenon is, however, rarely placed in the context of any formal model of supplier behavior or market functioning; it merely postulates that suppliers will wish to do more of whatever pays better. But if prices are endogenous and utilization is supplier-influenced, a consistent formalism becomes rather tricky, and requires an extended set of provider objectives.

Patients may of course vary the rate at which they <u>contact</u> the health services system in response to out-of-pocket costs; it would be rather surprising if they did not. But this is only one of many factors affecting overall levels of care utilization, and apparently not a very important one. In the United States, for example, physician visit rates and hospital days per capita have been stable for a number of years while servicing intensity has risen steadily. Prices could conceivably have an allocative effect if they influenced either the short-run willingness of providers to supply effort to the industry or the long-run rates of entry and exit. But excess demand for entry at current prices and incomes all over the world is at such a level that industry capacity is likely to depend for the foreseeable future on public decisions about medical school places (provision, as in Canada, or funding, as in the United States), and professional (or perhaps public) decisions about allowable technology, rather than on relative prices. Nor is there much evidence of short-run supply response; where prices are exogenous the supply curve appears, if anything, backward-bending.

In most jurisdictions, a significant share of the health-care industry does not display explicit prices for its products. Hospitals reimbursed on a budget-review basis receive annual grants to cover total operations, and per diems or dollars of expenditure per in-patient day are merely a synthetic ratio of heterogenous costs over a heterogenous (and incomplete) output measure. Hospitals reimbursed per unit of service may think of these as "prices" but they are hospital-specific "prices" per unit of inter-

mediate product. The overall "price" of an episode of care is
determined ex post from actual services used and negotiated production costs or charges. Thus, although there is clearly an implicit
"price" for any definition of output, this price is not explicitly
identified and does not serve as a critical input to resource allocation decisions at the micro level. Only for commodities such as
drugs or equipment, or for the component of professional services
reimbursed on fee-for-service, are explicit ex ante prices routinely
available. The latter, moreover, are less well defined if patients
self-pay and collection rates vary.

Emphasizing the income-generating rather than the market-clearing
role of (mostly implicit) health-care prices leads to the expectation that price levels will respond positively to levels of supply
in a market characterized by the typical pattern of agency and self-
government. This expectation rests upon complementary perceptions
of utilization as strongly supplier-influenced, and on a rather
gene?al formulation of supplier objectives. Profit-maximization is
of course generally recognized as an untenable objective for self-
employed entrepreneurs in imperfect competition, and net
income/leisure maximization is both unnecessarily restrictive and,
given what we know of health professionals, rather implausible. The
primary input to production is professional own time, with a marginal opportunity cost steeply rising in rate of use per time period.
But unless the utility function is separable, this opportunity cost
also depends on income, so price enters the cost curve. Effort and
output supply may then fall as price rises. Unless the output
market is competitive, of course, this marginal cost curve is not a
supply curve anyway; and most conventional models of health providers assume monopolistically competitive structure with limited
entry. Moreover short-run quasi-rents are necessary to reimburse
human capital costs, and human capital comes in discrete lumps. The
casual drawing of firm or industry supply curves, especially positively sloped ones, is thus rather suspect. But the demand curve, in
an agency world, is no more satisfactory as a central analytic
construct. The classical parrot, which once qualified as a political economist by virtue of its ability to say "supply and demand,"
now has laryngitis.

On the whole, the positive association of supply and price seems to
be at least as well supported empirically as the converse, though of
course any pattern of observations can be represented by a conventional demand curve with enough arguments. Nor is it easy to be
sure what is being priced--visits are simply not standard measures
of output over time, space, or firms.

The combined role of governments and insurers in all major health
care markets makes the behavior of prices in the abstract less
interesting (and less susceptible to testing). It does appear,
however, that received prices and incomes tend to advance more
rapidly, the more fragmented and/or provider-dominated the payment
process. When suppliers control insurance, or when insurance is
provided by a number of private firms at arm's length, explicit
price levels or unit costs rise more rapidly than if governments
integrate forward to control all insurance supply. When sources of
funding are multiple, first- and second-line suppliers can maintain
greater price-setting or budget-formulating independence because

their inherent monopoly power is not countered by monopsony and because direct charges to consumers are always available as a residual source of payment. So-called UCR fees for professionals in the United States seem to be the ultimate in price-setting freedom.

Correspondingly, servicing patterns seem to rise more rapidly in controlled price settings, as a more general model of suppliers would suggest. These increases are independent of changes in prices paid by users, if any, and reflect rather a change in the tradeoffs between income, leisure, and other physician objectives when price-setting behavior is constrained. Whether such increases in servicing imply either proportionately more resource inputs, or most importantly increases in health status, are critical but very difficult questions which can only be addressed at present in the context of particular illnesses and treatment protocols.

The income determination process remains rather obscure, however, in health care as in other industries. There is still ample evidence, of the unsatisfied-demand-for-entry and rate-of-return-on-investment sort, that physicians and dentists earn large rents. Rents in the not-for-profit hospital sector are more difficult to identify, showing up as costs, but here too there is evidence of earnings above opportunity cost. These take diverse forms: above-market salaries for employees, "perks" for physicians, the "quiet life" for administrators, or even supply contracts let to for-profit firms which are at less than arm's length. These persist not primarily as a result of entry barriers (rents can coexist with underemployment) but as a result of the conduct of firms in the industry, which again comes back to the structural issue: for and by whom are "firms" managed?

POLICY PARADOXES WITH STRUCTURAL ROOTS

The same structural issue underlies the very peculiar and ambiguous treatment of technological progress in health care. In general, rapid technological progress is a positive feature of any industry's performance. Yet in health care the primary policy interest seems to be in limiting and controlling the rate of advance. The resolution of this apparent paradox is to be found in the fact that the absorption of new technology is strongly motivated by its contribution to sales, or industry gross revenues, which society regards not as a benefit but as the cost of acquiring health. If utilization of a new service, via an assumption of consumer sovereignty, were prima facie evidence of its social utility, then the "proliferation of technology" could only be a benefit. But the assumption is untenable.

The problem of technology assessment is now generally recognized as simply a part of the broader issue: "Why are particular services provided in health care?" There is nothing special about sophisticated, or even expensive technology; simple laboratory tests in sufficient quantity can be even more expensive. The key question remains, Does the procedure lead to an increment in health status (a) at all, (b) sufficient to warrant its cost? The shift in

decision-making functions resulting from incomplete vertical
integration leads to decisions being taken as to the utilization of
both established and new technologies, on the basis of revenue
(cost) generation, not efficacy or cost effectiveness. This in turn
creates inappropriate incentives for the investment of resources in
new research. New information as to techniques which lower costs of
health care, by rendering some current workers unnecessary or
lowering their incomes, meets substantially greater resistance to
diffusion than advances which expand the revenue base. The structurally biased payoff to cost-enhancing advances and technological
add-ons suggests that new technology in health care is likely to
continue as a source of cost-inflation. The counterbalancing forces
depend on a reallocation of managerial functions--choice of technique or pattern of service use--away from providers and back toward
insurers and/or governments.

The focus on new technology, however, reflects one structural
peculiarity--the location of entry barriers. In most jurisdictions,
public agencies of various sorts have significantly more control
over the flow of new capacity to the industry than over the allocation of resources already there. Insofar as new technology is
embodied in capital equipment, systems which separate capital and
operating budgetary processes are able to limit technological proliferation as well as the overexpansion of conventional forms of
capital such as hospital space. Direct budgetary control seems to
be significantly more effective than regulation.

The most important form of direct public management of capital
availability, particularly in the longer run, is manpower policy.
The stock of human capital, skilled manpower, of particular types
and quantities exercises predominant influence over the critical
performance areas of what the industry will choose to supply, and
the mode of production it will choose. The arguments in many
countries for restriction of manpower supply assume that, in the
context of existing structure, such control provides the only,
albeit imperfect, lever for limiting overservicing and technological
inefficiency. Surgical capacity provides the best example of this
debate because the product, operations, is relatively well defined
and measured and because capacity is closely linked to numbers of
particular personnel available. Underutilized manpower is easily
observable, and underutilization is asserted to have negative cost
and quality implications. Clinicians argue that in the United
States, oversupply is reflected in rising prices and falling
workloads, but not falling incomes. Given the apparent magnitude of
the oversupply, if the conventional economic mechanism of falling
prices and incomes were at work, someone should have noticed.
Nevertheless the economic literature reaches no consensus. The
irony of the health manpower policy debate is that output restriction has shifted from being perceived as a professional tactic to
limit competition and maintain incomes, to a public policy to
improve resource allocation.

The debate over manpower policy highlights the structural pecu-
liarity of the health-care industry. Those who favor restriction
argue that a combination of agency, self-government, and
arm's-length or managerially ineffectual insurance enables suppliers
to prevent the outbreak of price competition when numbers are

increased. Prices as well as quantities supplied rise, so although
in the short run average incomes may fall, still total costs
increase substantially. At the same time, higher-cost modes of production are favored to provide employment for the "high-priced
help"--political resistance to less costly substitutes is both more
intense and more effective when "peak professionals" are plentiful.

Emphasis on the complexity of integration patterns indicates the
extent of the structural change that would be necessary to move to a
world in which supply increases had their conventional effects.
Modification of insurance packages (or as suggested in the United
States, the corporate income tax) does not change the locus of managerial decisions. At the very least, dismantling of self-
governmental controls over conduct and reallocation of authority
within hospitals and other second-line providers, together with
significant restructuring of insurance, would be necessary to induce
firms at either level to engage in price-competitive strategies
intended to expand their share of the market.

Whether such a shift would on balance improve welfare, however, is a
much more dubious question. Apart from the political feasibility of
such revolutionary change, the central problem of the agency relation persists. It is not exorcised with handwaving about (doubtless
desirable) increases in consumer information, least of all price
information. In practice, the observable alternatives for structural organization of the health-care industry can assign agency
responsibility entirely to providers (the "free enterprise"
approach) or to integrated provider/insurers (the HMO approach) or
to a limited degree to governments (intervening through limits on
performance or reimbursement of particular procedures, or restrictions on forms of capacity, or direct management of supply).
Alternative structures give different answers to the central medical
question, "Whose patient is this?" Hypothetical market models do
not. Improvements in the allocative and technical efficiency of the
health-care industry, for which there is substantial evidence of
feasibility in principle, seem to wait upon either the creation of
new institutions, or the more aggressive use of existing ones, to
reassign management functions, change the vertical integration pattern, so that incentives and resource allocation responsibilities
can better reflect available information.

Problems of industrial structure in health care thus take us back to
the fundamental social policy problem of economics: the design of
institutional frameworks so that resource-allocation decisions are
assigned to people or groups who both possess the necessary information to make optimal decisions (criteria of optimality are
necessarily a prior socio-political choice) and are under appropriate
incentives to ensure a correspondence of private and social objectives. The alternative structures outlined above represent different assignments of resource-allocation authority, reflecting the
inherent informational impactedness of health-care markets and the
perverse incentives created both by this characteristic and by
social responses to it.

To date the most effective (though far from perfect) means for
achieving this goal have been public, collective responses. The
nature of such responses varies markedly across countries. The

numerous theoretical attractions of private collective institutions
have been associated with some practical success in the United
States, but serious concerns about generalizability remain. Still,
there remains plenty of room for experiment in that country, since
the attempt to reallocate a portion of rents and of control over
utilization from private providers to the public sector through
national health insurance seems to be indefinitely stalled.
(Bill-paying is probably the least interesting aspect of public
insurance.)

In no society, however, are objectives and decision-making powers
within the health-care industry assigned to the sets of elementary
transactors (consumers, firms) on which conventional economic theory
is built. The characteristic patterns of incomplete vertical
integration, of "leaky" transactor boundaries, has made the application of economic methodology to health-care research particularly
difficult and frequently misleading. The task is in process of
becoming even more difficult, because the inherent tendency of
structural boundaries in the health-care industry to shift across
institutions does not stop at research. Since decision-making
powers are a form of property rights, their allocation is inherently
political. All transactors in the health industry have always
operated in the political as well as the economic domain, and from
this perspective research in general and economics in particular is
just a branch of public relations. Thus we now observe forward
integration of providers, either individual for-profit firms or
associations, into the economic research field in order to provide
pseudoscientific justification for structural patterns favorable to
their economic rental streams and/or decision-making authority. For
public relations purposes, economic analysis appears both effective,
and relatively cheap.

There is a bias towards defense of the status quo inherent in economic analysis, particularly in its most "scientific" forms.[11]
Predictive power is attained by the assumptions of simplified structure and minimal discretionary behavior in the objects of analysis.
When all transactors are subject to the "laws of the market," and
seek simple objectives under these well-defined constraints, then
the external analyst has the greatest opportunity to make unambiguous positive statements about aggregate behavior patterns. It
is an unfortunate coincidence that the structural assumptions which
best support technical, mathematical analysis are also those which
obscure the existence of discretionary power. Since the denial of
its existence is a traditional defense of political or economic
power in a democratic society, the needs of the status quo and the
predilections of the analyst are allied.[12]

This inherent conjunction emphasizes the importance of exploring the
structural linkages among the various transactors in health care,
and the channels whereby resource allocation decisions at one level
are in fact controlled from another. The task is rendered the more
difficult, insofar as the objects of analysis enter the analytic
process itself. Germs do not generally conduct or support bac-
teriological research, professional associations or private firms
do support economic research.

The structural framework suggested here is not presented with any illusion that it will prove adequate to embody all the complex conduct and performance issues which arise in different subindustries or national systems. But at least it permits one to raise and address a number of the issues which health-care analysts find important. In the simplified market model, too many important questions appear trivial, or cannot even be posed.

NOTES

[1]The literature relevant to industry structure is correspondingly broad, being drawn from economics, political science, sociology, and to a significant degree from epidemiology, clinical studies, and "health research" generally. To focus on the economic alone would again be incomplete and seriously misleading, but to survey the whole, impossible. Accordingly references will be to general categories or tendencies in the literature, illustrated by leading examples, with no pretense at representativeness (let alone completeness). Choices will be arbitrary and idiosyncratic--like everyone else's.

[2]These interactions are sometimes wrongly identified with concepts of complementarity or substitution, e.g., when physician stocks are inserted in equations "explaining" hospital use. But complementarity and substitution are features of utility or production functions, conditions on matrices of second derivatives, not relations among transactors.

[3]This concept of agency must not be confused with the "agent" in the literature on "principal-agent" problems--e.g., share-cropping, defense contracting. In the principal-agent problem, "selfish" transactors with independent utility functions participate in a non-zero-sum game where the principal's payoff depends on the agent's action but the principal can define the payoff framework. In the professional relationship, by contrast, the professional agent's objective function includes the client/patient's health, welfare, or other characteristics. The test question is, if an action is available to the agent which is totally undetectable, and which transfers wealth from principal to agent, will it be taken? In the "principal-agent" literature, yes; in the professional agency concept, no, or at least not always. Otherwise the concept of a professional has no meaning, and its special regulatory status no justification.

[4]The importance of the agency concept was clearly brought out early by Arrow (1963), but has dropped out of much subsequent work. The application of the label "uncertainty" both to unforeseeable future risks (insurable) and to incomplete present information (requiring agency) was unfortunate. Efforts have been made to support conventional demand analysis by assuming perfect agency--the consumer as physician-patient pair and thus informed--or "generalized" agency. Perfect agency, apart from the direct evidence against it, undercuts all economic theories of professionals qua principals. Generalized agency is a concept that havers between perfect agency and nonagency without committing to the critical notion of incomplete agency. Operationally, it seems indistinguishable from perfect agency.

[5]This point is central to the "supplier-induced utilization" strand of econo-

mic literature. The existence of such inducement has been hotly debated in economic literature, principally in the United States. It appears taken for granted in
the other health-care literature, especially clinical, and attention focuses
rather on the factors which motivate suppliers to recommend particular services.

[6]The literature appears to have gone full circle, as recent work harks back to
the earlier administrators' emphasis on the problem of multiple lines of
authority. Formal analytic models of hospitals are easy to write down, difficult
to justify or to learn from.

[7]Whether changes in the professional powers (and protections) conferred by
self-government, or privately monopolized insurance, could enable insurers to
monitor service provision effectively, is still an open issue. There do not yet
appear to be any examples of successful intervention by private insurers in a
pluralistic environment, except possibly for some components of dental care.

[8]The recent economic literature on the demand for health, not health care,
emphasizes the importance of this distinction, as does the literature on preventive versus curative services. Most of this literature implicitly treats the partial impact of health care (health stock constant) on utility as zero, a
constraint which seems unnecessary and difficult to justify. A negative effect is
more plausible. A more serious weakness, however, is the common but aggressively
counterfactual assumption that consumers possess full information about health
production functions. Yet uninformed consumers are not (fortunately) weeded out
of the market.

[9]This literature has two major subcategories, the "econometric," and the
"engineering." The former approach has the great strength that it reflects in
vivo not in vitro conditions, the field not the lab. But output definitions and
functional forms in econometric studies are of necessity appallingly simplistic.
Further, field experience is a blend of the technological and the behavioral,
under legal constraint. Substitutions which are technically possible may be (are)
legally barred; and behavior cannot in general be assumed cost-minimizing in
imperfect markets. In general, detailed engineering-type production studies
demonstrate much more severe inefficiencies in manpower use, though the econometric studies are rarely consistent with cost-minimization either.

[10]One is reminded of Schumpeter's contrast between an artillery bombardment
and forcing a door, in describing competitive styles. Econometric production studies could not reveal the possibility of such substitutions, let alone measure
their impact.

[11]Stigler (1959) has pointed out (with apparent approval) the conservative
bias of economic theory. If one starts from normative assumptions of consumer
sovereignty and positive assumptions of complete information, zero transactions
costs, and dynamic stability, one moves quickly to the position that whatever is,
is right, and the market like Pangloss's providence yields the best of all
possible worlds. Some technological questions must be finessed to get to competitive market structure, but if information really is perfect, and transactions
costs zero, then these problems can be sidestepped. The only villain in the piece
is government.

[12]Galbraith (1973, pp. 1-11), among others, has pointed to the usefulness of
this neoclassical approach in defending whatever power relationships and wealth
distributions are currently in existence; Unger (1978) is more brutal. He refers
to economics becoming "Despite the seeming agnosticism of its methods and assumptions ... a metaphysic for solid operators, a coat of armor for the prudent and
the passive, and a hocus-pocus in the vestibule of power."

HEALTH, ECONOMICS, AND HEALTH ECONOMICS
J. van der Gaag and M. Perlman (editors)
© North-Holland Publishing Company, 1981

MAJOR POLICY ISSUES IN THE ECONOMICS OF HEALTH CARE
IN THE UNITED STATES

Michael D. Intriligator

RECENT CHANGES IN THE ECONOMICS OF HEALTH CARE IN THE UNITED STATES

Several important and, in some cases, dramatic changes in the economics of health care in the United States and in the recent past must
be taken into account in evaluating national health policies.

First, there has been a great increase in the total cost of health
care. For example, in the years between 1965 and 1978 per capita
spending on health increased 397%, and per capita hospital spending
increased even faster, by 484% over the same period (see Gibson,
1979; Gibson and Mueller, 1977). This growth in spending on health
is even more impressive in view of the relatively large amounts
spent at the beginning of the period. The large initial amounts and
subsequent growth have led to truly remarkable levels of health
expenditures, which have made health care the third largest industry
in the United States. In 1978 national spending for health amounted
to $192 billion, representing $863 per capita and absorbing 9.1% of
the U.S. gross national product. By contrast, health expenditures
amounted to $12 billion, or 4.6% of gross national product, in 1950;
and as recently as 1970, they amounted to $69 billion, or 7.2% of
gross national product. From 1975 to 1978 alone, national health
expenditures rose from $118 billion to $192 billion, or from 8.3% to
9.1% of gross national product. Hospital spending itself amounted
to $76 billion, or 40% of total health expenditures, in 1978, making
hospitals the subject of considerable attention in terms of national
health policies.

Second, there has been an enormous increase in the price of health
services, particularly hospital services. For example, from 1950 to
1976 the average cost of a day of hospital care rose from $15.62 to
$172.70, or over 1000% (see Health Insurance Institute, 1979).[1]
Average annual increases in the cost of a day of hospital care
amounted to 14.8% from 1965 to 1970, 13.4% from 1970 to 1975, 13.4%
from 1975 to 1978, and 13.9% in the total period to 1978 (see
Freeland, Calat, and Schendler, 1980; U.S. DHEW, 1975). These price
increases have, over the last fifteen years, exceeded the rate of
inflation for virtually all other consumer goods and services. They
have also contributed in a significant way to the overall increase
in consumer prices.

Third, there has been no significant increase in the quantities of
health services provided the population. While some groups have

355

certainly received more care, and there have been clear improvements
in particular areas in the quality of care, the overall quantity of
care has increased at only a moderate rate. The total cost of
health services can be considered the product of an average price of
all health services times an average quantity of health services,
where health services include hospital services, physician services,
long-term care services, outpatient services, and other related services. Thus, while the total cost of health services has been
increasing at a dramatic rate in recent years, already noted as the
first trend, this increase is largely accounted for by price
increases, noted as the second trend, rather than by additional
quantities of health services. As a result, the substantially
higher health expenditures have not appreciably improved the health
status of the population. For example, aggregate measures of mortality and morbidity have not shown significant improvement in
recent years, and there has been no increase in life expectancy.[2]

Fourth, there has been a substantial increase in third-party payment
of health costs. In third-party payment the entity paying for
health care is neither the recipient of care (the consumer) nor the
provider of care (the hospital or physician) but a third party.
Traditionally, the third-party payers have been commercial insurance
companies, paying for part of the cost of health care of employees
covered under group health insurance or individuals enrolled in some
other health insurance plan. Government has encouraged such private
third-party payment by substantial tax subsidies. The individual
income tax allows deductions of the cost of health insurance up to a
certain amount. Furthermore, employer paid health benefits are not
included in taxable income, and these same benefits reduce the
taxable income of the employer. These tax subsidies amounted to
almost $6 billion annually in 1974 (Davis, 1975).[3] Since 1967
government has also played an increasingly important role as a third-
party payer in its own right. The federal government pays for a
substantial part of the cost of health care of individuals over 65
under the Medicare program, and federal and state agencies pay for a
substantial part of the cost of health care of low-income individuals under state Medicaid programs. Under both the Medicare and
the Medicaid programs providers of health services are reimbursed
for all reasonable costs borne in providing health services to
program beneficiaries. In 1965, before Medicare and Medicaid,
federal, state, and local governments paid 24.9% of total health
care costs; by 1978 this government share had risen to 40.6% and the
total share of all third-party sources exceeded 65%. The change in
payment of hospital costs is even more dramatic: the share of
hospital costs paid by the consumer declined from 49.6% in 1950 to
10.0% in 1978 (Gibson, 1979).[4]

Thus there have been four important changes in the recent United
States experience in the economics of health care that must be taken
into account in studying policy initiatives: a dramatic increase in
the cost of health care; enormous increases in the prices of health
services; no appreciable increase in the quantity of health care
provided; and a very large increase in third-party payment of health
costs. The purpose of this paper is to analyze these changes using
the basic economic tools of demand and supply and to discuss
possible national health policies in the light of this analysis.
The following section treats demand for care, and the next treats

supply of demand for health care. The last two sections discuss
possible health policies: first, partial policy responses involving
shifting supply or demand, and then a comprehensive policy response,
that of national health insurance.

THE SHIFTING DEMAND FOR HEALTH CARE

Health care involves a wide variety of health services, including
hospital services (measured, for example, by bed days of care) and
physician services (measured, for example, by visits to physicians).
An aggregate measure of these services--which would involve
appropriate weighting of hospital services, physician services, and
other services--is the total quantity of health services provided
the population. Multiplying this total quantity of health services
by a measure of the price of health services would yield the total
cost of health services, where the price of health services is an
appropriate average of the cost per hospital bed day, cost per physician visit, and so forth.[5]

The demand curve for health services, shown in Figure 1, summarizes
the total quantity of health care demanded at alternative prices for
these services.[6] The demand curve, D, in this figure exhibits two
distinctive features, which are worthy of discussion and which are
related to the concept of "need." First, there is a finite intercept on the quantity axis; this intercept is the amount of health
care demanded when the price falls to zero. Second, there is a
minimum level of health care which the demand curve approaches in an
asymptotic fashion as price increases to very high levels.[7]

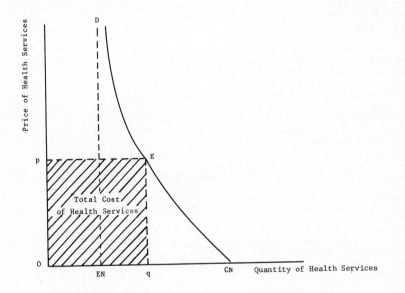

Figure 1. The demand curve for health services.

The first special feature of the demand curve is the finite intercept, labeled CN in Figure 1, which can be interpreted as <u>clinical</u>
<u>need</u>.[8]   This is the amount of care that a clinical expert might
recommend if there were no charge for care. Clearly this is larger
than the care demanded at a positive price, such as price p, for
which the quantity demanded is q, as shown at point E on the demand
curve. The quantity demanded at a zero price is, however, finite.
In particular, there is an upper limit to the amount of health care
that individuals will seek when its cost is zero, since there are
limits to the amount of health care that can be utilized. For
example, certain groups that receive free care, such as those in the
armed services and veterans, do not utilize infinite amounts of
health care.[9] Nor do physicians and their families. Yet another
example is extremely wealthy individuals for whom the price of
health care, relative to their income or assets, is very small.
Although such individuals may demand a large amount of care, it is
not an unlimited amount.[10]

The second special feature of the demand curve is the minimum asymptotic level, labeled EN in Figure 1, which can be interpreted as
<u>economic need</u>. This is the amount of care that the individual would
seek even if the price were very high (but still affordable, given
the income of the individual).[11] It is a measure of need, using
economic considerations of high price to exclude all health care
that is not considered essential by the individual. The level of
care provided at this point is, to a large extent, that minimum
needed to preserve life and basic health, all other health care
having disappeared in the face of an extremely high price of care.
The amount of health care labeled EN can be interpreted as the <u>mini-</u>
<u>mum need</u> , while that labeled CN can be interpreted as the <u>maximum</u>
<u>need</u>. The former is that level of care chosen as price rises very
high, while the latter is that level chosen as price falls to zero.
It might be noted that there is frequently some confusion when the
term "need" is used as to which of these two measures (or some
other) is meant.

The demand curve such as the one shown in Figure 1 may be relevant
at any one time, but over time the demand curve shifts as factors
other than price, which also affect the demand for health care,
change. In recent years probably the leading cause of the demand
curve for health care to shift has been the growth of health care
financing mechanisms, particularly third-party payment, which, as
has already been noted, is one of the significant changes in the
economics of health care in the United States. The result of such
third-party payment is a shift of the demand curve as shown in
Figure 2.[12] The effect of third-party payment is to reduce the net
price of health services paid by the consumer.[13] Consider, for
example, the consumer of health care at E, where price is p and
quantity is q on demand curve D_0. Suppose a third-party payment
mechanism that paid half the cost of care was established. From the
viewpoint of the consumer the cost is cut in half--to p/2. The
quantity associated with this net price is the new quantity demanded
at price p with 50% payment by third parties, as shown in the
figure. Considering all possible prices and quantities before this
establishment of a third-party payment mechanism and locating the
quantity associated with price after it is cut in half generates the
demand curve $D_{.5}$, where the .5 subscript refers to the 50% payment
by third parties. Similarly, $D_{.3}$ and $D_{.6}$ refer to 30% and 60%

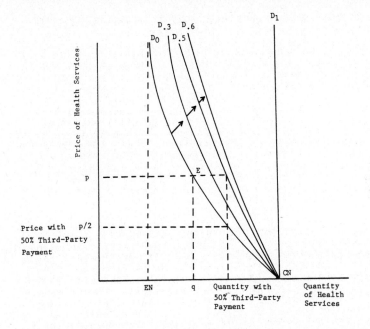

Figure 2. Shifts over time in the demand curve for health services due to third-party payment.

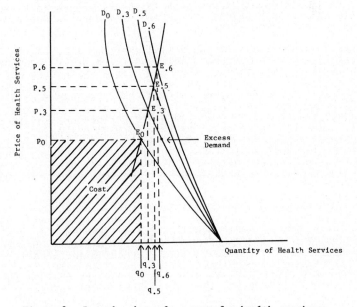

Figure 3. Demand and supply curves for health services.

payment by third parties, respectively, and the original demand
curve D_0 refers to no such third-party payment.

The recent shift of the demand curve in the United States has been
like that from $D_{.3}$ to $D_{.5}$ to $D_{.6}$, as there has been greater and
greater reliance on private and public third-party payment mechanisms. This shift is shown by the arrows in the figure. The result
of this shift is to increase the quantity demanded at any price by
shifting the demand curve closer and closer to D_1, which is the
limiting case as 100% of the cost of care is provided by third
parties.[14] This limiting demand curve calls for purchase of CN as
the amount of health care at any price, since others are paying the
full cost of care.

SUPPLY OF AND DEMAND FOR HEALTH CARE

The supply curve of health care, shown as S in Figure 3 together
with the shifting demand curves of Figure 2, summarizes the total
quantity of health services supplied at alternative prices. It
tends to be rather inelastic because of the difficulty of substituting other inputs for physicians and hospitals, the large expense
and long lags in the production of new physicians and hospitals, and
the difficulties in using new techniques and equipment.

Furthermore, unlike the demand curve, which has shifted outward
significantly over the recent past, the supply curve has tended to
be constant or nonshifting.[15] Thus the enormous expense of new
facilities and new health personnel, combined with the substantial
political, legal and economic constraints on the entry of new providers, has led to a supply curve that is both inelastic and constant,
exhibiting neither any significant responsiveness to price nor any
appreciable change over time.

Figure 3 also shows the shifting demand curves, which are shifting
largely as a result of increased third-party payment. Consider the
equilibrium at E_0, and assume there has been a shift of the demand
curve to $D_{.3}$, based on private and/or public third party payment of
30% of the cost of health care. Assume that the supply curve does
not shift. The result of the shift of the demand curve from D_0 to
$D_{.3}$ is that at the old equilibrium price p_0 there is an excess
demand (ED) and pressure for price to rise toward the new
equilibrium at $E_{.3}$, where price $p_{.3}$ is larger than the old
equilibrium price and where the quantity $q_{.3}$ is slightly larger than
the old equilibrium quantity, q_0. Similarly, the equilibrum rises
to $E_{.5}$ and $E_{.6}$ as a result of a shift of demand to $D_{.5}$ and $D_{.6}$,
respectively.

The process depicted in Figure 3 is very useful as a way of
understanding the recent changes in health care prices and costs.
Given a stable and inelastic supply curve, as demand has shifted out
over time because of increases in third-party payment, prices have
risen substantially, quantities have increased only slightly, and
total cost has risen dramatically (as shown in Figure 3 as the area
of the rectangle representing price times quantity such as that for
E_0). These four changes are precisely those summarized in the first

section of this paper as recent changes in the economics of health care in the United States.

An important aspect of this interpretation of the recent history of rising prices and substantial cost increases is its feedback nature. The dynamics of the process are such that, as prices and costs increase, there is more pressure for third parties, including the government, to pay a higher share of the cost of health care.[16] Thus, group health insurance becomes a more attractive fringe benefit for both employers and employees, and there is political pressure for government to pay a greater share of the cost of health care for populations already covered or for new population groups. The result is a further shift outward of demand as in Figure 3, and further increases in price and cost. The system tends not to correct itself, but to magnify initial price increases, with higher prices leading to greater third-party payment, which leads to yet higher prices. This process keeps increasing prices and costs over time, slowing down only as the percentage of costs paid by third parties approaches its maximum level.[17]

In addition to rising prices and substantial cost increases, other recent major changes in health care can be explained by the demand and supply curves of Figure 3, coupled with the dynamic feedback process of price and cost increases leading to greater third-party payments and to further outward shifts in demand. At $E_{.6}$, for example, where third-party payment amounts to 60% of health care costs, there is more health care provided, at a higher price and at much larger cost, than at $E_{.3}$, where third-party payment amounts to 30% of health care costs. In addition, however, the demand curve is more inelastic at $E_{.6}$ than at $E_{.3}$, meaning that consumers respond less to price increases. Consumers at the new equilibrium will seek longer hospital stays, more frequent visits to physicians, use of the latest (and most expensive) medical equipment, etc. Such behavior, which has become very much a part of current health care delivery in the United States, is quite understandable. Consumers are quite rational in seeking more and a higher quality health care when others, the third parties, are paying a substantial share of the cost of care.

PARTIAL RESPONSES THAT SHIFT SUPPLY OR DEMAND

What are appropriate policy responses to these changes in the economics of health care in the United States? This section treats some of the partial responses that involve shifting supply or demand; the next section treats a comprehensive policy response in the form of national health insurance.

One type of policy response is to foster policies that will shift out supply, as shown in Figure 4 in the shift from supply curve S to supply curve S'. With this shift in supply, the shift in demand from $D_{.3}$ to $D_{.6}$, as in Figure 3, is offset in terms of price, price remaining at $p_{.3}$ despite the shift in demand. While total cost of health care is greater at $E'_{.6}$ than at $E_{.3}$, it is less than it would have been at $E_{.6}$, if the supply curve had not shifted as shown.[18] In fact, government policy has in recent years attempted to shift

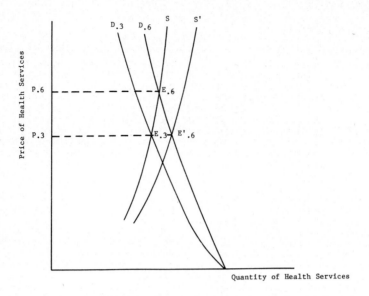

Figure 4. Shift in the supply curve for health services.

out supply as shown in the figure. Among such policies are substantial subsidies to hospital construction, subsidies for medical
school construction and expansion, and various attempts to encourage
greater efficiency in the delivery of health care. It should be
noted, however, that added hospital beds, more physicians, and other
supply increases will be utilized to some degree, adding to the cost
of health care. Thus there have been arguments advanced for
limiting hospital construction, expansion of medical schools, and so
forth. [19]

Another type of policy response would be a shift of demand inward,
e.g., from $D_{.6}$ to $D_{.3}$ in Figure 4, in order to reduce the price and
cost of health care. While this type of policy response has not
been as evident as that of fostering an outward shift of supply,
attempts have been made in this direction through measures regulating providers, such as stricter limits on Medicare and Medicaid
reimbursement and the development of Professional Standards Review
organizations (PSROs) to control hospital utilization. There have
also been proposals to reverse the mechanisms at work in Figure 3 by
substantially increasing the share of health care expenditures paid
by the patient by increases in coinsurance and in deductibles (see
M.S. Feldstein, 1971c). A change of this nature in the financing of
health care would, however, reverse the course of the recent past;
it could reduce access to health care for precisely those target
population groups for which government has sought to provide more
care, namely the elderly and the poor; and it would result in a
significant increase in the risk of severe financial loss as a
result of major illness, particularly for middle-income families.
These effects are politically unacceptable.[20]

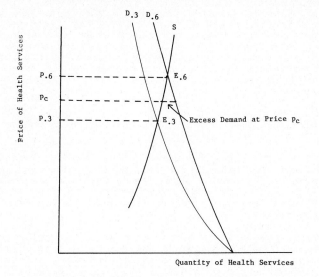

Figure 5. The result of setting a ceiling price, p_c.

A third type of policy response is to establish limits on the prices
of health care. This response is illustrated by the Economic
Stabilization Program, rate setting, rate review, and various
prospective reimbursement or prospective budgeting systems.[21] An
interpretation in terms of demand and supply curves is presented in
Figure 5. If the demand curve shifts from $D_{.3}$ to $D_{.6}$ in the face of
a constant supply curve, the equilibrium will shift from $E_{.3}$ to $E_{.6}$,
as in Figure 3. Suppose the government establishes a ceiling price
of p_c, which is, however, below $p_{.6}$. The result will be a dise-
quilibrium situation in which there is an excess of demand over
supply, as shown. The shortage of supply relative to demand will
lead to nonprice rationing, such as long delays in obtaining physician appointments or in obtaining a hospital bed, long waiting
periods for obtaining services, or to other systems of nonprice
rationing, which tend to redistribute health services to the poor.
Furthermore, to the extent that this limit on price applies only to
one category of consumer--limits, for example, on reimbursement
under Medicare and Medicaid--it will lead to substitution between
categories of consumers in favor of those for which no limit has
been set, a reduction in the quality of care provided the affected
population, and/or a shift of the cost of care from the affected
population to other populations--e.g., from the Medicare/Medicaid
population to private-paying patients. Finally, price setting (and
other forms of regulation) in a sector such as health care--
involving many diverse providers and involving services that are
difficult even to define--necessarily entails high cost, many exceptions, extensive case-by-case decision making, and political intervention, which tend to aggravate rather than solve the problem.[22]

A fourth type of policy response is to establish a ceiling price, as
in Figure 5, but using government health services, such as the
Veterans Administration hospitals, to handle the excess of demand
over supply. This type of policy has not been pursued, since most
government health services are intended for specific population
groups, such as veterans, Indians, and members of the armed services.

A COMPREHENSIVE POLICY RESPONSE: NATIONAL HEALTH INSURANCE

A comprehensive health policy would take into account demand,
supply, and their special features and dynamic behavior. Such a
policy could be established through the adoption of a system of
national health insurance, which would replace the present disorganized system based largely on fee-for-service by an integrated one
based on prepayment.[23]

A comprehensive national insurance system would recognize that it is
in the interest of both individuals and the society at large to provide the entire population with access, at low money and time price,
to certain minimal levels of health care. Above these minimums a
system of deductibles and coinsurance would restrain demand, with
some exemptions for low-income families. Thus, above the minimum
levels the consumer would pay all or part of the cost of care. The
traditional objection to national health insurance has been that the
system would boost demand and lead to substantial cost increases.
In recent years, however, such cost increases have occurred in the
absence of a national health insurance plan. Given the substantial
share of cost already paid by third parties, especially the federal
government, a comprehensive system of national health insurance may,
in fact, restrain, rather than promote cost increases. For example,
if current programs--representing a totally disorganized mixture of
programs, private and public--are replaced by a national system that
is universal, then everyone's access to health care could be
equalized, resulting in reduced benefits to some currently highly
favored groups, but increased benefits to those currently receiving
few, if any, benefits. In particular, low- and middle-income consumers would gain substantially, while those in the lowest income
group and in the older population would lose some benefits. Such
adjustments among population groups, comparable to "most-favored-
nation" treatment in international trade, would only be possible
under a comprehensive system of national health insurance. It would
also be more efficient, however, in that, with suitable deductibles
and coinsurance, all consumers would have an interest in reducing
the cost of care. By contrast, under the present system very few
consumers have such an interest, given the substantial benefits under
Medicare and Medicaid and under various private group health
insurance systems. Thus, far from accelerating health care cost
increases, national health insurance could restrain them.

In addition to providing a vehicle for making adjustments in
coverage between different population groups, a national health
insurance system could also be a vehicle for making adjustments of

other types, such as adjustments for catastrophic care, acute care, and preventive care. While there could be some provision for catastrophic coverage, it must be recognized that a few such cases can utilize vast amounts of health resources that could be utilized to provide acute and preventive care to many individuals. The proper balance between various types of care cannot be realized in the present disorganized system, but it could be realized under a comprehensive system. Similarly, the proper balance between long-term care and short-term care, among hospitals, nursing homes, and other facilities, and between older and newer medical technologies, which cannot be achieved in the present system, could be realized under a comprehensive system of national health insurance by means of regulations and incentives.

Another advantage of national health insurance would be a reorganization of health care delivery. This would have the effect of shifting out supply. Such reorganization could include, for example, large prepaid units with an integration of health delivery components, which can take advantage of scale economies in health care delivery. Other effects on supply through additional use of physician assistants, substitution of outpatient for inpatient care in hospitals, substitution of nursing home care for hospital care, and similar measures could also result from a comprehensive national health insurance plan. Those changes could lead to greater efficiency in the production and use of health care components.

Attention should be focused on the comprehensive nature of a system of national health insurance. Policy directed to health care delivery has thus far been both piecemeal and minimal. For example, some groups receive substantial coverage by the federal government through Medicare and Medicaid; others are not covered by those programs. Some groups receive a great variety of coverage through private insurance carriers, others have no coverage whatsoever. Similarly, some private groups such as the Kaiser Foundation have long provided care through large prepaid group plans. There have also been recent developments along these lines through Health Maintenance Organizations (HMOs). Altogether, however, those providers represent only a very small fraction of health care delivery, and there appear to be substantial political and economic barriers to the development of new HMO's. A national health insurance system, to the extent that it is comprehensive in treating all consumers and providers, could avoid the inequities and inefficiencies of piecemeal coverage and lead to more efficient modes of organization and operation.

Overall, then, a comprehensive system of national health insurance could be an important mechanism for improving both the efficiency and the equity of health care delivery.

NOTES

[1]For discussions of the inflation of health costs, particularly hospital costs, see M. S. Feldstein (1971a, 1971b, 1974, 1975), Klarman (1970), and Davis (1973, 1975).

[2]Fuchs (1975) points out that health in the United States has little to do with what is spent on health care. It has, instead, much to do with heredity, environment, and personal lifestyles.

[3]Approximately $3 billion is due to the exclusion of employers' contributions to health insurance plans from taxable income; about $2.6 billion is due to personal income tax deductions.

[4]See also M. S. Feldstein and Taylor (1977) and Gibson and Mueller (1977). The government share would be even larger if the government subsidies of private health insurance by means of tax reductions through deductions and exclusions were taken into account.

[5]To the extent that hospital expenditures account for a significant fraction of total health expenditures, a reasonable proxy measure of the price of health services is the average cost per hospital bed day.

[6]For empirical studies of demand, see P. Feldstein (1966), Rosenthal (1970), Joseph (1971), Newhouse and Phelps (1974), and Yett et al. (1975). See also the discussion in Intriligator (1978).

[7]Note that these two distinctive features are the opposite of those usually assumed for demand curves, the typical assumption being that the good or service is not purchased above a given price and that as price falls to zero the good or service is purchased in unlimited amounts.

[8]For a further discussion of this finite intercept see Yett et al. (1970, p. 35).

[9]Among other reasons for a finite demand at zero price for such groups is the time price of health care. While the money price may be zero, the time price, involving both the duration of care and waiting for care, may be high.

[10]Probably the most extreme case is the President of the United States, who has his own personal physician available at all times and has unrestricted access to hospital care. Even in this extreme case the demand for care is finite.

[11]Clearly, if price were large enough, the individual would have to reduce the quantity of care, since the cost would exceed his total income. The point at which all income is spent on health care is, however, never reached for most individuals.

[12]There are, in fact, other factors in addition to third-party payment which have resulted in the outward shift of demand. These include a greater role for physicians as the key decision makers in health care delivery, greater consciousness of health care, technical developments in the provision of health services, higher income levels, and many others. These other factors would result in even greater shifts of demand than those shown in Figure 2.

[13]See Klarman (1977) for a discussion of the "two-price system," in which the gross price of services exceeds the net price to the consumer. See also footnote 16, below.

[14]The increase in demand resulting from greater insurance coverage, which reduces the price to the consumer, is sometimes called "moral hazard." See Arrow (1974).

[15]In fact, adjusting for _quality_ of health care, the supply curve has if anything probably shifted upward because the cost of providing the same level of care has increased as a result of more sophisticated procedures, equipment, etc. Inflation in the prices of goods and services purchased by providers of health care also has the effect of shifting supply upward. These effects, which are ignored here, would further accelerate cost and price increases.

[16]If third parties pay a higher share of cost, the net price paid by the consumer will not increase as rapidly as the gross price. For example, M. S. Feldstein (1975) notes that in 1950 the average cost of a day of hospital care was about $16, but the consumer paid 63% of the cost of care, or about $10, as a net price. By 1974, the average cost had risen to about $125 but the consumer paid only 23%, or about $28.50, as a net price. Adjusting to 1950 prices, the net price rose to only $13, so in real terms the net cost rose only 30% in this 24-year period.

[17]A simple model of the effect of changing third-party payment on price consists of linear demand, supply, and change in the proportion of price paid by third parties:

$$q = a - bp(1-r),$$

$$q = vp - w,$$

$$\dot{r} = g(1-r).$$

Here q is quantity demanded (and supplied), p is price, and r is the proportion of price paid by third parties. The last equation represents the feedback effect of price on third-party payment, which increases at a rate proportional to the share paid by the consumer. This system implies that price rises over time as a logistic function, an s-shaped curve which rises at an increasing rate initially, then passes through an inflection point, and finally rises at a decreasing rate, asymptotically approaching the limiting value of $p_1 = (a+w)/v$ (corresponding to $r = 1$). Thus, assuming stable linear demand/supply relationships and assuming that the growth of third-party payment is proportional to the share paid by the consumer, the rate of change of price eventually falls to zero. Intuitively, the price change must diminish as the proportion of third-party payment approaches its limiting value of unity. Put another way, continued escalation of prices must eventually rely on nonlinearities and/or demand/supply curves shifting for reasons other than third-party payment.

[18]This reduction in expenditure due to an outward shift of the supply curve follows from the fact that the demand curve is inelastic.

[19]There has been a recognition recently that increasing hospital capacity may not, in fact, increase supply, given relatively low occupancy rates. Whatever the factors limiting supply are, they apparently do not include lack of hospital beds. Thus, policy on hospital capacity has reversed itself from the previous Hill-Burton program for financing of hospital construction to the present certificate-of-need requirement, under which a regulatory authority must issue a permit based on community needs before there can be an increase in hospital capacity. For discussions of the apparent lack of effectiveness of the certificate-of-need requirement, however, see Hellinger (1976a) and Salkever and Bice (1976).

For a discussion of the policy of limiting the production of physicians in order to contain costs, see Reinhardt (1977b).

[20]For example, proposals by the Nixon and Ford administrations to increase cost-sharing by Medicare beneficiaries did not even succeed in attracting a sponsor in Congress.

[21]On prospective reimbursement see Hellinger (1976b) and Gaus and Hellinger (1976). In such a system, rates are set prior to the delivery of services through budget review, application of formulas, negotiation, or some combination of these methods. Prospective budgeting systems, used in the United Kingdom and Canada, involve payment of a fixed share, e.g., 90%, of total cost.

[22]For further discussion of the inappropriateness of regulation of health care delivery, see Noll (1975) and Enthoven and Noll (1977).

[23]See discussions of national health insurance in Newhouse, Phelps, and Schwartz (1974), Rosett, ed. (1976), Enthoven (1978), and Yett et al. (1979).

HEALTH, ECONOMICS, AND HEALTH ECONOMICS
J. van der Gaag and M. Perlman (editors)
© North-Holland Publishing Company, 1981

REFERENCES

Abel-Smith, B., and Maynard, A. 1979. The organization, financing and cost of
    health care in the European community. Brussels: Commission of the European
    Communities, Social Policy Series, no. 36.

Acton, J. P. 1973. Demand for health care among the urban poor, with special
    emphasis on the role of time. Santa Monica, Cal.: Rand Corporation, Report
    R-1151 OEO/NYC.

Acton, J. P. 1975. Nonmonetary factors in the demand for medical service: Some
    empirical evidence. Journal of Political Economy, 83, 595-614.

Acton, J. P. 1976. Demand for health care among the urban poor, with special
    emphasis on the role of time. In R. N. Rosett, ed., The role of health
    insurance in the health services sector. Universities-NBER Conference Series
    No. 27. New York: Neale Watson.

Aday, L. A., and Eichhorn, R. 1972. The utilization of health services: Indices
    and correlates. Rockville, Md.: Department of Health, Education and Welfare,
    Publication (HSM) 73-3003.

Alchian, A. A. 1961. Some economics of property. Santa Monica, Cal.: Rand
    Corporation, Report P-2316.

Alchian, A. A., and Demsetz, H. 1972. Production, information costs, and economic
    organization. American Economic Review, 62, 777-795.

Alchian, A. A., and Kessel, R. 1962. Competition, monopoly, and the pursuit of
    money. In Aspects of labor economics: A conference of the Universities-
    National Bureau Committee for Economic Research. Princeton, N.J.: Princeton
    University Press.

Andersen, R. 1968. A behavioral model of families' use of health services.
    Research Series No. 25. Chicago: Center for Health Administration Studies,
    University of Chicago.

Andersen, R. O., and Benham, L. 1970. Factors affecting the relationship between
    family income and medical care consumption. In H. E. Klarman, ed., Empirical
    studies in health economics. Baltimore: Johns Hopkins Press.

Andersen, R., Kravits, J., and Anderson, O. W. 1975. Equity in health services.
    Cambridge, Mass.: Ballinger.

Anderson, J. G. 1973. Health services utilization: Framework and review. Health
    Services Research, 8 (Fall).

Anderson, O. W. 1972. Health care: Can there be equity? New York: John Wiley.

Arrow, K. J. 1963. Uncertainty and the welfare economics of medical care.
    American Economic Review, 53, 941-973.

Arrow, K. J. 1965. Reply. American Economic Review, 55, 155.

Arrow, K. J. 1971. Essays in the theory of risk bearing. Amsterdam:
    North-Holland.

Arrow, K. J. 1973. Welfare analysis of changes in health coinsurance rates.
    Santa Monica, Cal.: Rand Corporation, Publication No. R-1281-OEO.

Arrow, K. J. 1974. The economics of moral hazard. American Economic Review, 64, 253-272.

Ashford, J. R., and Pearson, N. G. 1970. Who uses the health services and why? Journal of the Royal Statistical Society, 133, 295-346.

Atkinson, A., and Stiglitz, J. 1976. The design of tax structure: Direct taxes versus indirect taxation. Journal of Public Economics, 6.

Auster, R., Leveson, I., and Sarachek, D. 1969. The production of health: An exploratory study. Journal of Human Resources, 4, 411-436.

Badgley, R. F., and Smith, R. D. 1979. User charges for health services. Toronto: Ontario Council of Health.

Balestra, P., and Nerlove, M. 1966. Pooling cross-section and time series data in the estimation of a dynamic model: The demand for natural gas. Econometrica, 34, 585-612.

Barer, M. L., Evans, R. G., and Stoddart, G. L. 1979. Controlling health care costs by direct charges to patients: Snare or delusion? Ontario Economic Council, Occasional Paper No. 10. Toronto: Ontario Economic Council.

Barer, M. L., Manga, P., Shillington, E. R., and Siegel, G. C. 1980. The OHIP family and hospital care: Benefit and utilization patterns under Ontario's Hospital Insurance Program. Research Report. Toronto: Ontario Economic Council.

Bashshur, R. L., Shannon, G. W., and Melzner, C. A. 1971. Some ecological differentials in the use of medical services. Health Services Research, 6 (Spring).

Bator, F. 1958. The anatomy of market failure. Quarterly Journal of Economics, 72.

Beck, R. G. 1974. The effects of co-payment on the poor. Journal of Human Resources, 9, 129-142.

Becker, G. S., and Lewis, H. G. 1973. On the interaction between the quantity and quality of children. Journal of Political Economy, 81.

Becker, M. H., Drachman, R. H., and Kirscht, J. P. 1974. A new approach to explaining sick-role behaviour in low-income populations. American Journal of Public Health, 64.

Berg, R. L., ed. 1973. Health status indexes. Chicago: Hospital Research and Educational Trust.

Berki, S. E., and Ashcraft, M. L. 1979. On the analysis of ambulatory utilization. Medical Care, 17 (12).

Berki, S. E., and Kobashigawa, B. 1978. Education and income effects in the use of ambulatory services in the United States. International Journal of Health Services, 8 (2).

Berlinguer, G. 1979. Lina riforma per la salute. Bari: De Donato.

Bishop, C. E. 1980. Nursing home cost studies: Implications for rate setting. Discussion Paper, Boston University Health Policy Consortium, Boston.

Blumberg, M. S. 1979. Rational provider prices: Provider price changes for improved health care use. In George K. Chacho, ed., Health handbook. Amsterdam: North-Holland.

Blumberg, M. S. 1980. Health status and health care use by type of private health care coverage. Milbank Memorial Fund Quarterly: Health and Society, 58.

Bombardier, C., Fuchs, V. R., Lillard, L., and Warner, K. 1977. Socio-economic factors affecting the utilization of surgical operations. New England Journal of Medicine, 297, 699-705.

Boutin, J. G., and Bisson, J. 1977. Les consommateurs et les coûts de la santé au Québec de 1971 à 1975. Quebec: Régie de l'Assurance-Maladie du Québec.

Brian, E. W., and Gibbens, S. F. 1974. California's Medi-Cal copayment experiment. Medical Care, 12, Supplement (December 12).

Brittain, J. A. 1972. The payroll tax for social security. Washington, D. C.: Brookings Institution.

Brook, R. H., Ware, J. E., Davies-Avery, A., Stewart, A. L., Donald, C. A., Rogers, W. H., Williams, K. N., and Johnston, S. A. 1979. Overview of adult health status measures fielded in Rand's health insurance study. Medical Care (Supplement), 17, 1-131.

Brown, J. A. C., and Deaton, A. S. 1972. Surveys in applied economics: Models of consumer behavior. Economic Journal, 82, 1145-1236.

Brunner, K. 1978. Reflections on the political economy of government: The persistent growth of government. Schweizerischen Zeitschrift für Volkswirtschaft und Statistik, 3, 619-679.

Buchanan, J. M., and Tullock, G. 1962. The calculus of consent. Ann Arbor: University of Michigan Press.

Buchanan, J. M., and Wagner, R. 1977. Democracy in deficit: The political legacy of Lord Keynes. New York: Academic Press.

Bunker, J. P., Barnes, B. A., and Mosteller, F., eds. 1977. Costs, risks and benefits of surgery. New York: Oxford University Press.

Burney, I. L., Schieber, G. J., Blaxall, M. O., and Gabel, J. R. 1979. Medicare and Medicaid physician payment incentives. Health Care Financing Review, 1 (Summer), 62-78.

Cairns, J. A., and Snell, M. C. 1978. Prices and the demand for care. In A. J. Culyer and K. G. Wright, eds., Economic aspects of health services. London: Martin Robertson.

Card, W. I., Rusenkiewicz, M., and Phillips, C. I. 1977. Utility estimates of a set of states of health. Methods of Information in Medicine, 16, 168.

Christensen, L. R., and Greene, W. H. 1976. Economies of scale in U.S. electric power generation. Journal of Political Economy, 84 (4), 655-676.

Christianson, J. B., and McClure, W. 1979. Competition in the delivery of medical care. New England Journal of Medicine, 301, 812-818.

Cochrane, A. L. 1972. Effectiveness and efficiency: Random reflections on health services. London: Nuffield Provincial Hospitals Trust.

Colle, A. D., and Grossman, M. 1978. Determinants of pediatric care utilization. Journal of Human Resources, 13, Supplement, 115-158.

Cragg, J. G. 1971. Some statistical models for limited dependent variables with application to the demand for durable goods. Econometrica, 39, 829-844.

Culyer, A. J. 1971a. Medical care and the economics of giving. Economica, 35, 295-303.

Culyer, A. J. 1971b. The nature of the commodity "health care" and its efficient allocation. Oxford Economic Papers, 23, 189-211.

Culyer, A. J. 1977. The quality of life and the limits of cost-benefit analysis. In L. Wingo and A. Evans, eds., Public economics and the quality of life. Baltimore: Johns Hopkins Press.

Culyer, A. J. 1978a. Measuring health: Lessons for Ontario. Chapter 5. Ontario Economic Council Research Series. Toronto: University of Toronto Press.

Culyer, A. J. 1978b. Needs, values and health status measurement. In A. J. Culyer and K. G. Wright, eds., Economic aspects of health services. London: Martin Robertson.

Culyer, A. J. 1979. Expenditure on real services: Health. Open University Course D323, Political Economy and Taxation, Unit 9. Radio broadcast (England).

Culyer, A. J. 1980. The political economy of social policy. London: Martin Robertson.

Culyer, A. J., Lavers, R. J., and Williams, A. 1971. Social indicators: Health. Social Trends, 2, 31-42.

Davis, K. 1973. Theories of hospital inflation: Some empirical evidence. Journal of Human Resources, 8, 181-201.

Davis, K. 1975. National health insurance: Benefits, costs and consequences. Washington, D.C.: Brookings Institution.

Davis, K., and Reynolds, R. 1976. The impact of Medicare and Medicaid on access to medical care. In R. Rosett, ed., The role of health insurance in the health services sector. New York: National Bureau of Economic Research.

Davis, K., and Russell, L. B. 1972. The substitution of hospital outpatient care for inpatient care. Review of Economics and Statistics, 54, 109-120.

Deacon, R., Lubitz, J., Gornick, M., and Newton, M. 1979. Analysis of variations in hospital use by medicare patients in PSRO areas, 1974-1977. Health Care Financing Review, 1 (Summer), 79-108.

DeAlessi, L. 1980. The economics of property rights: A review of the evidence. Research in Law and Economics, 2, 1-47.

Densen, P., Jones, E. W., Balamuth, E., and Shapiro, S. 1960. Prepaid medical care and hospital utilization in a dual choice situation. American Journal of Public Health and the Nation's Health, 50 (November), 1710-1726.

Densen, P., Shapiro, S., Jones, E. W., and Baldinger, I. 1962. Comparison of a group practice and a self-insurance situation. Hospitals, 36 (November).

Detsky, A. S. 1978. The economic foundations of national health policy. Cambridge, Mass.: Ballinger.

De Vos, A. F., and Bikker, J. A. 1978. A bivariate probit-regression model as an alternative to the tobit model. Faculty of Actuarial Science and Econometrics, Report No. 24, University of Amsterdam.

Donabedian, A. 1971. Social responsibility for personal health services: An examination of basic values. Inquiry, 8 (2), 3-19.

Downs, A. 1957. An economic theory of democracy. New York: Harper & Row.

Drummond, M. F. 1980. Principles of economic appraisal in health care. New York: Oxford University Press.

Drummond, M. F. 1981. Studies in economic appraisal in health care. New York: Oxford University Press.

Dyckman, Z. Y. 1978. A study of physicians' fees. Washington, D.C.: Council on Wage and Price Stability, Executive Office of the President.

Eckstein, H. 1964. The English health service. Cambridge, Mass.: Harvard University Press.

Edwards, L. N., and Grossman, M. 1978. Children's health and the family. New York: National Bureau of Economic Research, Working Paper No. 256.

Edwards, L. N., and Grossman, M. 1979a. Income and race differences in children's health. New York: National Bureau of Economic Research, Working Paper. No. 308.

Edwards, L. N., and Grossman, M. 1979b. The relationship between children's health and intellectual development. In S. Mushkin, ed., Health: What is it worth? Elmsford, N.Y.: Pergamon Press.

Edwards, L. N., and Grossman, M. 1980. Children's health and the family. In R. M. Scheffler, ed., Annual series of research in health economics, Vol. 2. Greenwich, Conn.: JAI Press.

Edwards, L. N., and Grossman, M. Forthcoming. Adolescent health, family background and preventive medical care. In I. Sirageldin and D. Salkever, eds., Annual series of research in human capital and development, Vol. 30. Greenwich, Conn.: JAI Press.

Eggers, P. 1980. Risk differential between Medicare beneficiaries enrolled and not enrolled in an HMO. Health Care Financing Review, 1, Winter, 91-99.

Eisen, M., Ware, J., Donald, C., and Brook, R. 1979. Measuring components of children's health status. Medical Care, 17, 9.

Ellwood, P. M., and McClure, W. 1976. Health delivery reform. Excelsior, Minn.: Interstudy. Mimeographed.

Enterline, P. E., Salter, V., McDonald, A. D., and McDonald, J. C. 1973. The distribution of medical services before and after "free" medical care—the Quebec experience. New England Journal of Medicine, 289, 1174-1178.

Enthoven, A. C. 1978. Consumer-choice health plan, parts I and II. New England Journal of Medicine, 298, 650–658, 709–720.

Enthoven, A. C. 1980a. Health plan: The only practical solution to the soaring cost of medical care. Reading, Mass.: Addison-Wesley.

Enthoven, A. C. 1980b. Note on Paul Eggers' December 1979 paper on GHC Puget Sound risk differential. Washington, D.C.: Hearings before Committee on Finance, United States Senate.

Enthoven, A. C., and Noll, R. G. 1977. Regulatory and nonregulatory strategies for controlling health care costs. Stanford, Cal.: Stanford Graduate School of Business.

Eurostat. 1977. Indicatori sociali per la Comunità Europea, 1960–1975. Brussels: Eurostat.

Evans, R. G. 1971. Behavioral cost functions for hospitals. Canadian Journal of Economics, 4, 198–215.

Evans, R. G. 1973. Price formation in the market for physicians' services in Canada, 1957–1969. Ottawa: The Queen's Printer.

Evans, R. G. 1974. Supplier-induced demand: Some empirical evidence and implications. In M. Perlman, ed., The economics of health and medical care. New York: John Wiley, London: Macmillan.

Evans, R. G. 1975. Beyond the medical market place: Expenditure, utilization and pricing of insured health in Canada. In S. Andreopoulos, ed., National health insurance: Can we learn from Canada? New York: John Wiley.

Evans, R. G. 1976a. Beyond the medical marketplace: Expenditure, utilization and pricing of insured health care in Canada. In R. N. Rosett, ed., The role of health insurance in the health services sector. New York: National Bureau of Economic Research.

Evans, R. G. 1976b. Review of M. Perlman, ed., The economics of health and medical care. Canadian Journal of Economics, 9 (3).

Evans, R. G. 1976c. Modelling the economic objectives of the physician. In R. D. Fraser, ed., Health economics symposium: Proceedings of the First Canadian Conference, September 4, 5, and 6, 1974. Kingston, Canada: Queens University, Industrial Relations Centre.

Evans, R. G., and Williamson, M. F. 1978. Extending Canadian National Health Insurance: Policy options for pharmacare and denticare. Ontario Economic Council Research Monograph Series #13. Toronto: University of Toronto Press.

Evans, R. G., and Wolfson, A. D. 1978. Moving the target to hit the bullet: Generation of utilization by physicians in Canada. Paper prepared for the National Bureau of Economic Research conference on the Economics of Physician and Patient Behavior, Stanford, January.

Fanshel, S., and Bush, J. W. 1970. A health status index and its application to health service outcomes. Operations Research, 18, 1021–1066.

Fein, R., and Weber, G. I. 1971. Financing medical education: An analysis of alternative policies and mechanisms. New York: McGraw-Hill.

Feldstein, M. S. 1967. Economic analysis for health services efficiency. Amsterdam: North-Holland.

Feldstein, M. S. 1970. The rising price of physician services. Review of Economics and Statistics, 52, 121-133.

Feldstein, M. S. 1971a. The rising cost of hospital care. Washington, D.C.: Information Resources Press.

Feldstein, M. S. 1971b. Hospital cost inflation: A study of nonprofit price dynamics. American Economic Review, 61, 853-872.

Feldstein, M. S. 1971c. A new approach to National Health Insurance. Public Interest, 23, 93-105.

Feldstein, M. S. 1973. The welfare loss of excess health insurance. Journal of Political Economy, 81, 251-280.

Feldstein, M. S. 1974. Econometric studies of health economics. In M. D. Intriligator and D. A. Kendrick, eds., Frontiers of quantitative economics, Vol. 2. Amsterdam: North-Holland.

Feldstein, M. S. 1975. How tax laws fuel hospital costs. Prism, April.

Feldstein, M. S. 1977. Quality change and the demand for hospital care. Econometrica, 45, 1681-1702.

Feldstein, M. S., and Friedman, B. 1977. Tax subsidies, the rational demand for insurance and the health care crisis. Journal of Public Economics, 7, 155-178.

Feldstein, M. S., and Taylor, A. 1977. The rapid rise in hospital costs. Washington, D.C.: Council on Wage and Price Stability, U. S. Executive Office of the President.

Feldstein, P. J. 1964. The demand for medical care. In Report of the Commission on the Cost of Medical Care, Vol. 1. Prepared by the American Medical Association. Chicago: American Medical Association.

Feldstein, P. J. 1966. Research on the demand for health services. Milbank Memorial Fund Quarterly, 44, 128-162.

Feldstein, P. J. 1973. Financing dental care: An economic analysis. Lexington, Mass.: D. C. Heath.

Fink, R. 1973. Analysis of utilization data. Medical Care, 11 (2).

Frech, H. E., III. 1976. The property rights theory of the firm: Empirical results from a natural experiment. Journal of Political Economy, 84 (1), 143-152.

Frech, H. E., III. 1980. Property rights, the theory of the firm and competitive markets for top decision-makers. Research in Law and Economics, 2, 48-68.

Frech, H. E., III, and Ginsburg, P. B. Forthcoming. Economics of nursing homes: Ownership and financing. Final Report, Department of Health, Education, and Welfare Grant No. HS 02675-02.

Freeburg, L. C., Lave, J. R., Lave, L. B., and Leinhardt, S. 1979. Health status, medical care utilization, and outcome: An annotated bibliography of empirical studies. Washington, D.C.: Government Printing Office, DHEW Publ. No. (PHS) 80-3263.

Freeland, M., Calat, G., and Schendler, C. E. 1980. Projections of national health expenditures, 1980, 1985, and 1990. Health Care Financing Review, 2, 1-28.

Freiberg, L., and Scutchfield, F. D. 1976. Insurance and the demand for hospital care: An examination of the moral hazard. Inquiry, 13, 54-60.

Friedman, B. 1974. Risk aversion and the consumer choice of health insurance option. Review of Economics and Statistics, 56, 209-214.

Friedman, M., and Kuznets, S. 1945. Income from independent profession practice. New York: National Bureau of Economic Research.

Fuchs, V. R. 1975. Who shall live? New York: Basic Books.

Fuchs, V. R. 1978. The supply of surgeons and the demand for operations. Journal of Human Resources, 13, Supplement, 35-56.

Fuchs, V. R. 1979. The economics of health in a post-industrial society. The Public Interest, 56.

Fuchs, V. R., Hughes, E. F. X., Jacoby, J. E., and Lewit, E. M. 1972. Surgical workloads in a community practice. Surgery, 71, 315-327.

Fuchs, V. R., and Kramer, M. J. 1972. Determinants of expenditures for physicians' services in the United States, 1948-68. New York: National Bureau of Economic Research, Occasional Paper No. 117.

Fuchs, V. R., and Newhouse, J. P. 1978. The conference and unresolved problems. Journal of Human Resources, 13, Supplement, 5-18.

Furubøtn, E. G., and Pejovich, S. 1972. Property rights and economic theory: A survey of recent literature. Journal of Economic Literature, 10:4, 1137-1162.

Galbraith, J. K. 1973. Power and the useful economist. American Economic Review, 63, 1-11.

Gaus, C. R., Cooper, B. S., and Hirschman, C. G. 1976. Contrasts in HMO and fee-for-service performance. Social Security Bulletin, 39, 3-14.

Gaus, C. R., and Hellinger, F. J. 1976. Results of prospective reimbursement systems in the United States. In Topics in health care financing. Germantown, Md.: Aspen Systems.

Gertman, P. M. 1974. Physicians as guides of health services use. In S. J. Mushkin, ed., Consumer incentives for health care. New York: Prodist.

Gibson, R. M. 1979. National health expenditures. 1978. Health Care Financing Review, 1, 1-36.

Gibson, R. M., and Mueller, M. S. 1977. National health expenditures, Fiscal Year 1976. Social Security Bulletin (April), 3-8.

Ginsburg, P. B., and Manheim, L. M. 1973. Insurance, copayment, and health services utilization: A critical review. Economics and Business Bulletin, 25, 142-153.

Ginzberg, E. 1951. Perspective on the economics of medical care. American Economic Review, 41, 617-625.

Gittelsohn, A. M., and Wennberg, J. E. 1977. On the incidence of tonsillectomy and other surgical procedures. In J. P. Bunker, B. A. Barnes, and F. Mosteller, eds., Costs, risks, and benefits of surgery. New York: Oxford University Press.

Glaser, W. A. 1970. Paying the doctor. Baltimore: Johns Hopkins Press.

Goldberg, L. E., and Greenberg, W. 1977. The effect of physician-controlled health insurance: U.S. v. Oregon State Medical Society. Journal of Health Politics, Policy and Law , 2, 48-78.

Goldman, F., and Grossman, M. 1978. The demand for pediatric care: A hedonic appraisal. Journal of Political Economy, 86, 259-280.

Goldstein, G., and Pauly, M. 1976. Group health insurance as a local public good. In R. N. Rosett, ed., The role of health insurance in the health services sector. New York: National Bureau of Economic Research.

Granger, C. W. J. 1969. Investigating causal relations by econometric models and cross-spectral methods. Econometrica, 37.

Great Britain, Department of Health and Social Security. 1976a. Priorities for health and personal social services. London: H. M. Stationery Office.

Great Britain, Department of Health and Social Security. 1976b. Sharing resources for health. Report of the Resource Allocation Working Party. London: H. M. Stationery Office.

Great Britain, Ministry of Health. 1944. A national health service. Command Paper 6502. London: H. M. Stationery Office.

Green, J. 1978. Physician-induced demand for medical care. Journal of Human Resources, 13, Supplement.

Greenlees, J. S., Marshall, J. M., and Yett, D. E. 1975. Setting nursing home rates under Medicare and Medicaid. Presented at the Joint Session of the American Economic Association and the Health Economics Research Organization, December.

Greenlick, M. R., Hurtado, A. V., Pope, C. R., Saward, E. W., and Yoshioka, S. S. 1968. Determinants of medical care utilization. Health Services Research, 3, Winter.

Griliches, Z. 1974. Errors in variables under other unobservables. Econometrica, 42 (November).

Griliches, Z. 1977. Estimating the returns to schooling: Some econometric problems. Econometrica, 45 (1).

Griliches, Z., Hal, B. H., and Hausman, J. A. 1978. Missing data and self-selection in large panels. Annales de l'INSEE, 30/31, 138-176.

Grossman, M. 1972a. The demand for health: A theoretical and empirical investigation. New York: Columbia University Press.

Grossman, M. 1972b. On the concept of health capital and the demand for health. Journal of Political Economy, 80, 223-255.

Grossman, M. 1975. The correlation between health and schooling. In N. E. Terleckyj, ed., Household production and consumption. New York: Columbia University Press, for the National Bureau of Economic Research.

Grubb, H. J. 1964. A statistical analysis of the dentists' supply company dental health plan. Chicago: Continental Casualty Company.

Guzick, D. S. 1978. Demand for general practitioner and internist services. Health Services Research, 13 (4).

Hadley, J., Holahan, J., and Scanlon, W. 1979. Can fee-for-service reimbursement coexist with demand creation? Inquiry, 16, 247-258.

Haggerty, R. J., Roghmann, K., and Pless, I. 1975. Child health and the community. New York: John Wiley.

Hall, C. P., Jr. 1974. Impact of cost sharing on consumer use of health services. In S. Mushkin, ed., Consumer incentives for health care. New York: Prodist.

Harberger, A. C. 1954. Monopoly and resource allocation. American Economic Review, 44, (May).

Harsanyi, J. 1955. Cardinal welfare, individualistic ethics and interpersonal comparisons of utility. Journal of Political Economy, 63, 309-321.

Health Insurance Institute. 1979. Source book of health insurance data, 1977-78. Washington, D.C.: Health Insurance Institute.

Heaney, C. T., and Riedel, D. C. 1970. From indemnity to full coverage: Changes in hospital utilization. Chicago: Blue Cross Association. Research Series 5.

Heckman, J. 1974. Shadow prices, market wages, and labor supply. Econometrica, 42, 679-694.

Heckman, J. 1976. The common structure of statistical models of truncation, sample selection and limited dependent variables and a simple estimator for such models. Annals of Economic and Social Measurement, 5, 475-492.

Heckman, J. 1979. Sample bias as a specification error. Econometrica, 47, 153-167.

Hellinger, F. J. 1976a. The effect of Certificate-of-Need legislation on hospital investment. Inquiry, 13, 187-193.

Hellinger, F. J. 1976b. Prospective reimbursement through budget review: New Jersey, Rhode Island, and Western Pennsylvania. Inquiry, 13, 309-320.

Helms, L. J., Newhouse, J. P., and Phelps, C. E. 1978. Copayments and demand for medical care: The California Medicaid experience. Bell Journal of Economics, 9, 192-208.

Hershey, J. C., Luft, H. S., and Gianaris, J. M. 1975. Making sense out of utilization data. Medical Care, 13.

Hill, D. B., and Veney, J. E. 1970. Kansas Blue Cross/Blue Shield outpatient benefits experiment. Medical Care, 8, 143-158.

Hill, J. D., Hampton, J. R., and Mitchell, J. R. A. 1978. A randomized trial of home versus hospital management for patients with suspected myocardial infarction. Lancet, 1, 837-841.

Hochman, H. M., and Rodgers, J. D. 1969. Pareto optimal redistribution. American Economic Review, 59, 542-557.

Holahan, J., Hadley, J., Scanlon, W., Lee, R., and Bluck, J. 1979. Paying for physician services under Medicare and Medicaid. Milbank Memorial Fund Quarterly: Health and Society, 57, 183-211.

Holtmann, A. G., and Olsen, E. O., Jr. 1976. The demand for dental care: A study of consumption and household production. Journal of Human Resources, 11, 546-560.

Hsiao, W. C., and Stason, W. B. 1979. Toward developing a relative value scale for medical and surgical services. Health Care Financing Review, 1, Fall, 23-28.

Hurst, J. W. 1977. Rationing social expenditure: Health and social services. In Posner, ed., Public expenditure--allocation between competing ends. London: Cambridge University Press.

Hutter, A. M., Jr., Sidel, V. W., Shine, K., and De Sanctis, R. W. 1973. Early hospital discharge after myocardial infarction. New England Journal of Medicine, 288, 1141-1144.

Hyman, J. 1971. Empirical research on the demand for health care. Inquiry, 8, 61-71.

Illich, I. 1976. Medical nemesis. London: Calder and Boyars.

INSEE. 1976. Tableaux démographiques et sociaux. Paris.

INSEE. 1979. Tableaux démographiques et sociaux. Supplement. Paris.

Intriligator, M. D. 1978. Econometric models, techniques, and applications. Englewood Cliffs, N.J.: Prentice-Hall, and Amsterdam: North-Holland.

Iuele, R. 1976. L'assistenza ospedaliera INAM nel periodo 1950-1974. I problemi della Sicurezza Sociale, 31.

Joereskog, K. G., and Van Thillo, M. 1973. LISREL: A general computer program for estimating a linear structural equation system involving multiple indicators of unmeasured variables. Uppsala: Department of Statistics, Research Report 73-5.

Jöreskog, K. G., and Sorbom, D. 1978. Estimation of linear structural equation systems by maximum likelihood methods: A Fortran IV program. Chicago: International Education Services.

Johnson, E. M., and Huber, G. P. 1977. The Technology of utility assessment. Transactions on Systems, Man and Cybernetics, SMC-7 (5), 311-325.

Joseph. H. 1971. Empirical research on the demand for health care. Inquiry, 8, 61-71.

Kaitaranta, H., and Purola, T. 1973. A systems-oriented approach to the consumption of medical commodities. Social Science and Medicine, 7.

Kane, R. L., Gardner, J., Wright, D. D., Snell, G., Sundwall, D., and Woolley, F. R. 1977. Relationship between process and outcome in ambulatory care. Medical Care, 15, 11.

Katz, S., Downs, T. D., Cash, H. R., and Grotz, R. C. 1970. Progress in development of the index of ADI. The Gerontologist, 10, 20-30.

Katz, S., Ford, A. B., Moskowitz, R. W., Jackson, B. A., and Jaffe, M. W.   1963.
The index of ADL: A standardized measure of biological and psycho-social
function. Journal of the American Medical Association, 185, 914-919.

Keeler, E. B., Morrow, D. T., and Newhouse, J. P.   1977. The demand for
supplementary health insurance, or do deductibles matter? Journal of
Political Economy, 85, 789-801.

Keeler, E. B., Newhouse, J. P., and Phelps, C. E.   1977. Deductibles and the
demand for medical care services: The theory of a consumer facing a variable
price schedule under uncertainty. Econometrica, 45, 641-655.

Kelly, J. E., and Sanchez, M. J.   1972. Periodontal disease and oral hygiene
among children. National Center for Health Statistics, U.S. Department of
Health, Education and Welfare, Public Health Publication Series 11, No. 117.

Keniston, K., and the Carnegie Council on Children.   1977. All our children: The
American family under pressure. New York: Harcourt Brace Jovanovich.

Kessel, R. A.   1958. Price discrimination in medicine. Journal of Law and
Economics, 1, 20-53.

Kimball, L. J., and Yett, D. E.   An evaluation of policy related research on the
effects of alternative health care reimbursement systems. Final Report to the
National Science Foundation under Grant No. GJ-39344. Mimeographed.

Kish, L., and Frankel, M. R.   1974. Influence from complex samples. Journal of
the Royal Statistical Society, 36, 1-37.

Klarman, H. E.   1965. The economics of health. New York: Columbia University
Press.

Klarman, H. E.   1970. Increases in the cost of physician and hospital services.
Inquiry, 7, 22-36.

Klarman, H. E.   1977. The financing of health care. Daedalus, 106, 215-234.

Kronenfeld, J. J.   1980. Sources of ambulatory care and utilization models.
Health Services Research, 15 (Spring).

Kruidenier, H. J.   1977. Afstand tot ziekenhuis van invloed op verwijspatroon.
Inzet, 1, 32-39.

Lairson, D. R., and Swint, J. M.   1978. A multivariate analysis of the likelihood
and volume of preventive visit demand in a prepaid group practice. Medical
Care, 16 (9).

Lairson, D. R., and Swint, J. M.   1979. Estimates of preventive versus nonpreventive medical care demand in an HMO. Health Services Research, 14 (1).

Lave, J., Lave, L., and Leinhardt, S.   1974. Modeling the delivery of medical
services. In M. Perlman, ed., The economics of health and medical care.
London: Macmillan.

Lee, L. F.   1979. Health and wage: A simultaneous equation model with multiple
discrete indicators. University of Minnesota, Department of Economics,
Discussion Paper No. 79-127.

Lee, M.   1978. Private and national health services. London: Policy Studies
Institute.

Lees, D. S. 1960. The economics of health services. Lloyds Bank Review, 56, 26-40.

Lees, D. S. 1961. Health through choice. London: Institute of Economic Affairs.

Lees, D. S. 1967. Efficiency in government spending—social services: Health. Public Finance, 22, 176-189.

Lees, D. S., and Rice, R. G. 1965. Comment on Arrow. American Economic Review, 55, 140-154.

Leffler, K. A. 1978. The economics of physician licensure. Journal of Law and Economics, 21, 165-186.

LeGrand, J. 1978. The distribution of public expenditure: The case of health care. Economica, 45, 125-142.

Lembcke, P. A. 1952. Measuring the quality of medical care through vital statistics based on hospital service areas: 1. Comparative study of appendectomy rates. American Journal of Public Health, 42, 276-286.

Lewis, C. E., and Keairnes, H. H. 1970. Controlling costs of medical care by expanding insurance coverage. New England Journal of Medicine, 282, 1405-1412.

Lewis, H. G. 1963. Unionism and relative wages in the United States: An empirical inquiry. Chicago: University of Chicago Press.

Lindsay, C. M. 1969. Medical care and the economics of sharing. Economica, 36, 351-362.

Lindsay, C. M. 1973. Real returns to medical education. Journal of Human Resources, 8.

Lindsay, C. M. 1976. A theory of government enterprise. Journal of Political Economy, 84.

Lindsay, C. M. 1980. National health issues: The British experience. New York: Hoffman La Roche.

Lloyd, C. 1971. The demand for medical care: A selective review of the literature. Working Paper No. 71-79, Bureau of Business and Economic Research, College of Business Administration, University of Iowa.

Loewy, E. 1980. Letter. New England Journal of Medicine, 302, 697.

Lohr, K. N., Brook, R. H., and Kaufman, M. A. 1980. Quality of care in the New Mexico Medicaid Program (1971-1975). Medical Care, 18 (1).

Luft, H. S. 1978. How do health maintenance organizations achieve their savings? New England Journal of Medicine, 298, 1336-1343.

Luft, H. S. 1979. HMOs, competition, cost containment and NHI. Paper presented at the American Enterprise Institute Conference, Washington, D.C.

Luft, H. S. Forthcoming. Health maintenance organizations: Dimensions of performance. New York: John Wiley.

Luft, H. S., Bunker, J. P., and Enthoven, A. C. 1979. Should operations be regionalized? The empirical relation between surgical volume and mortality. New England Journal of Medicine, 301, 1364-1369.

McKinlay, J. B. 1972. Some approaches and problems in the study of the use of services: An overview. Journal of Health and Social Behavior, 13.

McNeer, J. F., Wagner, G. S., Ginsburg, P. B., Wallace, A. G., McCantis, C. B., Conley, M. J., and Rosati, R. A. 1978. Hospital discharge one week after acute myocardial infarction. New England Journal of Medicine, 298, 229-232.

Maddala, G. S. 1971. The use of variance components models in pooling cross section and time series data. Econometrica, 39, 341-370.

Manning, W. G., Jr., Morris, C. N., Newhouse, J. P., Orr, L. L., Keeler, E. B., Liebowitz, A., Marquis, K. H., Marquis, M. S., and Phelps, C. E. 1980. A two-part model of the demand for medical care: Preliminary results from the health insurance study. Paper presented at the World Congress on Health Economics, Leiden, The Netherlands (see essay by Manning et al. in this volume).

Manning, W. G., Jr., Newhouse, J. P., and Ware, J. E., Jr. Forthcoming. The status of health in demand estimation. In V. R. Fuchs, ed., Economic aspects of health. Chicago: University of Chicago Press.

Manning, W. G., Jr., and Phelps, C. E. 1979. The demand for dental care. Bell Journal of Economics, 10, 503-520.

Marquis, K. H. 1979. Hospital stay response error estimates for the health insurance study's Dayton baseline survey. Santa Monica, Cal.: Rand Corporation, Publ. No. R-2535OHEW.

Marquis, K. H., Marquis, M. S., and Newhouse, J. P. 1976. The measurement of expenditures for outpatient physician and dental services: Methodological findings from the health insurance study. Medical Care, 14, 913-931.

Masson, R. T., and Wu, S. 1974. Price discrimination for physicians' services. Journal of Human Resources, 9, 64-79.

Mather, H. G., Morgan, D. C., Pearson, N. G., Read, K. L. Q., Shaw, D. B., Steed, G. R., Thorne, M. G., Lawrence, C. J., and Riley, I. S. 1976. Myocardial infarction: A comparison between home and hospital care for patients. British Medical Journal, 1, 925-929.

May, J. J. 1975. Utilization of health services and the availability of resources. In R. Andersen, J. Kravits, and O. Anderson, eds., Equity in health services. Cambridge, Mass.: Ballinger.

Maynard, A. 1975. Health care in the European Community. London and Pittsburgh: Croom Helm and Pittsburgh University Press.

Maynard, A. 1979a. Pricing, demanders and the supply of health care. International Journal of Health Services, 9, 121-137.

Maynard, A. 1979b. Pricing, insurance and the National Health Service. Journal of Social Policy, 8, 157-176.

Maynard, A. 1980. Medical care and the price mechanism. In K. Judge, ed., Pricing the social services. London: Macmillan.

Maynard, A., and Ludbrook, A. 1980a. Applying resource allocation formulae to constituent parts of the U.K. Lancet, 1, 85–87.

Maynard, A., and Ludbrook, A. 1980b. Budget allocation in the National Health Service. Journal of Social Policy, July.

Meiners, M. R. Summary of dissertation research project entitled "Nursing home costs: A statistical cost function analysis using national survey data." Office of Program Development, U.S. National Center for Health Services Research, unpublished paper.

Meltzer, A. H., and Richard, S. 1978. Why government grows (and grows) in a democracy. The Public Interest, 51.

Menchik, M. D. 1977. Hospital use under Medicaid in New York City. Santa Monica, Cal.: Rand Corporation, Report R-1955-NYC.

Mennemeyer, S. T. 1978. Really great returns to medical education? Journal of Human Resources, 13, 75–90.

Miller, M. K., and Stokes, C. S. 1978. Health status, health resources and consolidated structure parameters: Implications for public health care policy. Journal of Health and Social Behavior, 19, 263–279.

Mizrahi, A. 1978. Micro-économie de la consommation médicale. CREDOC publication no. 4637. Paris.

Moloney, T. W., and Rogers, D. E. 1979. Medical technology—A different view of the contentious debate over costs. New England Journal of Medicine, 301, 1413–1419.

Monsma, G. N., Jr. 1970. Marginal revenue and the demand for physician's services. In H. E. Klarman, ed., Empirical studies in health economics. Proceedings of the Second Conference on the Economics of Health. Baltimore: Johns Hopkins Press.

Mooney, G. H. 1977. The valuation of human life. London: Macmillan.

Moore, S. 1979. Cost containment through risk-sharing by primary-care physicians. New England Journal of Medicine, 300, 1359–1362.

Morcaldo, G., and Salvemini, G. 1978. Struttura ed evoluzione della spesa sanitaria. Rivista di Politica Economica, 68, 1584–1604.

Morehead, M. M., Donaldson, R., and Zanes, A. 1971. Dental service at Teamster comprehensive care program. Journal of the American Dental Association, 83, 601–606.

Morris, C. N. 1979. A finite selection model for experimental design of the health insurance study. In D. J. Aigner and C. N. Morris, Experimental design in econometrics. Journal of Econometrics, 11, 43–61.

Morris, C. N., Newhouse, J. P., and Archibald, R. W. 1979. On the theory and practice of obtaining unbiased and efficient samples in social surveys. In V. L. Smith, ed., Experimental economics, Vol. 1. Westport, Conn.: JAI Press. (Also in Evaluation Studies Review Annual, Vol. 5. Beverly Hills, Cal.: Sage Publications, 1980.)

Moscovice, I. 1977. A method for analyzing resource use in ambulatory care settings. Medical Care, 15 (12).

Mundlak, Y. 1978. On the pooling of time series and cross section data.
Econometrica, 46, 69-86.

Murphy, M. L., Hultgren, H. N., Detre, K., Thomsen, J., and Takaro, T. 1977.
Treatment of chronic stable angina: A preliminary report of survival data of
the randomized Veterans Administration cooperative study. New England Journal
of Medicine, 297, 621-627.

Mushkin, S. J. 1958. Towards a definition of health economics. Public Health
Reports, 73, 785-793.

National Center for Health Statistics (NCHS). 1967a. Plan, operation, and
response results of a program of children's examinations. Washington, D.C.:
U.S. Department of Education, and Welfare, Public Health Service Publication
No. 1000, Series 1, No. 5.

National Center for Health Statistics (NCHS). 1967b. A study of the achievement
test used in the health examination survey of persons aged 6-17 years.
Washington, D.C.: U.S. Department of Health, Education, and Welfare, Public
Health Service Publication No. 1000, Series 2, No. 24.

National Center for Health Statistics (NCHS). 1969. Plan and operation of a
health examination survey of U.S. youths 12-17 years of age. Washington,
D.C.: U.S. Department of Health, Education, and Welfare, Public Health
Service Publication No. 1000, Series 1, No. 8.

National Center for Health Statistics (NCHS). 1972. Subtest estimates of the WISC
full scale IQ's for children. Washington, D.C.: U.S. Department of Health,
Education, and Welfare, Vital and Health Statistics, Series 2, No. 47.

National Center for Health Statistics (NCHS). 1975. Selected operating and
financial characteristics of nursing homes: United States: 1973-1974
National Nursing Home Survey, Series 13, No. 22. Washington, D.C.: U.S.
Department of Health, Education, and Welfare (HRA) 76-1773.

National Center for Health Statistics (NCHS). 1979. The national nursing home
survey: 1977 summary for the United States, Series 13, No. 43. Washington,
D.C.: U.S. Department of Health, Education, and Welfare (PHS) 79-1794.

National Heart, Lung, and Blood Institute's Task Force on Blood Pressure Control
in Children. 1977. Report of the task force on blood pressure control in
children. Pediatrics, 59, Supplement.

Neutra, R. R., Fienberg, S. E., Greenland, S., and Friedman, E. A. 1978. Effect
of fetal monitoring on neonatal death rates. New England Journal of Medicine,
299, 324-326.

Newhouse, J. P. 1970. A model of physician pricing. Southern Economic Journal,
37, 174-183.

Newhouse, J. P. 1974. A design for a health insurance experiment. Inquiry, 11,
5-27.

Newhouse, J. P. 1978. Insurance benefits, out-of-pocket payments, and the demand
for medical care: A review of the literature. Health and Medical Care
Services Review, 1, 1,3-15.

Newhouse, J. P. 1979. The erosion of the medical marketplace. Santa Monica,
    Cal.: Rand Corporation. Publ. No. R-2141-1.

Newhouse, J. P., and Friedlander, L. J. 1977. The relationship between medical
    resources and measures of health: Some additional evidence. Santa Monica,
    Cal.: Rand Corporation, Report R-20660-HEW.

Newhouse, J. P., and Marquis, M. S. 1978. The norms hypothesis and the demand for
    medical care. Journal of Human Resources, 13, Supplement, 159-182.

Newhouse, J. P., Marquis, K. H., Morris, C. N., Phelps, C. E., and Rogers, W. H.
    1979. Measurement issues in the second generation of social experiments: The
    health insurance study. In D. J. Aigner, and C. N. Morris, eds., Experimental
    design in econometrics, Journal of Econometrics, 11, 117-129.

Newhouse, J. P., and Phelps, C. E. 1974. Price and income elasticities for medi-
    cal services. In M. Perlman, ed., The economics of health and medical care.
    International Economic Association. London: Macmillan, and New York: John
    Wiley.

Newhouse, J. P., and Phelps, C. E. 1976. New estimates of price and income
    elasticities of medical services. In R. N. Rosett, ed., The role of health
    insurance in the health services sector. Universities-NBER Conference Series
    No. 27. New York: Neale Watson.

Newhouse, J. P., Phelps, C. E., and Marquis, M. S. 1979. On having your cake and
    eating it too: An analysis of estimated effects of insurance on demand for
    medical care. Santa Monica, Cal.: Rand Corporation, Publ. No.
    R-1149-1-NC/HEW. (Also in Journal of Econometrics, 1980; see next entry.)

Newhouse, J. P., Phelps, C. E., and Marquis, M. S. 1980. On having your cake and
    eating it too: Econometric problems in estimating the demand for health ser-
    vices. Journal of Econometrics, 13, 365-390.

Newhouse, J. P., Phelps, C. E., and Schwartz, W. B. 1974. Policy options and the
    impact of national health insurance. New England Journal of Medicine, 290,
    1345-1359.

Newhouse, J. P., Rolph, J. E., Mori, B., and Murphy, M. 1978. An estimate of the
    impact of deductibles on the demand for medical care services. Santa Monica,
    Cal.: Rand Corporation, Publ. No. R-1661-HEW. (Also in Journal of the
    American Statistical Association, September 1980; see next entry.)

Newhouse, J. P., Rolph, J. E., Mori, B., and Murphy, M. 1980. The effect of
    deductibles on the demand for medical care services. Journal of the American
    Statistical Association, 75, 525-533.

Newhouse, J. P., and Taylor, V. 1971. How shall we pay for medical care? Public
    Interest, 23, 78-92.

Newhouse, J. P., Williams, A. P., Bennett, B., and Schwartz, W. B. 1979. The
    geographic distribution of physicians: Is the conventional wisdom correct?
    Paper presented at the American Economic Association meetings, Atlanta,
    Georgia.

Nelson, F. D. 1977. Censored regression models with unobserved, stochastic cen-
    soring thresholds. Journal of Econometrics, 6, 309-327.

Nerlove, M.   1965. Estimation and indentification of Cobb-Douglas production functions. Amsterdam: North-Holland.

Noll, R. G.   1975. The consequences of public utility regulation of hospitals.   In
Controls on health care. Washington, D.C.:   Institute of Medicine, National
Academy of Sciences.

Okun, A.   1975. Equality and efficiency: The big tradeoff. Washington, D.C.:
Brookings Institution.

Organization for Economic Cooperation and Development (OECD).   1977. Public expenditure on health.   (Studies in Resource Allocation, No. 4.) Paris: OECD.

Owen, J.   1969. The price of leisure. Rotterdam: Rotterdam University Press.

Patrick, D. L., Bush, J. W., and Chen, M. M.   1973. Methods of measuring levels of
well-being for a health status index. Health Services Research, 8, 229-244.

Pauly, M.   1968. The economics of moral hazard: Comment. American Economic
Review, 57, 231-237.

Pauly, M. V.   1969. A measure of the welfare cost of health insurance. Health
Services Research, 4 (Winter).

Pauly, M. V.   1971. Medical care at public expense. New York: Praeger.

Pauly, M. V.   1974. Economic aspects of consumer use. In Selma Mushkin, ed.,
Consumer incentives for health care. New York: Prodist.

Pauly, M. V.   1975. The role of demand creation in the provision of health services. Paper prepared for the annual meeting of the American Economic
Association, Dallas, December.

Pearson, D. A., and Abernethy, D. S.   1980. A qualitative assessment of previous
efforts to contain hospital costs. Journal of Health Politics, Policy, and
Law, 5, 120-141.

Petty, W.   1691. Verbum sapienti. London.

Phelps, C. E.   1973. Demand for health insurance: A theoretical and empiricial
investigation. Santa Monica, Cal.: Rand Corporation, Publ. No. R-1054-OEO.

Phelps, C. E.   1975. Effects of insurance on demand for medical care. In R.
Anderson et al., eds., Equity in health services. Cambridge, Mass.:
Ballinger.

Phelps, C. E.   1976. Demand for reimbursement insurance. In R. N. Rosett, ed.,
The role of health insurance in the health services sector. New York:
National Bureau of Economic Research.

Phelps, C. E., and Newhouse, J. P.   1972. Effects of coinsurance: A multivariate
analysis. Social Security Bulletin, 35, 20-29.

Phelps, C. E., and Newhouse, J. P.   1974. Coinsurance and the demand for medical
services. Santa Monica, Cal.: Rand Corporation, Publ. No. R-964-2-OEO/NC.

Phelps, C. E., and Newhouse, J. P.   1974. Coinsurance, the price of time, and the
demand for medical services. Review of Economics and Statistics, 56, 334-342.

Pratt, J. W. 1964. Risk aversion in the small and in the large. *Econometrica*, 32, 122–136.

Rafferty, J. A. 1971. Patterns of hospital use: An analysis of short-run variations. *Journal of Political Economy*, 79, 154–165.

Reinhardt, U. 1975a. Alternative methods of reimbursing noninstitutional providers of health care services. In Institute of Medicine, *Controls on health care*. Washington, D.C.: National Academy of Sciences.

Reinhardt, U. 1975b. Physician productivity and the demand for health manpower. Cambridge, Mass.: Ballinger.

Reinhardt, U. E. 1977a. Comment--monopolistic elements in the market for physicians' services. Paper presented at the Conference on Competition in the Health Care Sector, FTC, Washington, D.C.

Reinhardt, U. E. 1977b. Health manpower policy and the cost of health care. Paper presented at the National Health Leadership Conference, Washington, D.C., June 27–28.

Reinhardt, U. 1978a. Comment on Frank A. Sloan and Roger Feldman, Competition among physicians. In W. Greenberg, ed., *Competition in the health care sector*. Proceedings of a conference sponsored by the Bureau of Economics-Federal Trade Commission. Germantown, Md.: Aspen Systems Corp.

Reinhardt, U. E. 1978b. The physician as generator of health care costs. In Health care in the American economy: Issues and forecasts. Chicago: Health Services Foundation.

Richardson, W. C. 1970. Measuring the urban poor's use of physicians' services in response to illness episodes. *Medical Care*, 8.

Riker, W. H. 1962. The theory of political coalitions. New Haven: Yale University Press.

Roemer, M. I., Hopkins, C. E., Carr, L., and Gartside, F. 1975. Copayments for ambulatory care: Penny-wise and pound-foolish. *Medical Care*, 13, 457–466.

Roemer, M. I., and Shain, M. 1959. Hospital utilization under insurance. Chicago: American Hospital Association.

Roemer, M. I., and Shonick, W. 1973. HMO performance: The recent evidence. *Milbank Fund Quarterly: Health and Society*, 51, 271–317.

Rosen, S. 1974. Hedonic prices and implicit markets. *Journal of Political Economy*, 82, 34–55.

Rosenstock, I. M. 1966. Why people use health services. *Milbank Memorial Fund Quarterly*, 44 (July).

Rosenthal, G. D. 1964. The demand for general hospital facilities. Chicago: American Hospital Association.

Rosenthal, G. 1970. Price elasticity of demand for short-term general hospital services. In H. E. Klarman, ed., *Empirical studies in health economics*. Baltimore: Johns Hopkins Press.

Rosett, R. N., ed. 1976. The role of health insurance in the health services sector. New York: National Bureau of Economic Research.

Rosett, R. N., and Huang, L. F. 1973. The effect of health insurance on the demand for medical care. Journal of Political Economy, 81, 281-305.

Rosser, R. 1979. Issues of measurement in the design of health indicators: A review. Paper given at the University of York (England) European Workshop on Health Indicators, A. J. Culyer, chairman.

Rosser, R. M., and Kind, P. 1978. A scale of valuations of states of illness: Is there a social consensus? International Journal of Epidemiology, 7, 347-357.

Ruffin, R. J., and Leigh, D. E. 1973. Charity, competition, and the pricing of doctors' services. Journal of Human Resources, 8, 212-222.

Russell, A. L. 1956. A system of classification and scoring for prevalence surveys of periodontal disease. Journal of Dental Research, 35.

Russell, I. T., Brendon Devlin, H., Fell, M., Glass, N. J., and Newell, D. J. 1977. Day-case surgery for hernias and haemorrhoids. Lancet, 1, 844-847.

Russell, L. 1979. Technology in hospitals: Medical advances and their diffusion. Washington, D.C.: Brookings Institution.

Rutten, F. F. H. 1978. The use of health care facilities in The Netherlands: An econometric analysis. Ph.D. dissertation, Center for research in public economics, Leiden University, The Netherlands.

Salber, E. J., Feldman, J. J., Rosenberg, L. A., and Williams, S. 1971. Utilization of services at a neighborhood health center. Pediatrics, 47 (February).

Salkever, D. S., and Bice, T. W. 1976. The impact of Certificate-of-Need controls on hospital investment. Milbank Memorial Fund Quarterly: Health and Society, 54, 185-214.

Santé Securité Sociale (France). 1977. Problèmes de santé et inégalités sociales. No. 4, tome A. Paris.

Savings, T. R., Battalio, R. C., De Vany, A. S., Gramm, W. L., Mouse, D. R., and Kagel, J. H. 1978. Labor substitutes and the economics of the delivery of dental services. Washington, D.C.: Department of Health, Education, and Welfare, Bureau of Health Manpower, Final Report, Contract No. HRA 231-77-0135.

Scanlon, W., and Feder, J. 1980. Regulation of investment in long-term care facilities. Working Paper 1218-9. Washington, D.C.: Urban Institute.

Schwartz, W. B., and Joskow, P. L. 1978. Medical efficacy versus economic efficiency: A conflict of values. New England Journal of Medicine, 299:26, 1462-1464.

Scitovsky, A. A. 1964. An index of the cost of medical care--A proposed new approach. In S. J. Axelrod, ed., Proceedings of the conference on the economics of health and medical care. Ann Arbor: University of Michigan.

Scitovsky, A. A. 1967. Changes in the costs of treatment of selected illnesses, 1951-65. American Economic Review, 57 (December).

Scitovsky, A. A., and McCall, N.   1977. Coinsurance and the demand for physician
    services: Four years later. Social Security Bulletin, 40, 19-27.

Scitovsky, A. A., and McCall, N.   1980. Use of hospital services under two prepaid
    plans. Medical Care, 18, 30-41.

Scitvosky, A. A., and Snyder, N. M.   1972. Effect of coinsurance on use of physi-
    cian services. Social Security Bulletin, 35, 3-19.

Searle, S. R.   1971. Linear models. New York: John Wiley.

Sen, A. K.   1977. Rational fools. Philosophy and Public Affairs, 6, 317-344.

Shah, B. V.   1976. STDERR: Standard errors program for sample survey data.
    Preliminary Statistical Analysis System Version. Durham, N.C.: Research
    Triangle Institute. Mimeographed.

Shah, B. V., Holt, M. M., and Folsom, R. E.   1977. Inference about regression
    models from sample survey data. Paper presented at the International
    Association of Survey Statisticians Third Annual Meeting, New Delhi, December.

Shakotko, R. A.   1977. Health and economic variables: An empiricial investigation
    of the dynamics. Ph.D. dissertation, University of Minnesota.

Shakotko, R. A.   1979. Dynamic aspects of children's health, intellectual develop-
    ment, and family economic status. Paper presented at a session sponsored by
    the American Economic Association and the Health Economics Research
    Organization at the annual meeting of the Allied Social Science Association,
    Atlanta, Georgia, December. (See also next entry.)

Shakotko, R. A.   1980. Dynamic aspects of children's health, intellectual develop-
    ment, and family economic status. New York: National Bureau of Economic
    Research, Working Paper No. 451.

Silvey, S. D.   1975. Statistical inference. London: Chapman & Hill.

Simanis, J. G., and Coleman, J. R.   1980. Health care expenditures in nine
    industrialized countries, 1960-76. Social Security Bulletin, 43, 3-8.

Simon, J. L., and Smith, D. B.   1973. Change in location of a student health
    service: A quasi-experimental evaluation of the effects of distance on utili-
    zation. Medical Care, 11, 59-67.

Skinner, D. E., and Yett, D. E.   1973. Debility index for long-term care patients.
    In R. Berg, ed., Health status indexes. Chicago: Health Services Research
    and Educational Trust.

Sloan, F. A.   1970. Lifetime earnings and physicians' choice of specialty.
    Industrial and Labour Relations Review, 24.

Sloan, F. A.   1974. A microanalysis of physicians' hours of work. In M. Perlman,
    ed., The economics of health and medical care. London: Macmillan.

Sloan, F. A.   1976. Physician fee inflation: Evidence from the late 1960s. In
    R. N. Rosett, ed., The role of health insurance in the health services sector.
    New York: National Bureau of Economic Research.

Sloan, F. A., and Feldman, R. 1978. Competition among physicians. In W.
    Greenberg, ed., Competition in the health care sector. Proceedings of a con-
    ference sponsored by the Bureau of Economics, Federal Trade Commission.
    Germantown, Md.: Aspen Systems Corp.

Sloan, F., and Lorant, J. 1976. The allocation of physicians' services: Evidence
    on length of visit. Quarterly Review of Economics and Business, 16.

Sloan, F., and Lorant, J. 1977. The role of waiting time: Evidence from
    physicians' practices. Journal of Business, 50.

Smallwood, D. E., and Smith, K. R. 1975. Optimal treatment decisions, optimal fee
    schedules and the allocation of medical resources. Research and Analytic
    Report Series, No. 2/75. University of Wisconsin Health Economics Research
    Center, Madison, Wis.

Smith, M. C., and Garner, D. D. 1974. Effects of a Medicaid program on prescrip-
    tion drug availability and acquisition. Medical Care, 12, 571-581.

Solon, J. A., Rigg, R. D., Jones, S. H., Feeney, J. J., Lingner, J. W., and Sheps,
    C. G. 1969. Episodes of medical care: Nursing students' use of medical ser
    vices. American Journal of Public Health, 59 (June).

Solon, J. A., Sheps, C. G., and Lee, S. S. 1960. Delineating patterns of medical
    care. American Journal of Public Health and the Nation's Health, 50 (August),
    1105-1113.

Steinwald, B., and Sloan, F. A. 1974. Determinants of physicians' fees. Journal
    of Business, 47, 493-511.

Stevens, R. 1966. Medical practice in modern England: The impact of specializa-
    tion and state medicine. New Haven: Yale University Press.

Stigler, G. S. 1959. The politics of political economists. Quarterly Journal of
    Economics, 73, 522-533.

Stoddart, G. L. 1975. An episodic approach to the demand for medical care. Ph.D.
    dissertation, University of British Columbia: Department of Economics.

Sweeney, G. H. 1980. The market for physicians' services: Theoretical implica-
    tions and an empirical test of the target income hypothesis. Research paper
    Nashville, Tenn.: Vanderbilt University.

Thouez, J. P. 1979. Health measurement bibliography. Social Science and
    Medicine, 13D, 31-32.

Titmuss, R. M. 1968. Commitment to welfare. London: Allen & Unwin.

Tobin, J. 1958. Estimation of relationships for limited dependent variables.
    Econometrica, 26, 24-36.

Torrance, G. W. 1970. A generalised cost-effectiveness model for the evaluation
    of health programs. Research Report Series 101, Faculty of Business, McMaster
    University, Hamilton, Ontario.

Torrance, G. W. 1976. Towards a utility theory foundation of health status index
    models. Health Services Research, 11, 349-369.

Tuohy, C. J., and Wolfson, A. D. 1977. The political economy of professionalism: A perspective. In M. Trebilcock, ed., Four aspects of professionalism. Ottawa: Consumer Research Council.

Unger, R. 1978. Illusions of necessity in the economic order. American Economic Review, 68, 369-373.

U.S. Department of Health, Education, and Welfare (Social Security Administration, Office of Research and Statistics). 1975. Health care expenditures, prices, and costs: A background book. Washington, D.C.: DHEW Publication No. (SSA) 75-11909.

U.S. Department of Health, Education, and Welfare. 1979. New drug evaluation project: Briefing book. Rockville, Md.: Public Health Service, Food and Drug Administration, Bureau of Drugs.

U.S. General Accounting Office (GAO). 1978. Progress and problems in improving the availability of primary care providers in underserved areas. Washington, D.C.: Government Printing Office, Publ. No. HRO-77-135.

U.S. Senate. 1971. Health care crisis in America, 1971: Hearings before the subcommittee on health of the Committee on Labor and Public Welfare, Part 1; Feb. 22-3, testimony of Rashi Fein. Washington, D.C.: Government Printing Office.

van der Gaag, J. 1978. An econometric analysis of the Dutch health care system. Doctoral dissertation, Leiden University, The Netherlands.

van der Gaag, J., Rutten, F. F. H., and van Praag, B. M. S. 1975. Determinants of hospital utilization in the Netherlands. Health Services Research, 10, 264-277.

van der Gaag, J., and van de Ven, W. 1978. The demand for primary health care. Medical Care, 16, 299-312.

van de Ven, W. P. M. M., and van der Gaag, J. 1979. Health as an unobservable: A MIMIC-model for health-care demand. Madison, Wis.: Institute for Research on Poverty, Discussion Paper No. 544-79.

van de Ven, W. P. M. M., and van Praag, B. M. S. 1979. The demand for deductibles in private health insurance. Report No. 77.02.B. Center for Research in Public Economics, Leiden University. Forthcoming in Journal of Econometrics.

van de Ven, W. P. M. M., and van Praag, B. M. S. 1980. Risk aversion and deductibles in private health insurance: Application of an adjusted tobit model to health care expenditures. Report No. 80.12, Center for Research in Public Economics, Leiden University.

Vayda, E. 1973. A comparison of surgical rates in Canada and in England and Wales. New England Journal of Medicine, December 6.

Walker, A. 1980. Doctor manpower policy in Britain: A critical appraisal from the rate of return perspective. D. Phil. thesis, University of York.

Whitmore, G. A. 1973. Health state preferences and social choice. In R. L. Berg, ed., Health status indexes. Chicago: Hospital Research and Educational Trust.

Williams, A. 1979. One economist's view of social medicine. Epidemiology and Community Health, 33, 3-7.

392 References

Williams, R. 1966. A comparison of hospital utilization by costs and by types of coverage. Inquiry, 3, 28-42.

Williamson, O. E. 1969. Corporate control and the theory of the firm. In H. G. Mann, ed., Economic policy and the regulation of corporate securities. Washington, D.C.: American Enterprise Institute for Public Policy Research.

Wirick, G., and Barlow, R. 1964. The economic and social determinants of the demand for health services. In S. J. Axelrod, ed., Proceedings of conference on the economics of health and medical care. Ann Arbor: University of Michigan.

Wolfe, B. 1980. Children's utilization of medical care. Medical Care (December), 33-44.

World Health Organization and International Epidemiological Association. 1979. Measurement of levels of health. Copenhagen: WHO Regional Publications, European Series No. 7.

Wright, K. G. 1978. Output measurement in practice. In A. J. Culyer and K. G. Wright, eds., Economic aspects of health services. London: Martin Robertson.

Yett, D. E. 1978. Comment on F. A. Sloan and R. Feldman, Competition among physicians. In W. Greenberg, ed., Competition in the health care sector. Proceedings of a conference sponsored by the Bureau of Economics, Federal Trade Commission. Germantown, Md.: Aspen Systems Corp.

Yett, D. E., Drabek, L., Intriligator, M. D., and Kimbell, L. J. 1970. The development of a microsimulation model of health manpower supply and demand. In Proceedings and report of conference on a health manpower simulation model, Vol. 1. Washington, D.C.: Division of Manpower Intelligence, Bureau of Health Manpower Education, U.S. Department of Health, Education, and Welfare.

Yett, D. E., Drabek, L., Intriligator, M. D., and Kimbell, L. J. 1975. A microeconomic model of the health care system in the United States. Annals of Economic and Social Measurement, 4, 407-433.

Yett, D. E., Drabek, L., Intriligator, M. D., and Kimbell, L. J. 1979. A forecasting and policy simulation model of the health care sector. Lexington, Mass.: Lexington Books.

Zeckhauser, R. J. 1970. Medical insurance: A case study of the trade-off between risk spreading and appropriate incentives. Journal of Economic Theory, 2, 10-26.

Zellner, A., Kmenta, J., and Dreze, J. 1966. Specification and estimation of Cobb-Douglas production function models. Econometrics, 34, 784-795.

Zola, I. K. 1966. Culture and symptoms--An analysis of patients' presenting complaints. American Sociological Review, 31, 615-630.

Zweifel, P. 1980. Ein ökonomisches modell des ärztlichen verhaltens, Habilitationsschrift. (An economic model of physician behavior). Forthcoming.

Edwards, L. N., and Grossman, M.,
    291, 300, 309, 324n
Eggers, P., 183
Elasticities
    of coinsurance, 113-114, 121
    of demand, 85-87, 89, 100, 113,
        152, 154, 178, 203, 207
    of expenditures, 131, 132-137
    of income, 92-93, 95, 98, 117,
        121, 152, 153, 163, 199, 284
    of insurance, 85, 90
    of price, 85, 87, 88-92, 93, 95,
        96, 163, 173, 203, 251
    of utilization, 150, 152, 155,
        158, 178-179
Ellwood, P. M., and McClure, W., 185
England
    see Great Britain; United Kingdom
Enthoven, A. C., 338-339
Ethics
    and index of health, 276-277, 280
    medical, 245-265, 273
    professional, 18, 19-20
Evans, R. G., 168n, 170n, 178, 180,
    208, 216, 256
Expenditures
    for health care, 19, 33, 38-40,
        43, 125-146, 158, 173-174, 180,
        355
    for hospital care, 25, 28, 86, 99,
        174, 355
    as a measure of demand, 85-86,
        163
    for medical care, 20, 24-26, 33-
        34, 85-86, 88, 90, 91, 94-96,
        98, 105-121
    for nursing homes, 67
    for physician services, 174, 177,
        180
    see also Elasticities, of expendi-
        tures; Government, financing of
        nursing homes by; Health care,
        cost of; Hospital care, cost of,
        medical care, cost of

Fein, R., 86
Fein, R., and Weber, G. I., 48-49
Feldstein, M. S., 46, 76, 87, 89, 158,
    180, 246, 256, 266n, 367n
Feldstein, P. J., 159, 169n
Fink, R., 169n
France
    health-care system of, 22, 25, 45,
        52-64
Freiberg, L., and Scutchfield, F. D.,
    87
Friedman, B., 145, 146n, 148n
Friedman, M., and Kuznets, S., 48-49

Fuchs, V. R., 18, 94, 101n, 179, 180,
    181, 366n
Fuchs, V. R., Hughes, E. F. X.,
    Jacoby, J. E., and Lewit, E. M.,
    99
Fuchs, V. R., and Kramer, M. J., 89,
    90, 177, 178, 179, 190, 191, 197
Fuchs, V. R., and Newhouse, J. P.,
    215

Galbraith, J. K., 354n
Germany
    health-care system of, 22, 26, 28
Gittelsohn, A. M., and Wennberg,
    J. E., 174
Goldberg, L. E., and Greenberg, W.,
    338
Goldman, F., and Grossman, M., 96-97
Government
    financing of nursing homes by,
        67-77
    intervention of, in health-care
        industry, 15-16, 33-43, 45-50,
        53-64, 346, 348, 356, 361, 364
    regulation of health-care industry
        by, 27-31, 49-50, 53, 68, 99,
        178, 330, 333, 334-335, 337
    role of, in provision of health
        care, 15-31, 51-53, 333-334,
        338-339, 340, 343, 345, 346,
        356
    see also Medicaid program;
        Medicare program
Granger, C. W. J., 307
Great Britain
    health-care system of, 25, 26,
        28, 29, 45, 51-52, 53-64, 175
    see also United Kingdom
Greenlees, J. S., Marshall, J. M.,
    and Yett, D. E., 74
Griliches, Z., 323n
Griliches, Z., Hal, B. H., and
    Hausman, J. A., 147n
Grossman, M., 10, 92, 95, 151, 152,
    153, 163, 170n, 286-287, 319
Grubb, H. J., 88
Guzick, D. S., 168n

Hadley, J., Holahan, J., and Scanlon,
    W., 94
Haggerty, R. J., Roghmann, K., and
    Pless, I., 300
Health
    and cognitive development, 305-
        320
    index of, 8, 276-277, 280, 283,
        301-302, 303
    measures of, 273-274, 283, 293,

CONTRIBUTORS

HENRY J. AARON, Senior Fellow, The Brookings Institution, and Professor of Economics, University of Maryland, College Park.

MORRIS L. BARER, Associate Director, Division of Health Services Research and Development, Health Sciences Center, University of British Columbia, Vancouver, B.C., Canada.

A. J. CULYER, Professor of Economics and Deputy Director, Institute of Social and Economic Research, University of York, England.

NAIHUA DUAN, Statistician, The Rand Corporation, Santa Monica, California.

LINDA N. EDWARDS, Associate Professor of Economics, Queens College and Graduate School of the City University of New York, and Research Associate, National Bureau of Economic Research, New York.

ALAIN C. ENTHOVEN, Marriner S. Eccles Professor of Public and Private Management, Graduate School of Business, Stanford University, Palo Alto, California.

ROBERT G. EVANS, Professor, Department of Economics, University of British Columbia, Vancouver, B.C., Canada.

DOMENICANTONIO FAUSTO, Professor of Public Finance, University of Naples, Italy.

H. E. FRECH III, Associate Professor of Economics, University of California, Santa Barbara.

PAUL B. GINSBURG, Head Analyst, Health, U.S. Congressional Budget Office, Washington, D.C.

MICHAEL GROSSMAN, Professor of Economics, Graduate School of the City University of New York, and Research Associate, National Bureau of Economic Research, New York.

MICHAEL D. INTRILIGATOR, Professor of Economics, University of Caifornia, Los Angeles.

EMMETT B. KEELER, Mathematician, The Rand Corporation, Santa Monica, California.

MARIO LECCISOTTI, Professor of Public Finance, University of Naples, Italy.

ARLEEN LEIBOWITZ, Economist, The Rand Corporation, Santa Monica, California.

ANNE LUDBROOK, Research Fellow, Institute of Social and Economic Research, University of York, England.

WILLARD G. MANNING, Economist, The Rand Corporation, Santa Monica, California.

KENT H. MARQUIS, Economist, The Rand Corporation, Santa Monica, California.

M. SUSAN MARQUIS, Economist, The Rand Corporation, Santa Monica, California.

ALAN MAYNARD, Senior Lecturer in Health Economics, University of York, England.

CARL N. MORRIS, Professor of Mathematics, University of Texas, Austin.

JOSEPH P. NEWHOUSE, Economist, The Rand Corporation, Santa Monica, California.

LARRY L. ORR, Director, Office of Technical Analysis, Office of the Assistant
    Secretary for Policy, Evaluation, and Research, U.S. Department of Labor,
    Washington, D.C.

CHARLES E. PHELPS, Economist, The Rand Corporation, Santa Monica, California.

J. RICHARDSON, Research Fellow, Health Research Project, Australian National
    University, Canberra, ACT.

LOUIS F. ROSSITER, Senior Researcher, National Center for Health Services
    Research, Hyattsville, Maryland.

ROBERT A. SHAKOTKO, Assistant Professor of Economics, Columbia University, and
    Research Associate, National Bureau of Economic Research, New York.

GREG L. STODDART, Assistant Professor, Department of Clinical Epidemiology and
    Biostatistics, Associate Member, Department of Economics, McMaster
    University, Hamilton, Ontario, Canada.

JACQUES VAN DER GAAG, Research Associate, Institute for Research on Poverty,
    University of Wisconsin, Madison.

WYNAND P. M. M. VAN DE VEN, Research Associate, Centre for Research in Public
    Economics, Leiden University, The Netherlands.

BERNARD M. S. VAN PRAAG, Professor of Economics, Centre for Research in Public
    Economics, Leiden University, The Netherlands.

ALAN WILLIAMS, Professor of Economics, University of York, England.

BARBARA L. WOLFE, Assistant Professor, Department of Economics and Preventive
    Medicine, and Research Affiliate, Institute for Research on Poverty,
    University of Wisconsin, Madison.

GAIL ROGGIN WILENSKY, Senior Research Manager, National Center for Health
    Services Research, Hyattsville, Maryland.

PETER ZWEIFEL, Lecturer, Swiss National Science Foundation/University of Zurich,
    Zurich, Switzerland.